Textbook of
Neuroanatomy
with Clinical Orientation

Textbook of
Neuroanatomy
with Clinical Orientation

DR Singh

MBBS MS (Anatomy) PhD (Anatomy) FIANS FFASI

Emeritus Professor
Department of Anatomy
King George's Medical University
Lucknow, UP

Former Professor and Head
Department of Anatomy
King George's Medical College
Lucknow, UP

Recipient, MCI's Hari Om Ashram Alembic Research Award and
Prof. Indarjit Dewan Life Time Achievement Award of
Anatomical Society of India

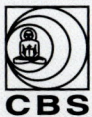

CBS

CBS Publishers & Distributors Pvt Ltd

New Delhi • Bengaluru • Chennai • Kochi • Kolkata • Mumbai
Bhopal • Bhubaneswar • Hyderabad • Jharkhand • Nagpur • Patna
• Pune • Uttarakhand • Dhaka (Bangladesh) • Kathmandu (Nepal)

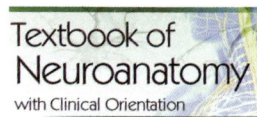

ISBN: 978-93-89688-50-4

Published by Satish Kumar Jain and produced by Varun Jain for

CBS Publishers & Distributors Pvt Ltd
4819/XI Prahlad Street, 24 Ansari Road, Daryaganj, New Delhi 110 002
Ph: 011-23289259, 23266861, 23266867   Fax: 011-23243014   Website: www.cbspd.com
                                                                e-mail: delhi@cbspd.com; cbspubs@airtelmail.in

Corporate Office: 204 FIE, Industrial Area, Patparganj, Delhi 110 092
Ph: 011-4934 4934   Fax: 011-4934 4935   e-mail: publishing@cbspd.com; publicity@cbspd.com

Branches

- **Bengaluru:** Seema House 2975, 17th Cross, K.R. Road, Banasankari 2nd Stage, Bengaluru 560 070, Karnataka
  Ph: +91-80-26771678/79   Fax: +91-80-26771680   e-mail: bangalore@cbspd.com
- **Chennai:** 7, Subbaraya Street, Shenoy Nagar, Chennai 600 030, Tamil Nadu
  Ph: +91-44-26260666, 26208620   Fax: +91-44-42032115   e-mail: chennai@cbspd.com
- **Kochi:** 42/1325, 1326, Power House Road, Opp KSEB Power House, Eranakulam 682 018, Kochi, Kerala
  Ph: +91-484-4059061-67   Fax: +91-484-4059065   e-mail: kochi@cbspd.com
- **Kolkata:** No. 6/B, Ground Floor, Rameswar Shaw Road, Kolkata-700014 (West Bengal), India
  Ph: +91-33-2289-1126, 2289-1127, 2289-1128   e-mail: kolkata@cbspd.com
- **Mumbai:** 83-C, Dr E Moses Road, Worli, Mumbai-400018, Maharashtra
  Ph: +91-22-24902340/41   Fax: +91-22-24902342   e-mail: mumbai@cbspd.com

Representatives

• **Bhopal**	0-8319310552	• **Bhubaneswar**	0-9911037372	• **Hyderabad**	0-9885175004
• **Jharkhand**	0-9811541605	• **Nagpur**	0-9421945513	• **Patna**	0-9334159340
• **Pune**	0-9623451994	• **Uttarakhand**	0-9716462459	• **Dhaka (Bangladesh)**	01912-003485
• **Kathmandu (Nepal)**	977-9818742655				

Printed at Nutech Print Services, Faridabad, Haryana, India

in loving memory of

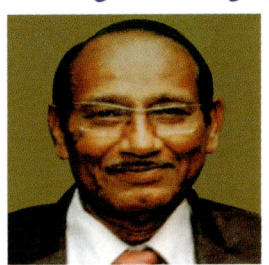

(Late) Dr SHM Abdi
Professor, Department of Anatomy
JN Medical College, AMU, Aligarh
my friend and colleague

Preface

Neuroanatomy is essential, in particular, for the localization of the site of lesion in the neurological disorders. Much of the appreciation of the subjects of neurophysiology, neurology and neurosurgery depends upon a good knowledge of the anatomy of nervous system. To majority of medical students, however, neuroanatomy appears quite 'boring' and 'complicated' as well due to the fact that most of the nuclei, tracts, and connections, etc. described in almost every component of the nervous system are not visible to the naked eye. This sometimes can be more disappointing during the dissection of brain.

There are two categories of books available for the study of the neuroanatomy. First, is a large, standard reference book which treats mainly the detailed account of central and peripheral nervous systems contents. The second category of book is a very concise book made easy and simple, which focuses directly on the essential fundamentals, eliminating those aspects of the subject which have little clinical bearing and emphasize only those aspects of the different subdivisions of the extensive neuroanatomical literature which are of applied interest.

The *Textbook of Neuroanatomy* is intended to fall in the second category of books. It provides brief, up-dated and easy to understand neuroanatomy to the medical students in their undergraduate courses. In addition to the conventional central nervous system, dealing with different approach to the brain and spinal cord, the chapters in lecture notes included in the present book deal emphatically with the autonomic and enteric components of the nervous system that still remain largely unexplored. It cannot be too emphatically stated that the 'clear concepts' in neuroanatomy are only imaginative. Hence, a good understanding of these concepts make the neuroanatomy most interesting.

In preparing this book the text has been supplemented from the latest editions of standard books of the neuroanatomy and made an attempt to present the knowledge in a simplified form. The book has been designed to cover the subject in the minimal possible space keeping in mind the predicament of the already over-burdened medical students. No compromise has, however, been made when it came to the number of illustrations. Simple and self-explanatory line diagrams have been, therefore, liberally incorporated. The diagrams are largely based on the author's self-designed outlines assisted by the ones drawn by Prof Nafis Faruqui, JN Medical College, Aligarh. All efforts to have text diagrams simple and reproducible in the examination have been kept in mind wherever possible.

I feel confident that present textbook will be useful not only to the undergraduate students but also to the postgraduates and young faculty members interested to teach their students with this crucial part of the human anatomy. The mnemonics (designed to aid memory) and humor used in these lecture notes do not intend any disrespect for the original investigators, rather they are employed as an educational device—because as it is well known that the best memory techniques involve the use of simple associations (unfortunately not attempted more frequently) in medical education. The text hopefully will be useful reading before or during the examination course, which will enable the students to rapidly revise overall facts about the clinical neuroanatomy.

I am conscious of my limitations and many errors might have escaped my scrutiny. Discerning readers are requested to inform me to my failings and forward me their critical comments as also their suggestions for improvement of the book.

DR Singh

Acknowledgments

The idea for writing this textbook was the constant suggestions from my present and former students. It is difficult to name all of them so I begin with expressing my gratefulness collectively. Indeed I learnt the subject of anatomy in general, and neuroanatomy in particular from my students of more than fifty years of my teaching. I should like to name a few of my former students, now colleagues, who were unhesitant in discussing with me their personnel teaching experiences.

I am indebted to Dr Punita Manik a devoted teacher and presently the Head, Department of Anatomy. Prof Anita Rani, of the department, has been very cooperative for any help I required during the preparation of this book.

It is a special pleasure to acknowledge the inspiration for hard work and constant encouragement which I received from YN Arjuna, Senior Vice President—Publishing, Editorial, and Publicity. He deserves my special thanks and sincere regards for his many helpful suggestions and whole heartedly cooperation throughout the completion of this book. I also appreciate the meticulous drawings made by Mr Ram Murti, Artist, CBS Publishers and Distributors Pvt Ltd, who worked extremely hard to finalize the illustrations, many of which were drawn initially by Prof. Nafis Faruqui, JN Medical College, Aligarh Muslim University, Aligarh.

The help rendered by Mr Mukund Kumar (Proofreader) and Mrs Jyoti Kaur (DTP Operator) is thankfully acknowledged for organizing the galley-proofs.

I put on records my full appreciation to my revered teachers in my alma mater, (Late) Prof Dharam Narayan, (Late) Prof AC Das, and (Late) Prof Mahdi Hasan who taught me anatomy during my undergraduate medical carrier.

Finally, I owe much to my life-partner Rekha, my children, and my daughter-in-law Supriya who always encouraged me in all my academic pursuits.

DR Singh

Contents

Section II: Peripheral Nervous System

Central Nervous System

Organs and Tissue of Central Nervous System

ORGANS OF CENTRAL NERVOUS SYSTEM

The *central nervous system* (CNS) consists of two organs: the *brain* (encephalon) and the *spinal cord* (medulla spinalis). Median in position, these two organs constitute the *neuraxis* and are connected with all other parts of the body through the *peripheral nerves* (12 pairs of cranial and 31 pairs of spinal nerves). The brain lies within the *cranial cavity* and the spinal cord occupies the *vertebral* (or *spinal*) canal. Both the parts of CNS are enveloped by three fibrous membranes called *(meninges* or *coverings)* the *pia mater*, the *arachnoid mater* and the *dura mater*, named from within outwards. The space between the arachnoid and pia mater *(subarachnoid space)* is filled with the *cerebrospinal fluid* (CSF). The CSF also fills the cavities *(ventricles)* within the brain.

The *midbrain, pons* and the *medulla oblongata* together constitute the *brainstem*. The brainstem and the spinal cord have an outer white matter (made up of nerve fibres) and an inner grey core (made up of nerve cell bodies). The *cerebellum* and *cerebrum* have an additional outer layer of grey matter called the *cortex.* Isolated masses of grey matter within the white matter of CNS constitute the *nuclei* or *ganglia,* e.g. the *basal nuclei* (erroneously called *basal ganglia*) in the cerebral hemispheres.

BRAIN

The brain, in adults, comprises the following parts in respect to the total brain weight:
   i. Cerebral hemispheres—83.0%
  ii. Cerebellum (little or small brain)—10.5%

iii. Brainstem—4.5%
   a. Interbrain or diencephalon (thalamus and hypothalamus)—1.9%
   b. Midbrain—0.8%
   c. Pons—1.3%
   d. Medulla oblongata—0.5%

Cerebral Hemispheres

The cerebral hemispheres are two in number, and together they constituent the largest and most prominent part of the brain (Fig. 1.1). They together overlap the diencephalon and midbrain parts. Sometimes, the term cerebrum is used (particularly by clinicians), which includes both cerebral hemispheres together with the midbrain. The right and left cerebral hemispheres, (each actually not a hemisphere but only a quarter of a sphere), are separated by a longitudinal cerebral fissure.

Cerebellum

The *cerebellum* (little or small brain) is the second largest part of the brain and is characterised by the presence of large numbers of closely set folia, separated by transversely running parallel fissures. It lies below the occipital lobes of the cerebrum and consists of two cerebellar *hemispheres* joined by a median portion called the *vermis.*

The inferior surface of each cerebellar hemisphere is convex and occupies the floor of the posterior cranial fossa. The depression between the two cerebellar hemispheres (*cerebellar vallecula*) presents parts of the *inferior vermis* of the cerebellum. More anteriorly the pons (a bridge) arches across the midline connecting the two cerebellar hemispheres.

The *cerebellum* and *cerebrum* have an additional outer layer of grey matter called the *cortex.* Isolated masses of grey matter within the white matter of CNS constitute the nuclei or *ganglia,* e.g. the *basal nuclei (ganglia)* in the cerebral hemispheres.

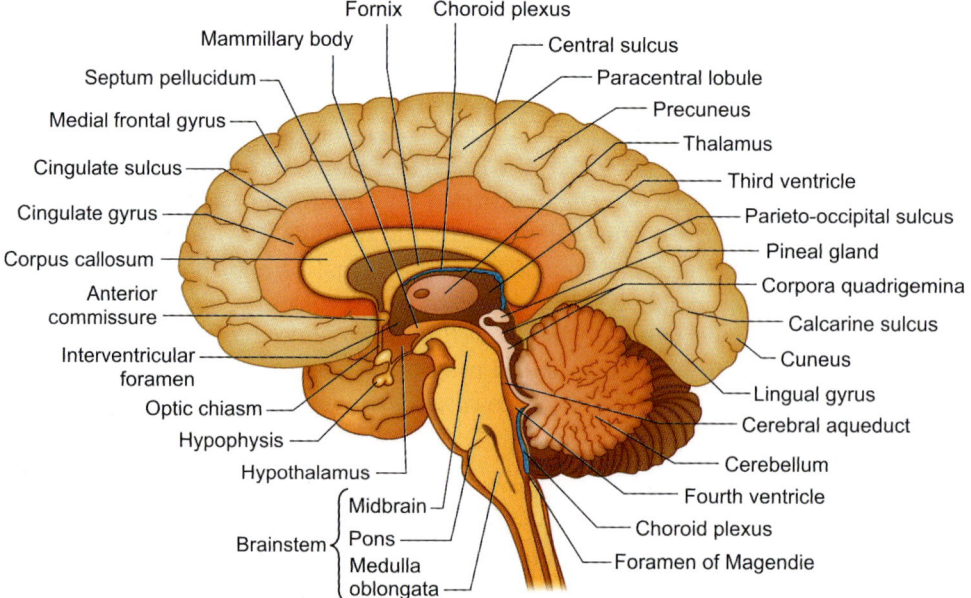

Fig. 1.1: Median sagittal section of the brain showing its main parts

Brainstem

The *brainstem* consists of: *midbrain, pons* and the *medulla oblongata.* The brainstem and the spinal cord have an outer white matter (made up of nerve fibres) and an inner grey core (made up of nerve cell bodies). Because the cerebral and cerebellar hemispheres are present on the sides of the central axis of the neural tube—the forerunner of the central nervous system, some authors include the most rostral part of the brain axis—the diencephalon also as a component of the brainstem. Hence, in the strict sense the brainstem consists of *four* anatomical parts which are from the rostral to caudal aspect: diencephalon (thalamus and hypothalamus), mesencephalon (midbrain), metencephalon (pons), and myelencephalon (medulla oblongata). In the present textbook, however, only the three conventional components of the brainstem are described.

SPINAL CORD

The spinal cord is cylindrical in shape and occupies the upper two-thirds of the vertebral canal. It is about 45 cm long and extends from the level of the upper border of atlas vertebra to the lower border of the body of L1 vertebra. It presents two enlargements, a cervical and a lumbar, corresponding to the regions where the large nerves of the upper and lower limbs, respectively, are attached (Fig. 1.2). The **cervical enlargement** extends from the level of C3 to T1 vertebrae (maximum diameter, 14 mm, opposite C6 vertebra).

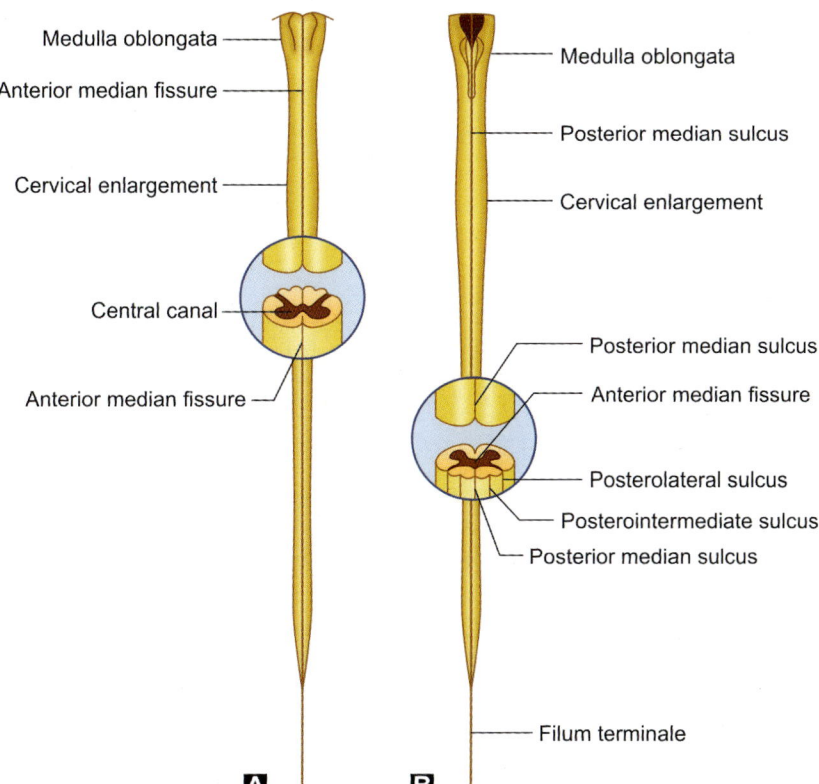

Fig. 1.2: Diagrams of the spinal cord (medulla spinalis): **A.** from anterior or ventral aspect, **B.** from posterior or dorsal aspect

The **lumbar enlargement** extends from T10 to T12 (maximum diameter 12 mm opposite T12). The lumbar enlargement tapers rapidly to form the conus medullaris. From the tip of the conus, a thread-like fibrous structure called the filum terminale extends downwards to be attached to the back of coccyx.

The spinal cord presents an **anteromedian** *fissure* anteriorly, a *posteromedian sulcus* posteriorly and on either side, a *posterolateral* sulcus. Thirty-one pairs of *spinal nerves* are attached to the spinal cord by *dorsal* and *ventral nerve roots*. The **dorsal nerve roots** are attached in the posterolateral sulcus. The **ventral nerve roots** are attached a short distance away from the anterior median fissure. The nerve roots join at the intervertebral foramina to form the *nerve trunks*. The upper spinal nerve roots are short and have a horizontal course in the vertebral canal on their way to the respective intervertebral foramina. The lower nerve roots are long and descend vertically from the conus medullaris in a bundle called the *cauda equina,* which occupies the lower part of the vertebral canal.

Spinal Segments

The portion of the spinal cord to which one pair of spinal nerves is attached is called a *spinal segment*. Accordingly there are 31 spinal segments (8 cervical, 12 thoracic, 5 lumbar, 5 sacral and 1 coccygeal). These segments do not correspond to the vertebral segments (vertebral bodies) and it is important clinically to know their relationship (Table 1.1).

Table 1.1: Interrelationship between spinal cord segments and vertebral bodies	
Spinal segments	*Corresponding vertebral bodies*
Cervical 1 to 8	Cervical 1 to 6
Upper 6 thoracic	Cervical 6 to thoracic 3
Lower 6 thoracic	Thoracic 4 to 9
Lumbar, sacral and coccygeal (L1 Co1)	Thoracic 10 to lumbar 1

STRUCTURE OF NERVOUS TISSUE

The nervous tissue is composed of two distinctive cell types: (1) the *neurons* (excitable cells) and (2) the *neuroglia* (non-excitable, supportive cells).

Neuron

The neuron (Fig. 1.3) is the structural, functional and developmental unit of the nervous system. It is specialised for the reception of stimuli and generation and propagation of nervous impulses. It has a *cell body (soma* or *perikaryon)* and commonly two types of processes, namely the *dendrites* and the *axon*. The dendrites are the receiving processes and conduct impulses towards the cell body. The axon is the efferent process and conducts impulses away from the cell body (axon–away). Usually, there are many dendrites but only a single axon. The axon acquires a fatty *myelin sheath* and together with it forms the *nerve fibre*. The cell bodies and the dendrites acquire no myelin sheath. Thickly myelinated fibres collect into bundles to form the *tracts* or *fasciculi* in the CNS, making up its *white matter*. The *grey matter,* on the other hand, is made up of neuron soma, dendrites and unmyelinated nerve fibres. The grey strip covering cerebrum and the cerebellum is called the *cortex*. Isolated masses of grey matter within the white matter constitute the *nuclei* (within the CNS) or *ganglia* (outside the CNS).

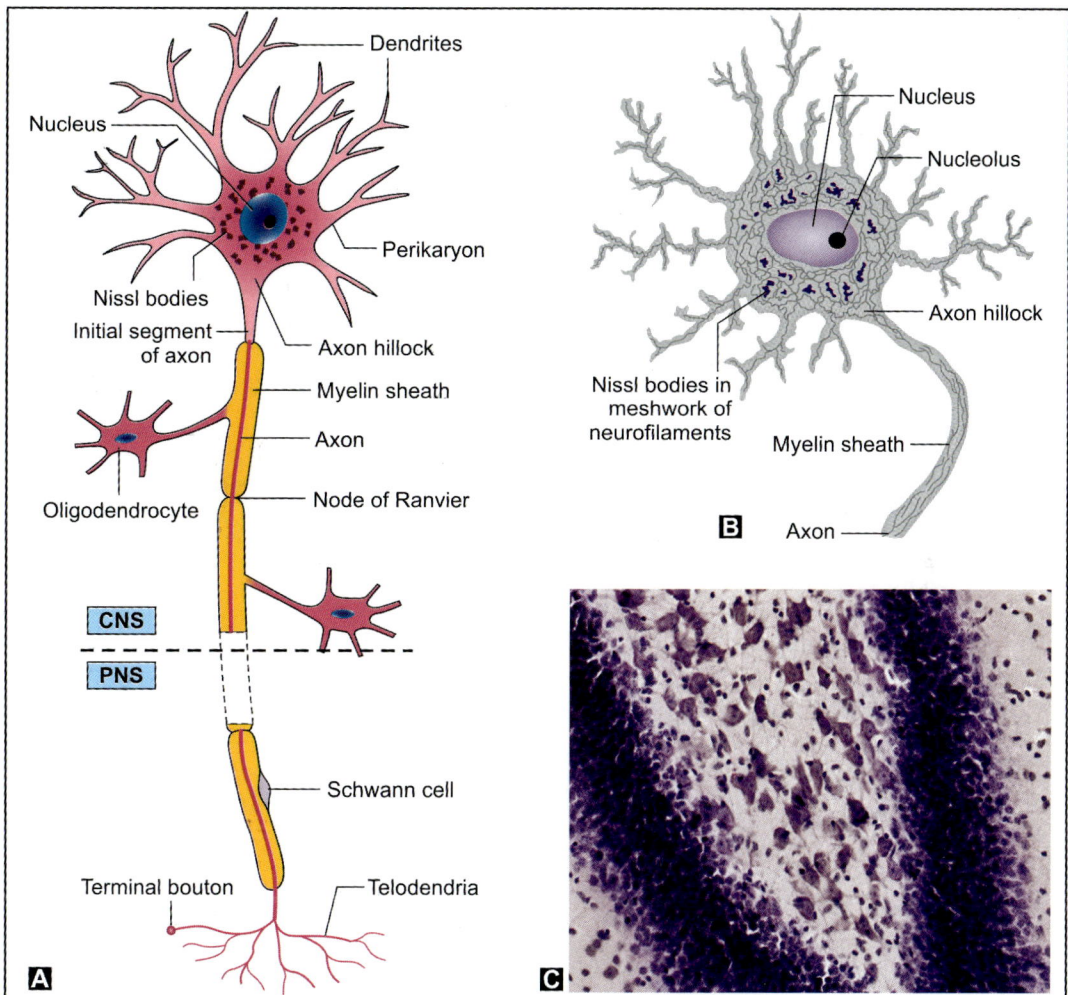

Fig. 1.3: Diagrams of a multipolar neuron: **A.** the CNS and PNS, **B.** several dendrites and a single axon covered by the myelin sheath, **C.** microscopic view of a part of neuron showing Nissl substance

Classification of Neurons

There are millions of neurons in the CNS; which may be classified mainly on the basis of two main criteria:

1. Number of Processes arising from Perikaryon (Fig. 1.4)

On the basis of the number of processes, the neurons may be classified into the following subtypes:

Unipolar neurons: These give out a single process that soon divides into two branches, one of which functions as a dendrite and the other as the axon, e.g. spinal ganglion and trigeminal ganglion cells and cells in the mesencephalic nucleus of trigeminal nerve.

Bipolar neurons: These are fusiform cells giving a single dendrite at one pole and an axon at the other pole, e.g. olfactory receptor cells, retinal bipolar cells and cells of spiral and vestibular ganglia.

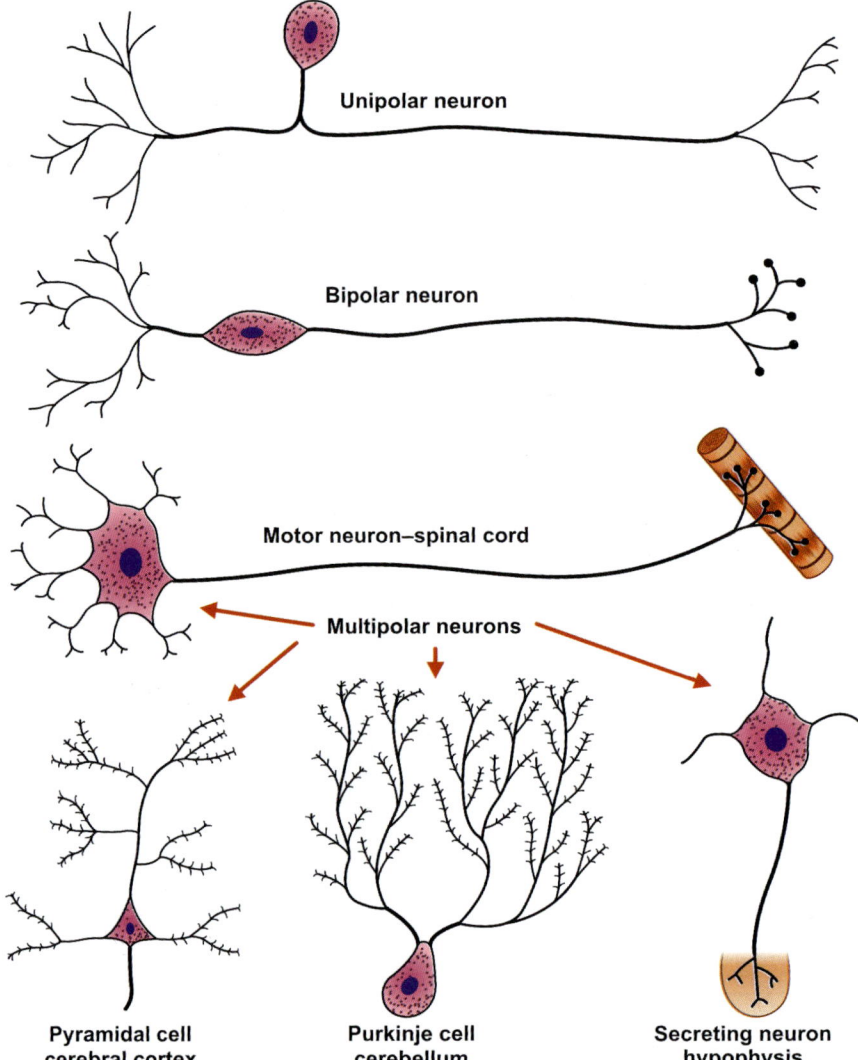

Fig. 1.4: Diagrams of different types of neurons (described in the text). Below are shown the drawings of multipolar neurons in the cerebral cortex, cerebellum, and secreting neuron from the pituitary gland

Multipolar neurons: These are the commonest type of neurons, which have several dendrites and an axon and are pyramidal or stellate in shape. Amacrine cells of retina though grouped as multipolar, however, have several dendrites but are without an apparent axon.

2. Size of Cell Bodies and Length of Axon

On the basis of size of the neuronal cell bodies, and the length of axon; the neurons are classified into the following subtypes:

Golgi type I neurons: These are neurons with large somata and long axons.

Golgi type II neurons: These are microneurons with short axons, which terminate in the neighbourhood of their cell bodies. These neurons are often **inhibitory** in nature. Amacrine neurons of the retina, which are without an apparent axon, are also included in this category.

Microscopic Structure of Neuron

Perikaryon

The *perikaryon* (*peri* = around; *karyon* = nucleus) or the cell body (soma) is the bulbous end of a neuron containing the cell nucleus. The soma contains many organelles, including granules called Nissl granules, which are composed largely of rough endoplasmic reticulum and free polyribosomes. The perikaryon varies greatly in shape and size. It may be stellate, pyramidal, pyriform, round or spindle shaped. The cell size varies from 5 to 120 µm in diameter. Under the light microscope, it presents a large rounded centrally placed nucleus with a prominent nucleolus. The cytoplasm shows large number of Nissl bodies (or granules), which stain deeply with basic dyes (e.g. thionine, methylene blue, and cresyl violet).

Dendrites

The dendrites extend in the form of several branching and tapering processes from the cell body. These bear dendritic spines on the surface and contain Nissl granules in their cytoplasm. The dendrites share many features of the cell body, e.g. they have large numbers of mitochondria, stacks of smooth and rough endoplasmic reticulum, aggregates of free and attached ribosomes, microtubules and neurofilaments.

Axon

The axon is often a long process with a uniform diameter. It does not give branches close to its cell body, though a few *collaterals* sometimes arise from its proximal part. The short pyramidal region of the cell body, from where the axon arises, is called the *axon hillock*. The Nissl granules do not extend into the axon hillock and are absent from the axon. The axon is enveloped in the myelin sheath except at its termination. The myelin sheath is interrupted at regular intervals *(nodes of Ranvier)*. Nodes of Ranvier, also known as *myelin-sheath gaps*, occur along a myelinated axon where the axolemma is exposed to the extracellular space. Nodes of Ranvier are uninsulated and highly enriched in ion channels, allowing them to participate in the exchange of ions required to regenerate the action potential. Nerve conduction in myelinated axons is referred to as saltatory conduction (from the Latin *saltare* "to hop or to leap") due to the manner in which the action potential seems to "jump" from one node to the next along the axon. This results in faster conduction of the action potential. An axon with a thick myelin sheath *(myelinated nerve fibre)* appears white while those with a thin sheath *(thinly myelinated/unmyelinated nerve fibre)* appear grey.

A typical myelinated nerve fibre has a central core of axon and a surrounding myelin sheath derived from the spiralling round of a flap of plasma membrane of a Schwann cell *(oligodendrocyte in CNS)*. Several turns of this plasma membrane flap provides a lamellated appearance to the myelin sheath as seen under electron microscope. Axons of several non-myelinated nerve fibres invaginate into a single Schwann or oligodendrocyte cell (Fig. 1.5). These include the smaller of the CNS axons, peripheral autonomic ganglionic axons and fine *(nociceptive)* sensory fibres.

At its termination, the axon loses its myelin sheath and divides into several branches called the *axon terminals* or the *telodendria* (*telo* = distant; *dendria* = branches). Each of these branches ends in a bulbous enlargement called the *terminal bouton* (bouton terminaux). The boutons establish specialised contacts called the *synapses* (synapse = to clasp) with dendrites, soma or the axon of another neuron. *Axodendritic, axosomatic* or *axoaxonic* types of synapses are thus formed. The synapses are the sites where a nerve impulse carried by one neuron is passed on to another neuron.

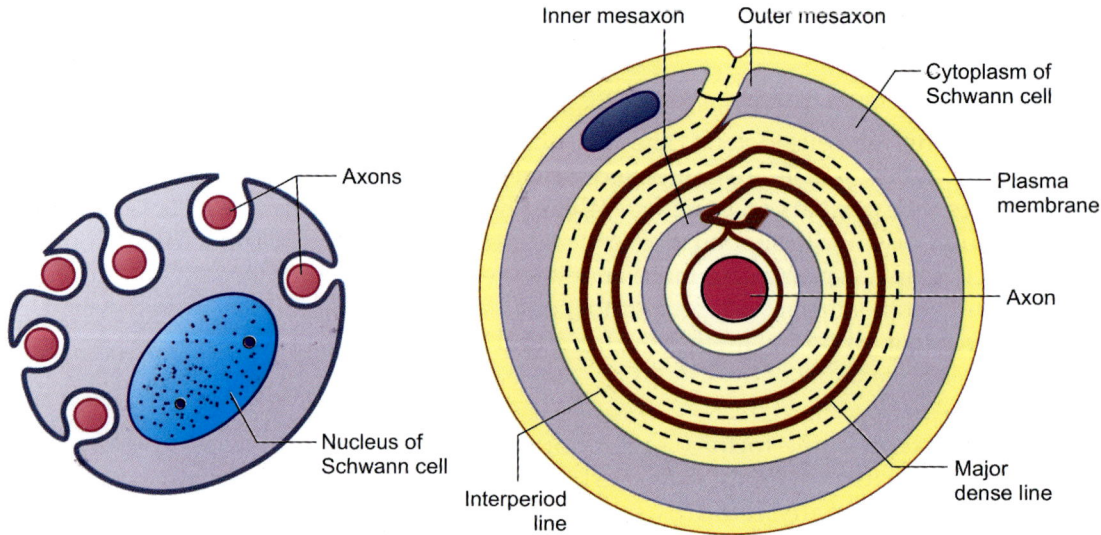

Fig. 1.5: Diagrams showing the process of myelination of axon (red) in the peripheral nervous system by a Schwann cell which wraps around axons (see text). The diagram on the right side shows the consequences of the wrapping—the formation of outer and inner mesaxons. In central nervous system, the myelination is taken by oligodendrocytes (*Courtesy:* Nafis Ahmad Faruqi)

The two major functions of axons are: (i) impulse conduction and (ii) axonal transport. Axonal transport occurs within and impulse conduction on its surface. Axonal injury results in dissolution of Nissl bodies, cytoplasmic swelling and nuclear eccentricity is called *chromatolysis*.

The axon is similar to the dendrites except that normally it does not contain Nissl body. The mitochondria are elongated and microtubules are fewer as compared to the dendrites. The axon is almost completely filled with the neurofilaments (Table 1.2).

Table 1.2: Comparison between dendrites and axon		
Features	*Dendrites*	*Axon*
Number	Usually several (only one in bipolar neuron)	Only one given by a neuron (absent in amacrine neurons)
Shape	Broad base tapering ends	Uniform diameter
Length	Short	Long
Branchings	Near the cell body	At a distance from cell body
Spines	Dendritic spines present	Absent
Myelin sheath	Absent	Present
Nissl granules	Present	Absent
Electron Microscopic Features		
Mitochondria	Usual shape	Elongated
Ribosomes	Present	Absent
Microtubules	Large numbers	Fewer
Functions	Conduct impulses towards the cell body	Conduct impulses away from cell body

Ultrastructure of Neuron

Cytoplasm

The following organelles are seen in the cytoplasm.

- *Endoplasmic reticulum:* The cytoplasm is rich in both smooth and rough endoplasmic reticulum. Stacks of rough endoplasmic reticulum (also aggregates of free ribosomes) constitute the strongly basophilic Nissl granules seen under the light microscope. Stacks of the smooth endoplasmic reticulum constitute the Golgi apparatus, often forming distinct groups in different parts of the cell body.
- *Ribosomes:* Both free and attached ribosomes are found in plenty and indicate a high protein synthesizing activity.
- *Mitochondria:* These are found in fairly large numbers and indicate greater energy demands of cell. A mitochondrion (*plural* mitochondria) is a membrane-enclosed organelle (Fig. 1.6) found in most eukaryotic cells—which generate most of the cell's supply of adenosine triphosphate (ATP), used as a source of chemical energy. In addition, mitochondria are involved in a range of other processes, such as cellular differentiation, cell death, as well as the control of the cell cycle and cell growth.
- *Lysosomes:* These are often a prominent feature of the cell body. These contain hydrolytic enzymes required for degradative reactions.
- *Golgi apparatus:* It is a conspicuous element of the neuron and is made up of clusters of flattened cisternae and small vesicles. It provides membranes for packing secretions, contributes glycogen moiety to proteins and is the source of lysosomes.
- *Neurofilaments:* These are protein filaments, 10 nm in diameter. Groups of neurofilaments can be seen even with light microscope, in silver stained sections.
- *Microtubules:* These are 24 nm in diameter and help in the bi-directional, rapid (400 mm/day) transport of proteins and enzyme substance of low molecular weight along them, e.g.

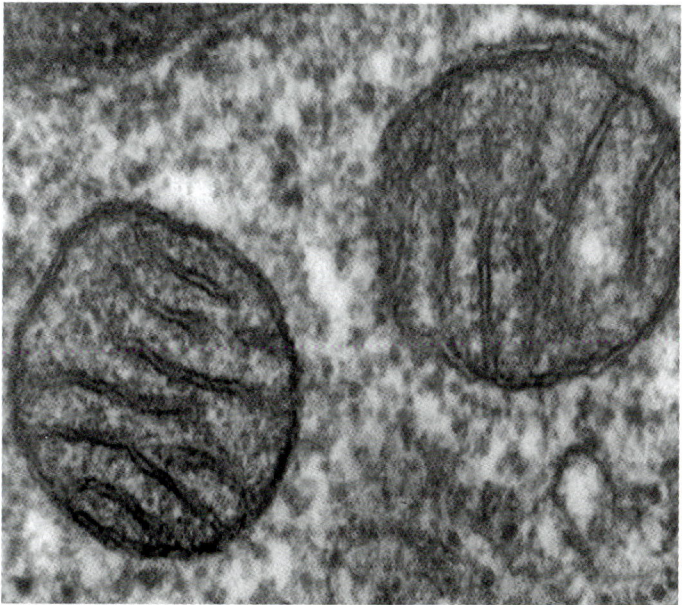

Fig. 1.6: Electron micrograph showing two mitochondria from a neuron. Notice double membrane of cristae

horseradish peroxidise (HRP). Slow transport involves bulk movement of cytoplasm at a speed of 14 mm/day, is independent of microtubules and is only anterograde.

- *Centrioles:* Long believed to be absent from mature neurons, they have now been demonstrated in almost all types of neurons. These are made up of microtubules.
- *Pigment granules:* Several neurons show pigment in their cytoplasm, e.g. cells in the substantia nigra and locus coeruleus contain melanin. Lipofuscin, a yellowish brown pigment, accumulates in the cytoplasm with age and is often prominent in the cell of the hippocampus and the spinal ganglia.

Nucleus

In cell biology, the nucleus (pl. *nuclei*; from Latin *nucleus* or *nuculeus*, meaning *kernel* or *seed*) is a membrane-enclosed organelle found in eukaryotic cells. Eukaryotes usually have a single nucleus, but a few cell types, such as mammalian red blood cells, have no nuclei, and a few others including osteoclasts have many. The neuron has a large, centrally located euchromatic (open faced) nucleus with one or more prominent nucleoli (Fig. 1.7). The large size of the nucleus is associated with high rate of protein synthesis.

Nuclei contain most of the genetic material, organised as multiple long linear DNA molecules in a complex with a large variety of proteins, such as histones, to form chromosomes. The nucleus maintains the integrity of genes and is, therefore, the control centre of the cell. The main structures making up the nucleus are the nuclear envelope, a double membrane that encloses the entire organelle and isolates its contents from the cellular cytoplasm, and the nuclear matrix that adds mechanical support, much like the cytoskeleton, which supports the cell as a whole.

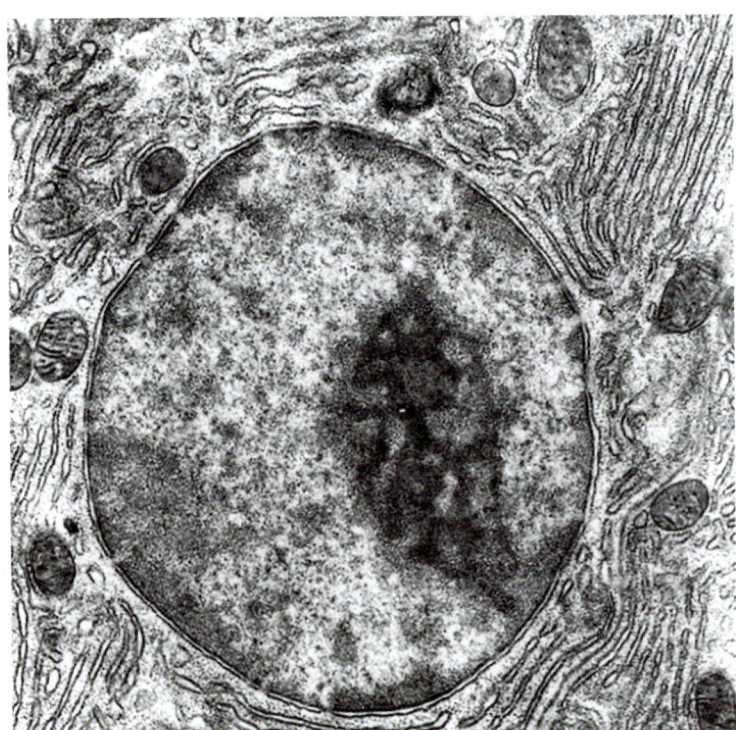

Fig. 1.7: An electron micrograph of a nerve cell nucleus showing the darkly stained nucleolus

Because the nuclear envelope is impermeable to large molecules, nuclear pores are required to regulate nuclear transport of molecules across the envelope. Movement of large molecules such as proteins and RNA through the pores is required for both gene expression and the maintenance of chromosomes. The nucleolus (Fig. 1.7) is mainly involved in the assembly of ribosomes. After being produced in the nucleolus, ribosomes are exported to the cytoplasm where they translate mRNA.

Nuclei per cell may result into two categories of cells:

i. *Anucleated cells*—contain no nucleus and the cell is, therefore, incapable of dividing to produce daughter cells. The best-known anucleated cell is the mammalian red blood cell, or erythrocyte, which also lacks other organelles such as mitochondria, and serves primarily as a transport vessel to ferry oxygen from the lungs to the body's tissues.

ii. *Multinucleated cells*—contain multiple nuclei. In humans, skeletal muscle cells, called myocytes and syncytium, become multinucleated during development; the resulting arrangement of nuclei near the periphery of the cells allows maximal intracellular space for myofibrils. Other multinucleate cells in the human are osteoclasts a type of bone cell. Multinucleated and binucleated cells can also be abnormal in humans, e.g. cells arising from the fusion of monocytes and macrophages, known as giant multinucleated cells, sometimes accompany inflammation.

Neuroglia

The neuroglial cells (Fig. 1.8) are the non-excitable supportive cells in the CNS. These are smaller cells and outnumber the neurons 5 to 10 times. They comprise about half the total volume of the brain and spinal cord. They include the *macroglia* (astrocytes and oligodendrocytes) and the ependymal cells, which are ectodermal in origin and the *microglia* derived from the mesoderm.

There are six types of neuroglia—four for the CNS (central nervous system) and two in the PNS (section 2). These glial cells are involved in many specialized functions apart from support of the neurons. Neuroglia in CNS include astrocytes, microglial cells, ependymal cells, and oligodendrocytes. In the PNS, satellite cells and Schwann cells are the two kinds of neuroglia.

Astrocytes

The astrocytes as suggested by their name are star-shaped and have many processes. Two types of astrocytes are described, (1) *protoplasmic astrocytes* (found in grey matter) and (2) *fibrous astrocytes* (present in the white matter). The astrocyte processes: (i) form *end-feet* on

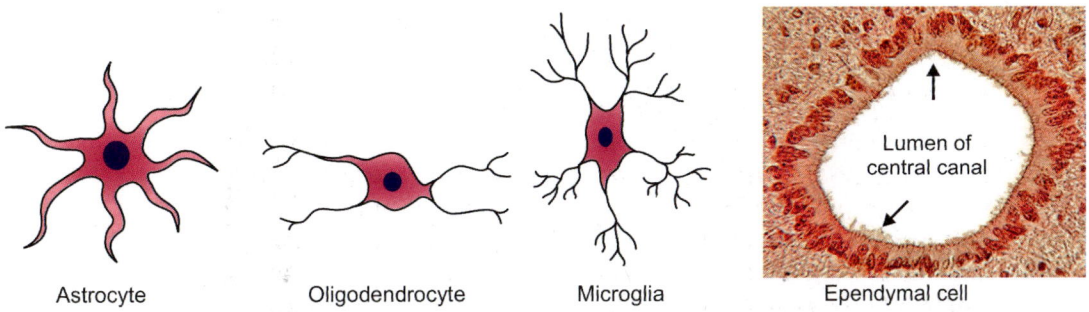

| Astrocyte | Oligodendrocyte | Microglia | Ependymal cell |

Fig. 1.8: Drawings of different neuroglial cells present in the central nervous system

the capillary wall providing the glial component of the blood–brain barrier, (ii) form a *subpial membrane* on the surface of the brain, (iii) interconnect the vascular tree within the brain and together with them from a meshwork to support the neurons and their process, and (iv) transport metabolites from the capillaries to the neuron. In the event of injury to the brain astrocytes proliferate (gliosis) and act as phagocytes to clear the cellular debris.

Oligodendrocytes

The oligodendrocytes, as their name suggests, have only a few processes (oligos = few). They are found as satellites to neurons (perineuronal cells) or in the vicinity of nerve fibres (intrafascicular). The oligodendrocytes form myelin sheath in the CNS. Their processes encircle a number of neighbouring axons in separate sheaths, unlike Schwann cells, which form a sheath for only one axon (in the peripheral nervous system).

Microglia

These are small spindle-shaped cells with polar processes, scanty cytoplasm and an elongated deeply staining nucleus. The cytoplasm shows large number of lysosomes. In the grey matter they are located close to neurons and blood vessels. In the white matter they follow the course of nerve fibres. The microglia are phagocytic in function and are concerned with the removal of both intraneuronal debris and the remains of degenerated neurons.

Ependymal Cells

These cells line the ventricles of brain and the central canal of spinal cord. Adjacent ependymal cells are held together by gap junctions and occasional desmosomes. Their free faces bear numerous microvilli and cilia. Colloid substances injected into the ventricles of brain have been shown to pass through the intercellular junction of the ependymal layer into the interstices between the cells of the CNS. These are, however, prevented from entering the capillaries in the brain parenchyma by: (1) the lack of fenestration, (2) presence of endothelial tight junctions, and (3) absence of a well-developed vesicular transport system in the capillary wall. Thus a very effective barrier exists permitting the diffusion of only small molecules across the capillary wall.

SYNAPSE

A synapse is a specialised region of close junction between two neurons, i.e. where the axonal end arborizations of one neuron come in contact with the cell body or dendrites or axon of another; and may involve contact between almost any parts of the two neuronal surfaces (synapse = to clasp); as an example when two persons shake their hands, the hands are in contact with a minimal space intervening. The most common synapse is, however, between an axon and a dendrite or soma. The opposing plasma membranes are called the pre- and *post-synaptic membranes* and are separated by a 20 nm wide *synaptic cleft* (Fig. 1.9). The increased electron density of the cytoplasm immediately underlying both these membranes clearly outlines a synapse. The postsynaptic density is more prominent and it often forms an uninterrupted *subsynaptic web*. The presynaptic density is usually broken up. The synaptic bag contains mitochondria and many synaptic vesicles enveloping neurotransmitter substances. The following morphological types of synaptic vesicles (Fig. 1.10) have been described.
1. *S type* or spherical vesicles (excitatory).
2. *F type* or flat vesicles (inhibitory).

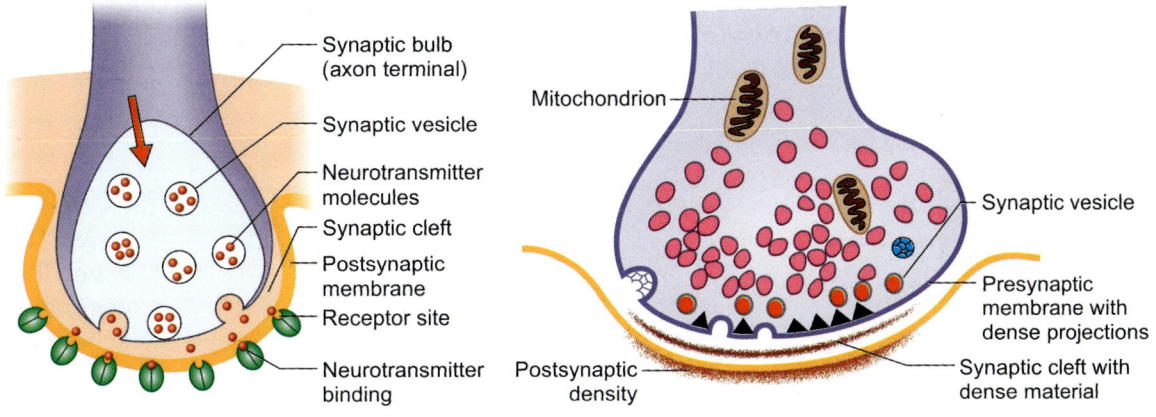

Fig. 1.9: Drawing of a synaptic bulb at the presynaptic axon terminal (red arrow). Receptor sites are present on the cell membrane of a postsynaptic neuron in the central nervous system (*Courtesy:* Nafis Ahmad Faruqi)

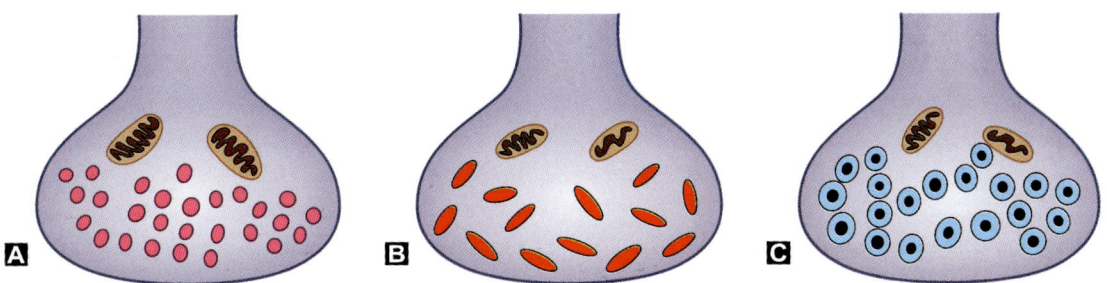

Fig. 1.10: Morphological types of the synaptic vesicles: **A.** excitatory with spherical synaptic vesicles, **B.** inhibitory with flat vesicles, **C.** both excitatory and inhibitory with dense-cored vesicles

3. *C type* are large, dense cored, noradrenaline containing vesicles. These can be both excitatory and inhibitory.

Transmission at the synapses involves release of a neurotransmitter, which causes an alteration of the resting potential of the postsynaptic membrane. The net result for the transmitter release is depolarisation of the presynaptic membrane on the arrival of a nerve impulse and the subsequent uptake of calcium ions in the cytoplasm of the terminal. At excitatory synapses permeability to most ions is increased and the postsynaptic membrane is depolarised. At inhibitory synapses there is increased permeability for chloride ions and the postsynaptic membrane is hyperpolarised. The transmitter substance acts for a short period only. The time restriction is achieved by the enzymatic destruction as of acetylcholine by acetylcholinesterase or by taking them back in the nerve terminal for future use as with catecholamines and possibly other transmitters. There are two types of synapses found in the body: Chemical synapses and electrical synapses.

• *Chemical synapses:* At the end of a neuron's axon is an enlarged region of the axon known as the axon terminal. The axon terminal is separated from the next cell by a small gap known as the synaptic cleft. When an axon potential reaches the axon terminal, it opens voltage-gated calcium ion channels. Calcium ions cause vesicles containing chemicals known as neurotransmitters (NT) to release their contents by exocytosis into the synaptic cleft. The

NT molecules cross the synaptic cleft and bind to receptor molecules on the cell, forming a synapse with the neuron. These receptor molecules open ion channels that they may either stimulate the receptor cell to form a new action potential or may inhibit the cell from forming an action potential when stimulated by another neuron.

- *Electrical synapses:* Electrical synapses are formed when two neurons are connected by small holes called gap junctions. The gap junctions allow electric current to pass from one neuron to the other so that an action potential in one cell is passed directly onto the other cell through the synapse.

2

Development of Central Nervous System

- Central Nervous System
  - Primary brain vesicles and flexures
  - Further development of the brain vesicles
  - Developmental defects in central nervous system
  - Developmental defect in brain
- Histogenesis of CNS
  - Myelination and postnatal development of brain

CENTRAL NERVOUS SYSTEM

The *central nervous system* (CNS) develops from the outer embryonic layer—the ectoderm, which is exposed to the surroundings. About the 16th day of development, the central region of ectoderm on the dorsal aspect of embryonic disc thickens (presumably under the inductive influence of the developing notochord) to from the *neural plate* (Fig. 2.1). Shortly thereafter the neural plate folds to from the *neural groove* (Fig. 2.2). The elevated edges of the groove the *(neural folds)* approach each other, meet and fuse to from the *neural tube* in such a manner that the junctional region is pinched off to form the *neural crest* (Table 2.1). The surface ectoderm is restored and the neural tube along with the neural crest masses is buried under it.

Neurulation is the process of **forming** the **neural tube**, which will become the brain and spinal cord. In **humans**, it begins in the 3rd week after fertilization and requires that the top layers of the **embryonic** germ disc elevate as folds and fuse in the midline.

The fusion of the neural folds to form the neural tube (Fig. 2.2) commences in the future cervical region and extends both rostrally and caudally.

Primary Brain Vesicles and Flexures

The rostral portion of the neural tube expands to form the *brain (encephalon).* The remaining portion of the tube develops into the *spinal cord.* The developing brain forms *three* primary brain vesicles: *prosencephalon* (forebrain), *mesencephalon* (midbrain) and *rhombencephalon* (hindbrain), separated by two constrictions (Fig. 2.3).

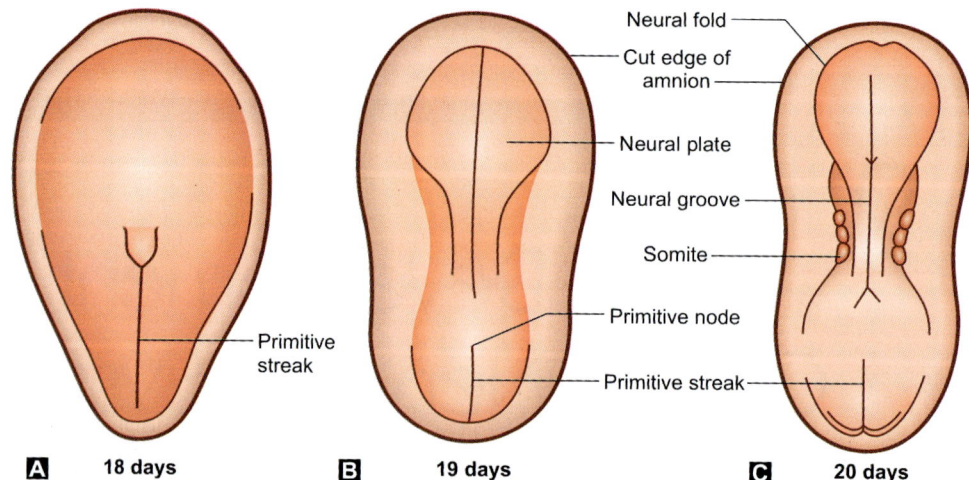

Fig. 2.1A to C: Growth of the embryonic disc (viewed from the dorsal aspect). Notice that the ingress of epiblast through the primitive streak results in an expansion of the embryonic disc at the cranial end of the embryo. The cells begin to differentiate in the cranial end of the embryo while in the caudal end they continue to undergo gastrulation

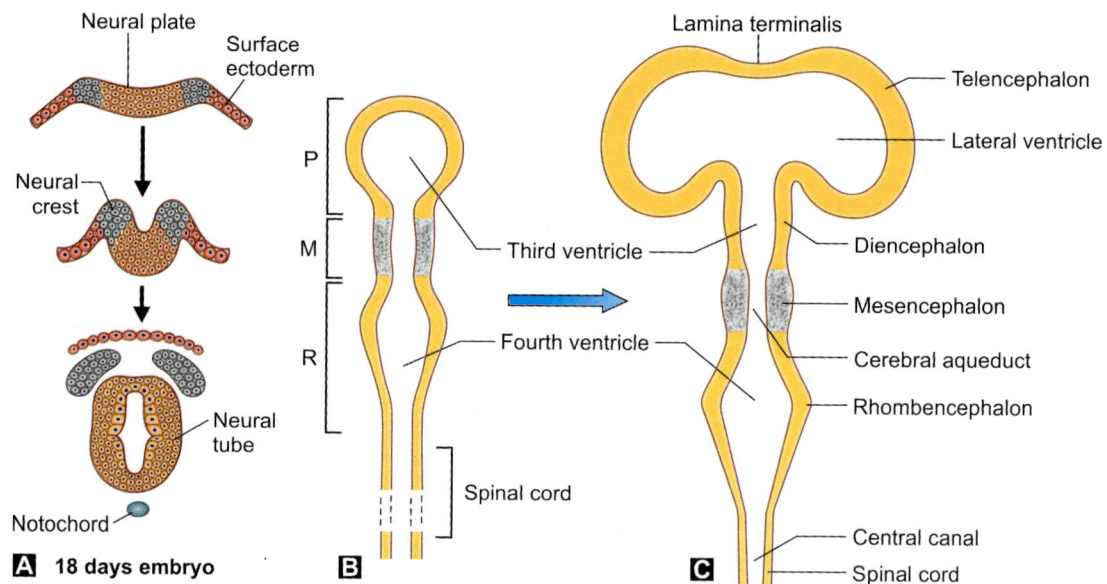

Fig. 2.2A to C: The three primary brain vesicles and their derivatives. P—prosencephalon or forebrain; M—mesencephalon or midbrain; and R—rhombencephalon or hindbrain

Further Development of the Brain Vesicles

The rostral portion of prosencephalon forms the *telencephalon* (end brain), which develops two lateral outpouchings. These outpouchings develop into the cerebral hemispheres with their cavities forming the *lateral ventricles* (Fig. 2.4).

The rostral end of the neural tube forms the *lamina terminalis*, in which all the *commissures* joining the two cerebral hemispheres develop (e.g. anterior commissure and the corpus callosum).

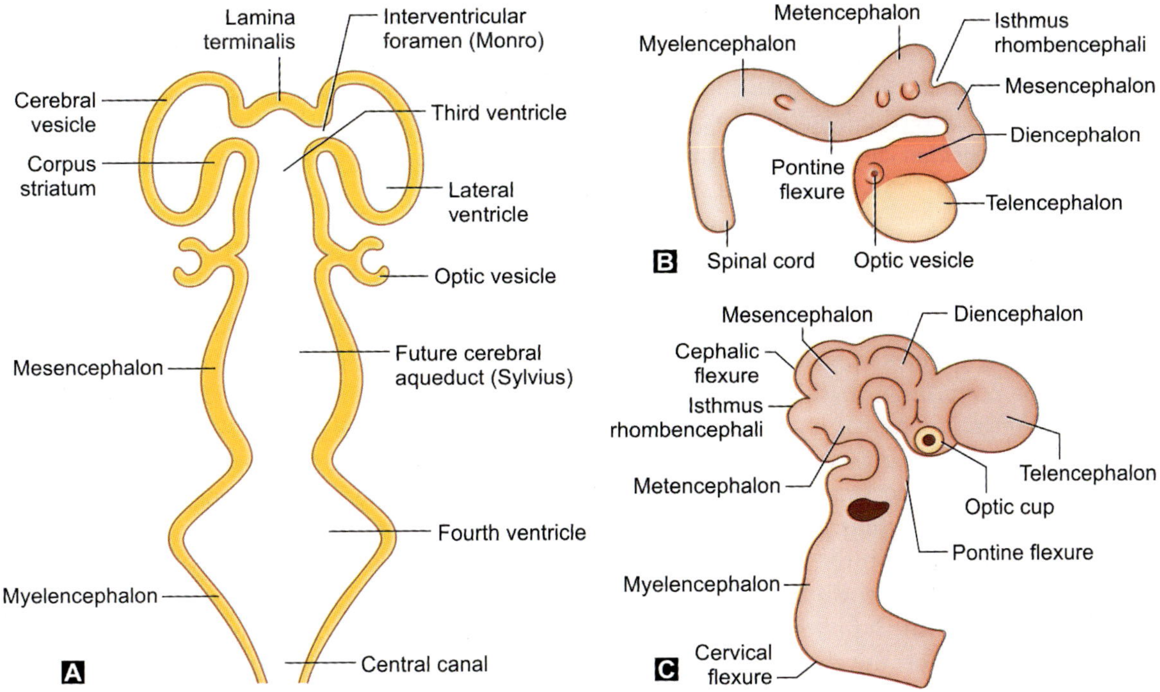

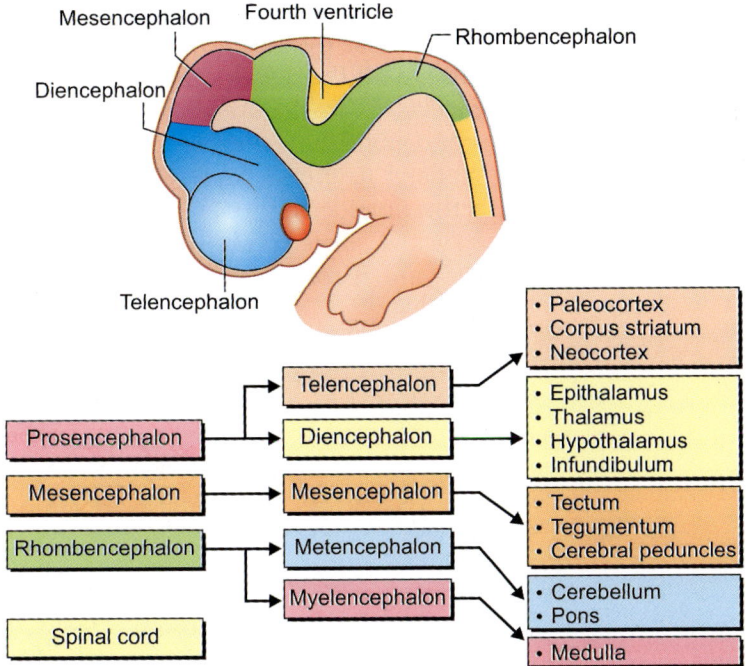

Fig. 2.3A to C: Lateral view of developing brain showing the three brain flexures and the derivatives of the brain vesicles (*Courtesy:* Nafis Ahmad Faruqi)

Fig. 2.4: Sequential development of the regions of the neuroectodermal neural tube forms the central nervous system consisting of the brain and the spinal cord

The caudal part of the *prosencephalon* forms the *diencephalon* and its cavity forms the *third ventricle*. Its roof remains essentially non-nervous. *Pineal body* developing in the posterior part of the roof constitutes the *epithalamus*. The lateral walls are largely occupied by the *thalamus* except below where the *hypothalamic structures* (which also occupy the floor) develop.

The *mesencephalon* develops into the midbrain and its cavity is greatly reduced to form the cerebral aqueduct. In its dorsal region called the *tectum* (roof) develop the *corpora quadrigemina* while the ventral portion develops into the *cerebral peduncles*.

The *isthmus rhombencephali* is the constricted portion between the mesencephalon and the rhombencephalon. It forms the *superior medullary velum* and the *superior cerebellar peduncles*.

With the development of the pontine flexure the *rhombencephalon* gets divided into the cranially sloping *metencephalon* and the caudally sloping *myelencephalon*. From the *metencephalon* develop the *cerebellum* dorsally and the *pons* ventrally. From the *myelencephalon* develops the *medulla oblongata*. The cavity of the rhombencephalon forms the *fourth ventricle*. Its roof is stretched out and is attached to the dorsal edges of the (rhomboidal) floor of the ventricle. These edges form the *superior* and the *inferior rhombic* lips. The floor of the *fourth ventricle* presents a sulcus *limitans*. It separates medially placed motor (efferent) cell columns of the *basal lamina* (plate) from the laterally placed sensory (afferent) cell columns of the *alar lamina*.

The portion of the neural tube caudal to the cervical flexure forms the *spinal cord*. Its cavity is narrowed to form the *central canal*. In the embryo, the spinal cord occupies whole of the vertebral canal. After the third month, the vertebral canal grows more rapidly than the spinal cord. As a result, the lower end of the spinal cord shifts higher. It lies opposite the third lumbar vertebra at birth and opposite the lower border of the first lumbar vertebra in the adult.

Developmental Defects in Central Nervous System

The rostral and caudal portions of the neural tube remain open for a short period as the *rostral* and *caudal neuropores*. Both pores, however, close by the end of the fourth week. A failure of the rostral neuropore to close will interfere with the development of the brain (especially the cerebral hemispheres), resulting in *anencephaly*. Non-closure of the caudal neuropore will result in myelocele or *rachischisis*. Both these conditions are associated with defects in the overlying bone, and the neural tissue may be exposed to the surface. The associated bony defect in anencephaly is *cranium bifidum* and in the myelocele it is *spina bifida* (Fig. 2.5). Less severe forms of *spina bifida* include *spina bifida occulta, meningocele* (meninges project through defect in vertebral arches) and *meningomyelocele* (spinal cord lies within a meningeal sac).

Table 2.1: Derivatives of the neural tube		
Primary brain vesicles	*Subdivisions of brain vesicles*	*Derivatives*
Prosencephalon	Telencephalon	Cerebral hemisphere
	Diencephalon	Thalamus
		Hypothalamus
		Epithalamus
Mesencephalon	—	Midbrain
Rhombencephalon	Metencephalon	Pons cerebellum (small or little brain)
	Myelencephalon	Medulla oblongata
Rest of the neural tube	—	Spinal cord (medulla spinalis)

Note: Some neural crest derivatives are: (1) Sensory ganglia of cranial nerves 5th, 7th, 8th, 9th and 10th; (2) Spinal ganglia; (3) Sympathetic and parasympathetic ganglia; (4) Schwann cells; (5) Adrenal medulla; and (6) Pia-arachnoid.

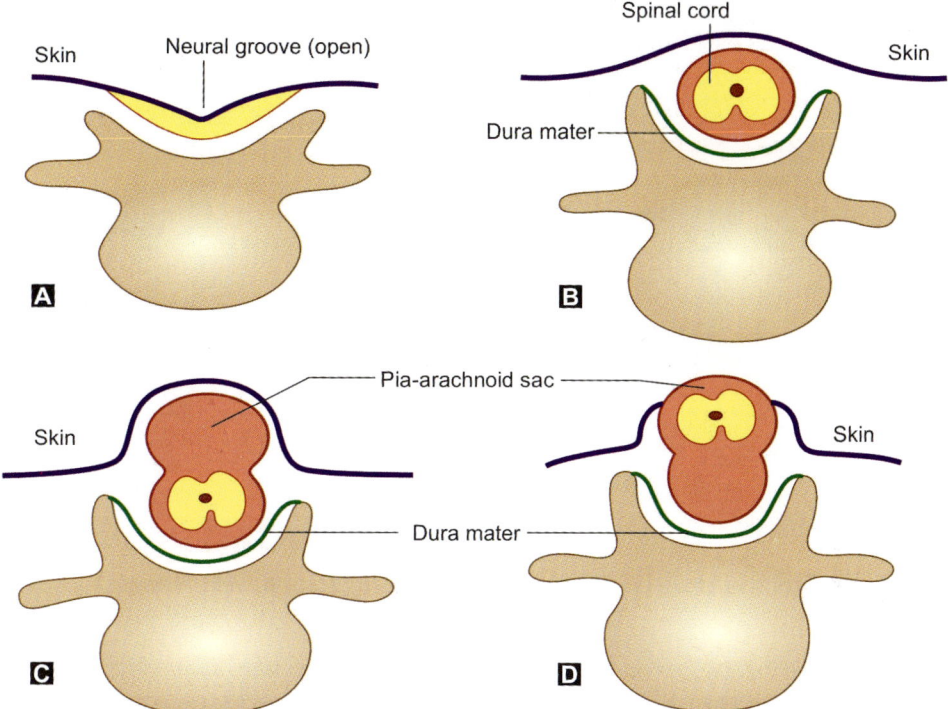

Fig. 2.5: Congenital anomalies of spinal cord: **A.** rachischisis, **B.** spina bifida occulta, **C.** meningocele, **D.** meningomyelocele

Developmental Defects in Brain

1. *Anencephaly* is a defect caused by failure of closure of the neural groove in the region of the developing brain, often associated with degeneration of the exposed neural plate tissue. But the degeneration occurs after the differentiation of the cranial nerves—these nerves and eyes are present in anencephalic fetuses.
2. *Hydrocephalus*—a condition produced due to:
   - Complete or partial blockage of the ventricular system
   - Imbalance between production and absorption of CSF
   - After operations of spina bifida cystica—not as a complication of the operation itself, but due to Arnold-Chiari malformation commonly termed Chiari malformation displacement of rhombencephalon and herniation of cerebellar tonsils in the subarachnoid space which produces hydrocephalus. In type II Chiari malformation, both the cerebellum and the brainstem extend into the foramen magnum (Fig. 2.6B).
3. *Congenital idiocy*—results due to faulty development or differentiation of cerebral cortex.
4. *Spastic mono* or *diplegia*—occurs if motor cortex is involved
5. *Congenital palsy*—due to faulty development or differentiation of brainstem.

HISTOGENESIS OF CNS

The early neural tube wall consists of a single layer of columnar cells, extending from the *internal* to the *external limiting membrane*. The nuclei of these cells are clustered close to the

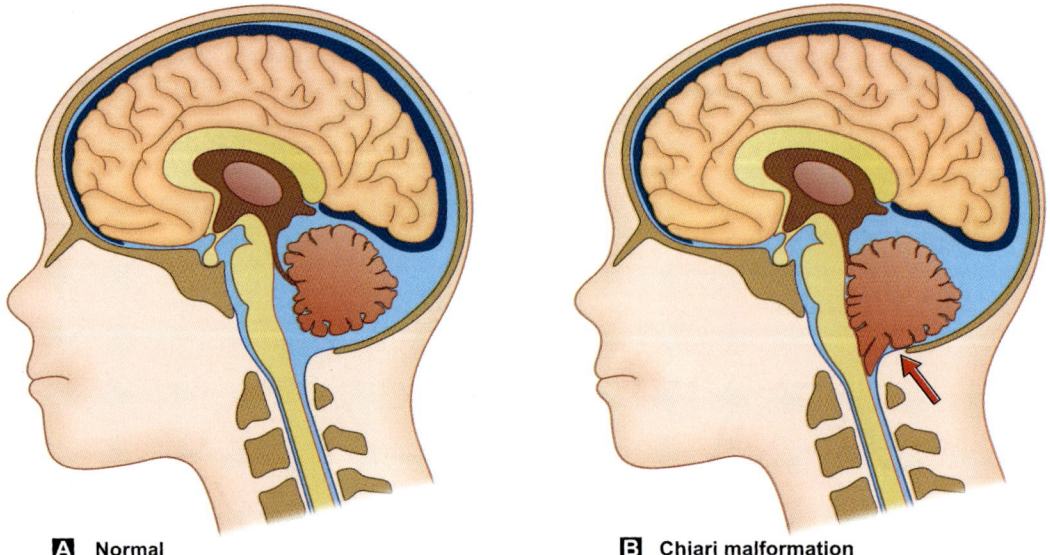

A Normal   B Chiari malformation

Fig. 2.6: Two drawings of the development of the brain: **A.** normal, **B.** with Arnold-Chiari malformation defect

internal limiting membrane, over a region called the *ventricular zone* (Fig. 2.6) . The outer nonnucleated portions of the cells, drawn out as cytoplasmic processes, constitute the *marginal zone.*

Several of these cells detach from the external membrane, become rounded, lie against the internal membrane and undergo repeated mitosis. The daughter cells migrate outwards to from an *intermediate (mantle) zone* between the ventricular and the marginal zones (Fig. 2.7).

The early migrants to the mantle zone form the *neurons*, which send their axonal sprouts into the marginal zone. The later migrants form the *neuroglia*. The embryonic CNS now consists of *three* zones: *ventricular, intermediate* and *marginal,* named from within outwards. The structures of the spinal cord and most brainstem regions are derived from these three zones, giving rise, respectively to the ependymal linings of their cavities, inner mass of grey matter including the nuclei and the outer white matter (Fig. 2.8). The white matter of the spinal cord and the brainstem are invaded at first by intersegmental fibers. Later, long ascending and descending fibers grow into them. In the developing *cerebrum, midbrain tectum* and the *cerebellum,* the neurons continue their migration beyond the mantle zone to from the *cortical plate* and *subplate* in the superficial parts of the marginal zone. An additional source of the migratory neurons is the subventricular *zone of* proliferating neurons. In the developing cerebrum the following zones may now be defined: marginal zone, cortical plate, subplate, intermediate, subventricular and the ventricular zones. The marginal zone forms the most superficial cortical layer (molecular layer). The remaining cortical layers are derived from the cortical plate and subplates. The intermediate zone transforms into the white matter. As proliferation ceases in the ventricular and subventricular layers the remaining cells in these zones differentiate into the *ependymal* cells, *tanycytes* and *subependymal glial* cells.

Myelination and Postnatal Development of Brain

Myelination of fibers in the brain begins in the sixth foetal month but progress is slow so that the brain is largely unmyelinated at birth. There is very little cerebral function and motor

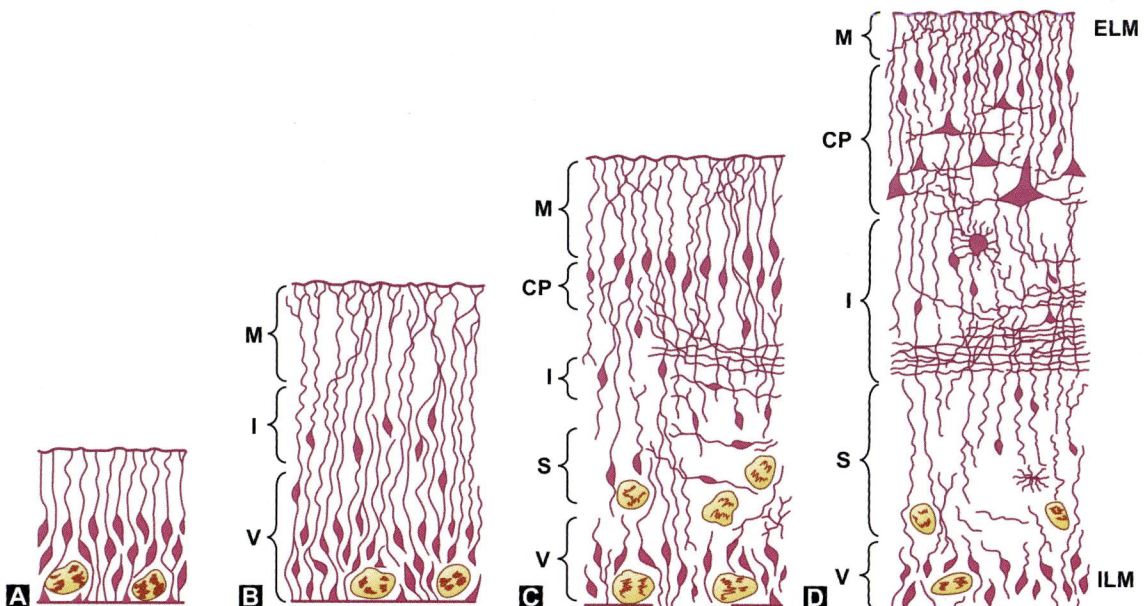

Fig. 2.7: Histogenesis of the CNS. Figures (A) to (D) indicate the stages during the development of the wall of neural tube and the differentiation of its zones: V: Ventricular zone, S: Subventricular zone, I: Intermediate zone, M: Marginal zone. Abbreviations: CP: Cortical plate, ELM: External limiting membrane, ILM: Internal limiting membrane

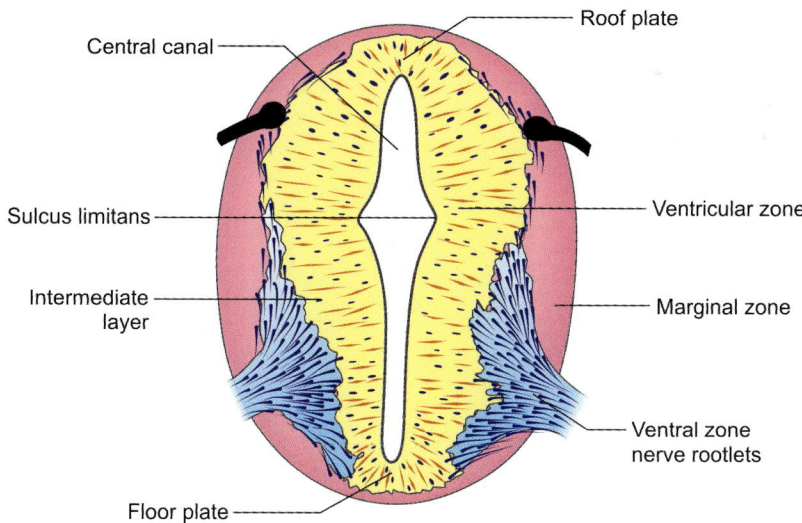

Fig. 2.8: Developing spinal cord shows the three principal zones in its wall

activities such as respiration, sucking and swallowing are essentially *reflex* in nature. The volume of the brain at birth is approximately 25% of its volume in the adult. The greater part of the increase occurs in the first year (Table 2.2). Acquisition of myelin sheath is largely responsible for this rapid early growth.

Table 2.2: Brain weight at different age-periods

Age-period	Weight of brain (g)	Remarks
Foetal month (3rd)	4	—
Foetal month (7th)	100	—
At Birth	300	20% of adult brain weight
1 year	600	2 times the birth brain weight
3 years	900	3 times the birth brain weight
6 years	1050	75% of adult brain weight
16 years	1400–1500	Adult brain weight
50 years	—	Decline in brain weight
70 years	—	30% loss in brain weight

Myelination does not occur simultaneously in all the fibre bundles. The main sensory pathways: visual, auditory and somatic, become myelinated first, and the motor fibers later. The corticospinal fibers start to myelinate at about 6 months after birth and the process is completed by the end of second year. Functional maturity in nervous system appears to depend upon myelination of the associated nerve fibers. Interestingly, however, the newborn opossum is precociously active and capable of many behavioral functions at a time when hardly any myelinated fibers are present in its brain and spinal cord.

Spinal Cord or Medulla Spinalis

DEVELOPMENT OF SPINAL CORD

Normal Development

Phylogenetically, the spinal cord appears in stage III of the development of the nervous system, when there is still no brain. Hence, it has centres for the control of all processes in the organism, both vegetative (autonomic) and animal (visceral and somatic). In the animals which have no limbs (e.g. snakes), the spinal cord is uniformly developed along its whole length and has no thickenings. Animals that use limbs develop two thickenings:

i. The anterior or cervical thickening predominates if the anterior or forelimbs are more developed (e.g. wings of birds).

ii. The posterior or lumbar thickening is larger if the posterior or hindlimbs are developed better. Both thickenings are equally developed in animals that use both the fore- and hind-limbs in walking (e.g. quadruped mammals). In man, the cervical thickening is differentiated more highly than the lumbar thickening because of the more complex activity of the hand.

The spinal cord develops from the posterior segment of the neural tube (the anterior segment gives rise to brain). The ventral part of the neural tube gives rise to the anterior (ventral) grey matter forming the cell bodies of the motor neurons and the adjacent bundles of the longitudinal nerve fibres and the processes of these neurons form the motor nerve roots. From the dorsal part are derived the posterior (dorsal) grey matter forming the cell bodies of the sensory neurons and the processes of the sensory neurons. As a result of a reduction of the caudal part of the spinal cord, a thin strand of nerve tissue forms the filum terminalae. Initially in the third month of intrauterine life, the spinal cord occupies the entire vertebral canal. Due to the fact that the vertebral column grows faster than the spinal cord, the end of the spinal cord moves cranially. At the time of birth it reaches at the level of L3 vertebra while in the adult it reaches the level of the L1 or L2 vertebra. Due to such 'ascent' of the spinal cord the nerve roots arising from it take an oblique direction.

In the developing spinal cord the neural tube wall shows ventricular, intermediate and marginal zones (*see* Fig. 2.8) from which are derived, respectively, the ependymal lining of the central canal, grey matter and the white matter of the spinal cord. The sulcus limitans divides the lateral wall of the developing spinal cord into the *basal* and *alar* laminae. The neuroblasts of the basal lamina form motor neurons of the *anterior* and *lateral grey* columns (horns), while the cells of the alar lamina form interneurons that receive sensory fibres from the dorsal root ganglion. The cavity of the neural tube, slit like at first, becomes diamond-shaped. Later its dorsal and ventral portions obliterate to form the narrow *central canal*. With the development of the anterior horns the floor plate sinks into a median groove, which later deepens to form the anterior *median fissure*. The posterior *median septum* is ependymal in origin and neuroglial in nature.

The earliest axonal sprouts invading the marginal zone of the developing spinal cord are the short *intersegmental fibres* (end of first month of IUL). *Long intersegmental fibres invade* in the third month and the *corticospinal fibres* during the fifth month of IUL. All the fibres are at first unmyelinated. Myelination beings at variable times, e.g. in dorsal and ventral nerve roots about the fifth month and in corticospinal fibres after ninth month. Myelination start at fourth month and continue during first postnatal period and it formed by oligodendrocytes.

Abnormal Development

The abnormal development of the spinal cord produces **congenital defects** (Fig. 3.1); and occurs due to:
- Genetic and environmental factors
- Alterations in the morphogenesis (histogenesis) of nervous tissue—intrinsic factors
- Failure in mesodermal structures related to early nervous system—extrinsic factors
  - Asyntaxia dorsalis—failure of closure of neural groove
- Extending along whole length—posterior rachischisis
- Limited in localised portion—myelocele
  - Spina bifida—failure to closure in spinal cord region—involves one vertebra as a rule.

The vertebral arch is not formed; more frequent in females:
- Most common in lumbosacral region
- May be complete or incomplete.

Spina bifida occulta is a condition caused by faulty development of the spinal cord that is characterized by a gap in the vertebral arch on only one vertebra; the gap is filled by fibrous tissue which may be adherent to the spinal cord. As a rule, there is no projection of the defect on the surface. Skin overlying it is intact. Sometimes, a local patch of hair, or a dimple, or a tumor frequently marks the site of defect. *Of the visible and outward manifestation, the most important is dimple*—caused by a fibrous cord called **membrana reunieus** which unites the deep layers of the skin to the spinal theca.

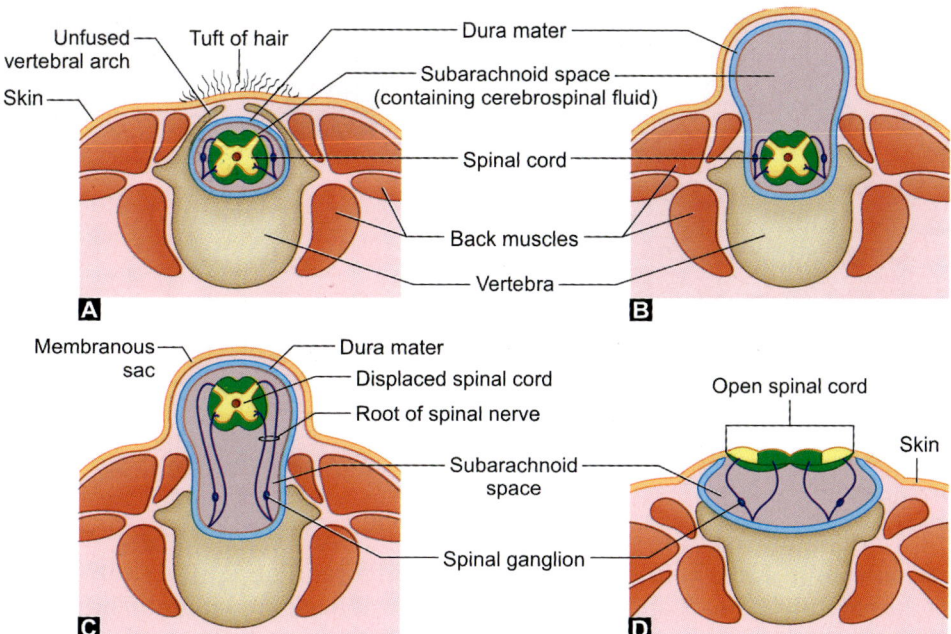

Fig. 3.1: Abnormal development of the spinal cord: **A.** spina bifida occulta with a tuft of hairs, **B.** spina bifida with a closed sac containing CSF in the subarachnoid space, **C.** spina bifida with the membranous sac containing displaced spinal cord with roots of spinal nerves, **D.** extreme condition where the defect consists of open spinal cord exposed dorsally. (see text for details)

The main complaints are:
- Backache
- Footdrop
- Talipes equinovarus—a congenital defect in the foot
- Nocturnal enuresis (only sometimes).

The other variety of spina bifida is **spina bifida cystica** (forming a cyst 80%). Neurological symptoms are present. These may vary according to three subtypes (Fig. 3.2) as described below:

 i. **Spina bifida with meningocele**—protrusion of sac containing meninges and CSF.

 ii. **Spina bifida with meningomyelocoele**—protrusion of sac containing meninges with spinal cord and/or nerve roots.

iii. **Spina bifida with myeloschisis**—spinal cord is open due to failure of neural folds.

When a dimpling occurs very early in the fetal life—at birth a pit of varying depth is noticeable. This condition is known as **congenital sacrococcygeal sinus**. The cause of non-closure of the neural groove is not known. But in most cases it is due to an abnormality in the mechanism of induction of the neural plate by the underlying notochord and mesoderm.

Spina bifida is frequently found in association with faulty differentiation of notochord and the vertebral bodies (e.g. in Klippel-Feil syndrome). Klippel-Feil syndrome (KFS) is a congenital, musculoskeletal condition (Fig. 3.2) characterized by the fusion of at least two vertebrae of the neck. Common symptoms include a short neck, low hairline at the back of the head, and restricted mobility of the upper spine. Klippel-Feil fusion of the cervical vertebrae may include any 2 or more of the 7 vertebrae.

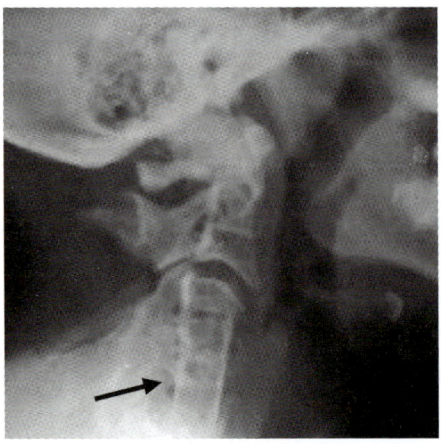
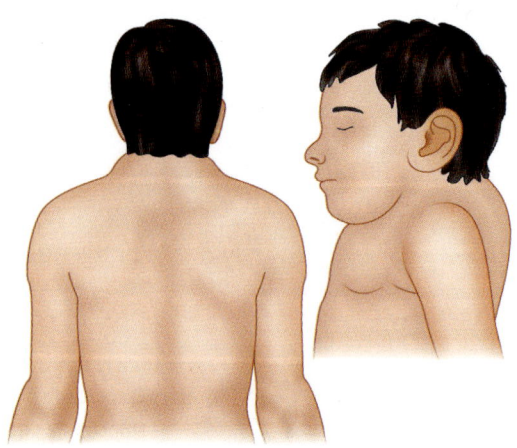

Fig. 3.2: Klippel-Feil syndrome—short neck, low hair-line, and fusion of some cervical vertebrae seen in the radiograph (arrow)

Three significant features result from this fused vertebra in neck: (i) a **short neck**, (ii) a **low hairline** at the back of the head, and (iii) a **limited range of neck movement**. The fused vertebrae in the neck can limit the neck movement and lead to chronic headaches and muscle pain in the neck and back. Over time, in Klippel-Feil syndrome can develop a narrowing of the spinal canal in the neck, which can compress the spinal cord. In addition, people with Klippel-Feil syndrome have abnormal side-to-side curvature of the spine (scoliosis); the fusion of additional vertebrae below the neck may also occur.

GROSS FEATURES OF THE SPINAL CORD

The spinal cord is a nearly cylindrical structure (average length in males is 45 cm) occupying the upper two-thirds of the vertebral canal. It extends from the foramen magnum to the lower border of L1 vertebra. A *posteromedian* and on its either side a *posterolateral sulcus* mark its dorsal surface. Both of these sulci are very shallow. An *anterior median fissure* and a *posterior median septum* incompletely divide the spinal cord into two symmetrical parts (Fig. 3.3).

Two enlargements or swellings are found in the spinal cord: an upper or *cervical enlargement* (from C3 to T2) and a lower or *lumbar enlargement* (from T9 to L2) externally. The lumbar enlargement reaches its maximum circumference opposite the T12 vertebra, below which it tapers rapidly into the *conus medullaris*. A delicate, long filament (about 20 cm) known as *filum terminale* continues downwards from the apex of the conus medullaris. Its upper part—*filum terminale internum* is continued within a tubular sheath of dura and arachnoid mater and extends up to the lower border of the second piece of sacrum. Its lower part—*filum terminale externum* descends from the dural sheath and is attached to the back of the first segment of the coccyx.

INTERNAL STRUCTURE OF SPINAL CORD SEEN IN TRANSVERSE SECTIONS

The spinal cord sections show an external layer of white matter enclosing a central core of grey matter. The right and left halves of the spinal cord are separated by the *anterior median fissure* dipping from the front and the *posterior median* septum, which dips from the posterior *median sulcus* (Fig. 3.4).

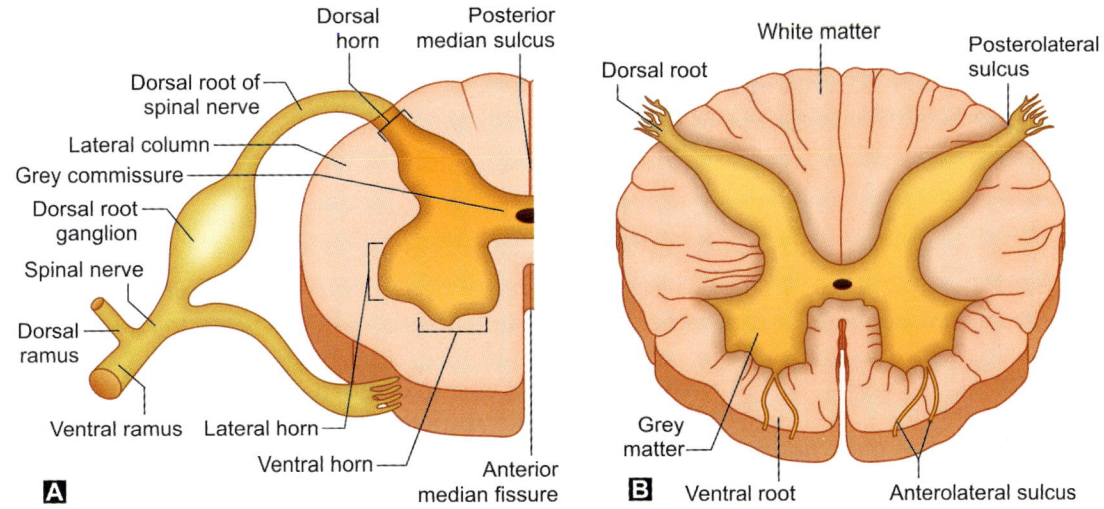

Fig. 3.3: Internal structure of the spinal cord seen in transverse sections: **A.** shows the dorsal and ventral roots of a spinal nerve arising from respective grey horns, **B.** is a section depicting symmetrical halves each having an inner grey matter surrounded by the white matter. In the centre is seen an oval central canal extending throughout the entire length of the spinal cord

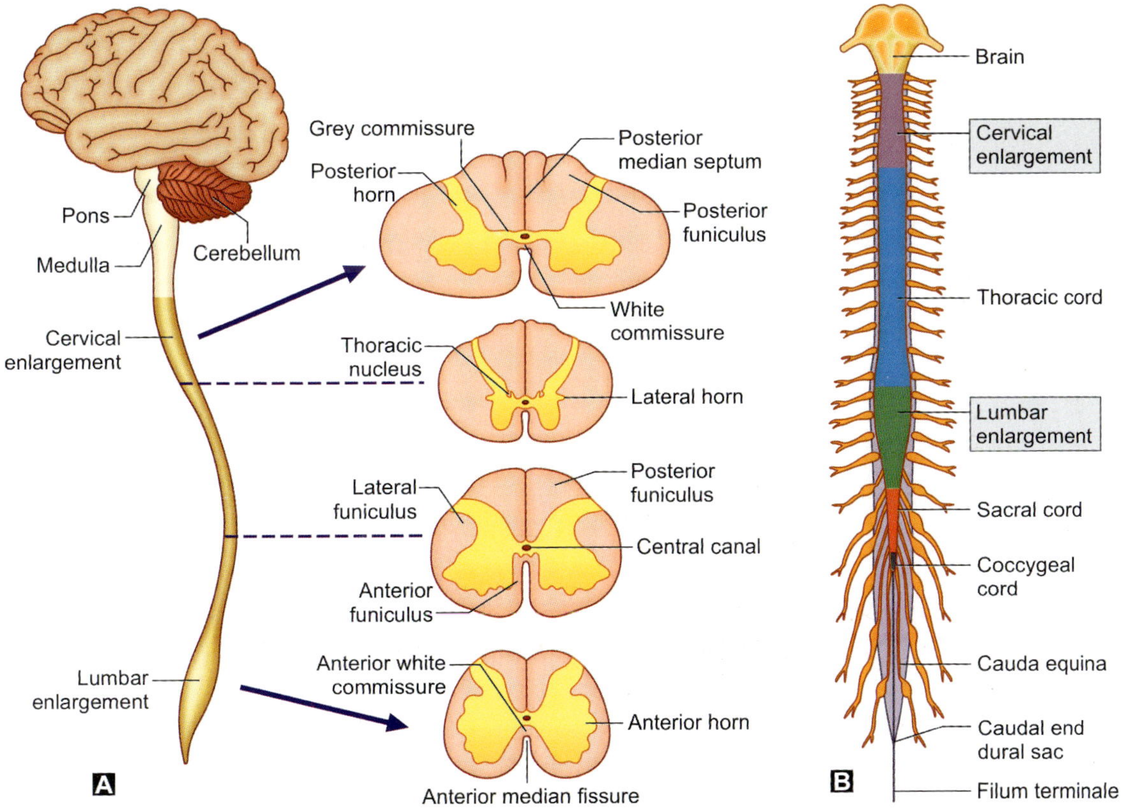

Fig. 3.4: A. External appearance of the brain and spinal cord with relative amount and shape of grey and white matters as seen in transverse sections cut at the levels shown; **B.** a schematic sketch of different regions of the spinal cord shown with different colors. Notice cauda equina and filum terminale

The peripheral white matter, on each side, consists of: (1) the *posterior funiculus* between the posterior median septum and the posterior grey horn, (2) the *anterolateral funiculus* (often divided into lateral and anterior funiculi) between the posterior horn and the anterior median fissure, and (3) the *white commissure,* lying in front of the grey commissure.

The grey matter core appears H-shaped in transverse sections. It consists of: (1) a *grey commissure,* traversed by the *central canal of the spinal cord,* (2) a pair of *posterior horns,* (3) a pair of *anterior horns,* and (4) a pair of *lateral horn* exclusively in the thoracic and upper two lumbar segments of the spinal cord. The **posterior grey horn** consists *of head, neck* and the *base.* The *apex* of the head is separated from the posterolateral sulcus by the *Lissauer's tract.* In this tract (mainly composed of propriospinal fibres) many fibres of the posterior nerve root, ascend (mostly) for 1–2 segments before entering the posterior grey horn. The **anterior grey horn** is short and broad and fails to reach the surface of the spinal cord. Axons of the motor neurons in the anterior horn form the *ventral nerve roots.*

TS at Different Vertebral Levels

Spinal cord sections from different regions present distinctive features (Fig. 3.4).

Cervical Region

The section is relatively large and oval in outline. The posterior grey horns are narrow but the anterior horns are broad. The relative amount of white matter is maximal.

Thoracic Region

The section is small and circular. Both the anterior and posterior grey horns are narrow. A short lateral horn is also present.

Lumbar Region

The section is relatively large and circular. Both the anterior and posterior grey horns are broad. The amount of white matter is relatively less.

Sacral Region

The section is small and circular. Both grey horns are broad. The white matter is reduced to a thin outer rim.

Terminal or Fifth Ventricle

The **terminal ventricle** (of **Krause**), also known as the **5th ventricle** (Fig. 3.5), is an ependyma-lined fusiform dilatation of the terminal central canal of the spinal cord, positioned at the transition from the tip of the conus medullaris to the origin of the filum terminale. The average size of the terminal ventricle is approximately $22 \times 4.1 \times 4.2$ mm. It represents the canalisation and retrogressive differentiation of the caudal end of the developing spinal cord and regresses in size during the first weeks after birth. Rarely, the terminal ventricle may dilate and cause significant clinical symptoms. MRI is useful in the detection and diagnosis of the terminal ventricle.

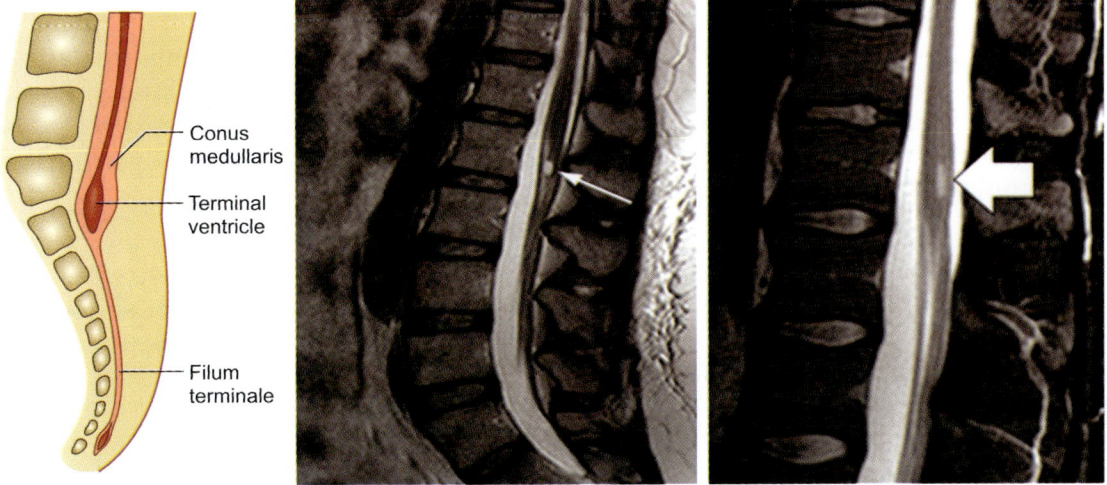

Fig. 3.5: The terminal or fifth ventricle is a dilated portion of the central canal of the spinal cord in the lower vertebral canal

Nuclei in Spinal Grey Matter

The nuclei or nerve cell groups present in the spinal grey matter (Fig. 3.6) are as follows:

Nucleus Postero Marginalis

Capping the apex of the posterior horn, it contains both small and large neurons. The large neurons contribute axons to the opposite lateral spinothalamic tract.

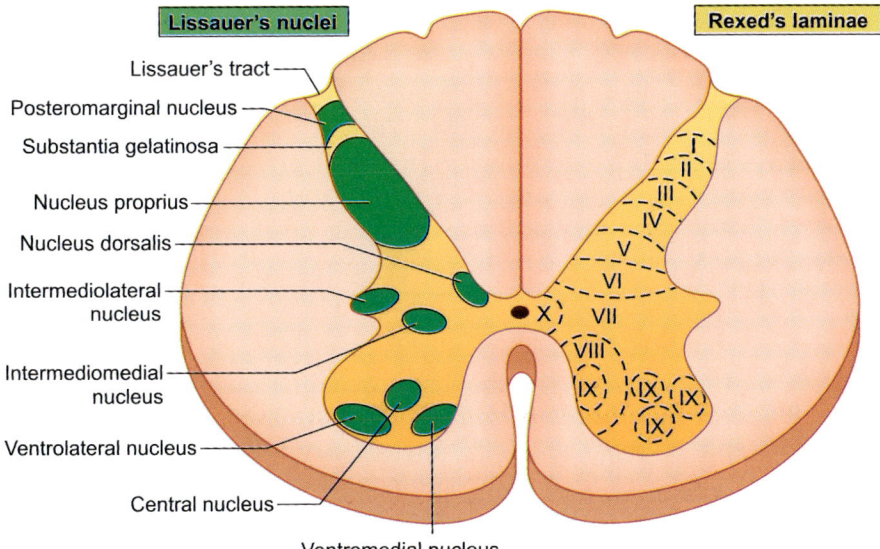

Fig. 3.6: Internal structure of the spinal cord seen in transverse section is composed of peripheral white nervous matter (in light brown) and centrally located grey matter, which consists of right and left symmetrical portions connected by a transverse grey commissure (depicted in yellow color here) and bearing a resemblance to the letter H. In the left half of the section are shown the main nuclei (green) in the grey column; on the right side of the grey neural matter are shown location of ten Rexed's laminae described in the text

Substantia Gelatinosa of Rolando

It is a compact mass of small cells forming the apex of posterior horn. Afferents are derived from collaterals of dorsal root axons and also descending reticulospinal fibres. Efferents make contact with cells in the dorsal grey horn. Its cells (inhibitory) are supposed to control the 'gate' for incoming painful impulses and can be stimulated by tactile sensations (e.g. rubbing of skin) to inhibit pain.

Nucleus Proprius

It forms the head of the posterior horn. Axons of these cells cross the midline to enter the opposite spinothalamic tract. These conduct pain, temperature, crude touch and pressure.

Nucleus Thoracicus (Clarke's Column)

This nucleus is discernible only in the thoracic and upper 3 or 4 lumbar regions where it projects from the medial side of the base of the posterior horn. It receives collaterals from the tracts in the dorsal funiculus. Axons of these cells join the ipsilateral dorsal spinocerebellar tract. These conduct unconscious proprioceptive impulses, necessary for muscular coordination and tone.

Intermediate Group Nuclei

Neurons in these nuclei (intermediolateral group in particular) produce the lateral horn in the thoracic and upper two lumbar segments and are preganglionic sympathetic motor neurons. Corresponding cells at the sacral 2, 3 and 4 levels constitute parasympathetic motor neurons.

Anterior Horn Cell Groups

These consist of large (a) and small (g) motor neurons whose axons form the ventral nerve roots and are distributed to the striated muscles. Three basic groups—medial, central and lateral are recognized. The medial group innervates axial muscles (of neck and trunk). The lateral group supplies limb muscles while the central group is represented by the phrenic nucleus in the cervical cord. The spinal accessory nucleus also found in the cervical region is more ventrally placed.

Rexed's Laminae

Rexed (1964) described 10 laminae in the grey matter of spinal cord, based on the cytoarchitecture (Fig. 3.6). Six laminae (laminae I to VI) occupy the posterior horn. The nucleus posteromarginalis corresponds to the lamina I, the substantia gelatinosa corresponds to the laminae II and III, and nucleus proprius to the laminae IV to VI.

- Laminae I–IV receive all types of cutaneous stimuli and give rise to *spinothalamic tracts*.
- Laminae V and VI receive proprioceptive impulses and also *corticospinal projections*.
- Lamina VII includes Clarke's nucleus whose cells connect extensively with the midbrain and cerebellum (via the *spinocerebellar, spinotectal* and *spinoreticular tracts*).
- Laminae V to VII are involved in the regulation of posture, movements and autonomic functions.

- Cells in lamina VIII are mostly interneurons receiving *vestibulospinal* and *reticulospinal fibres.* Their axons influence motor neurons in the anterior horn.
- Lamina IX contains motor neurons whose axons terminate on motor end plates and motor neurons, which supply *intrafusal muscle fibres* in muscle spindles.
- Lamina X surrounds the central canal.

Interneurons

Majority of the neurons in the grey matter of spinal cord are interneurons. These neurons are intercalated in various reflex loops and neuronal circuits. A spinal interneuron, found in the spinal cord, relays signals between (afferent) sensory neurons, and (efferent) motor neurons. Different classes of spinal **interneurons** are involved in the process of sensory-motor integration. These neurons also serve as intermediaries between the primary afferent neurons and the second order neurons giving rise to the long ascending fibre bundles (e.g. spinothalamic tracts). Other interneurons are interposed between the long descending fibres (e.g. corticospinal tracts) and the motor neurons in the anterior horn. Through the interneurons the motor neurons are influenced by dorsal root afferents (for spinal reflexes) and several descending tracts from the brain for the control of motor activity.

Funiculi or Tracts in White Matter

The white matter of the spinal cord is made up of bundles of myelinated nerve fibres (tracts or fasciculi). Some of the tracts are ascending, i.e. conducting impulses to the higher regions of the neuraxis while others descend from the higher centres (Fig. 3.7). The posterior funiculus of the spinal cord has *ascending tracts* while the anterolateral funiculus has both *ascending* and *descending tracts.* There are also propriospinal fibres forming intersegmental tracts that connect neurons in the adjacent as well as more distantly placed segments. The *dorsolateral tract (of*

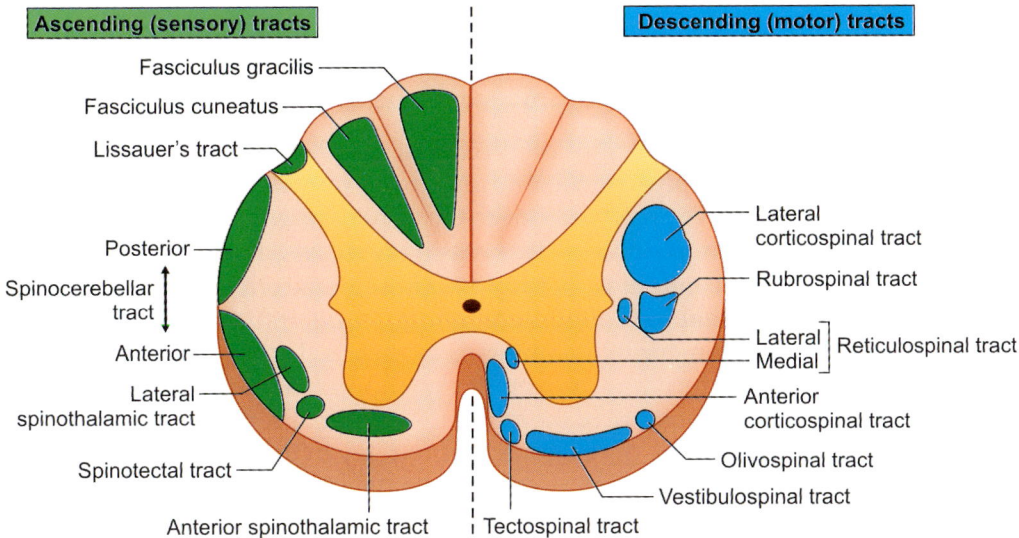

Fig. 3.7: TS of spinal cord showing the ascending or sensory tracts (green) on the left side and descending or motor tracts (blue) on the right side

Lissauer) opposite the apex of the posterior horn is essentially a propriospinal tract even though pain fibres are also supposed to ascend in this tract for a segment or two.

Tracts in the Posterior Funiculus

The dorsal funiculus includes the *fasciculi gracilis* and *cuneatus* which contain long ascending fibres derived from ipsilateral spinal ganglion cells (primary afferent neurons) and about 15% secondary neurons from the ipsilateral posterior horn cells. These large diameter nerve fibres carry the sense of fine touch, position (static position as well as kinesthesia, i.e. sense of movement), vibration, tactile discrimination and stereognosis.

Fasciculus Gracilis

This is placed medially, commences at the caudal limit of the spinal cord and carries impulses from the lower limb and the abdominal regions.

Fasciculus Cuneatus

This lies laterally, commences at the mid-thoracic level and carries impulses from the thorax, upper limb and cervical regions. The fibres in both these tracts ascend through the spinal cord to terminate in the *nuclei gracilis* and *cuneatus* present in the medulla oblongata.

Tracts in the Anterolateral Funiculus

The anterolateral funiculus that can be subdivided into the anterior and the lateral funiculi (*plural* of funiculus) by the ventral root fibres have both ascending and descending tracts. In general the *ascending tracts* occupy a more superficial position than the *descending tracts* (Fig. 3.7).

Ascending Tracts

Posterior spinocerebellar tract: This tract is situated at the periphery of the posterior region of the lateral funiculus. Its fibres are derived from the *ipsilateral* thoracic nucleus, which in turn, receives exteroceptive (touch and pressure) and proprioceptive impulses through the collaterals and terminals derived from the long ascending tracts in the dorsal funiculus. The tract passes to the cerebellum through the inferior cerebellar peduncle.

Anterior spinocerebellar tract: This tract lies in front of the above tract and begins about the same level. It contains crossed fibres, which originate from the cells of the laminae V to VII of the *contralateral* posterior horn. The tract ascends to the upper pons and passes to the cerebellum through the superior cerebellar peduncle after crossing a second time.

Both spinocerebellar tracts conduct proprioceptive impulses from the muscles and joints of the lower limbs to the ipsilateral half of the cerebellum. These informations are essential for posture and muscle coordination during voluntary movements. The posterior tract is concerned with fine coordination of posture and movement of individual muscle. The anterior tract coordinates the movement and posture of the entire lower limb. Proprioceptive impulses from the upper limb are conducted in the dorsal funiculus to relay in the accessory cuneate nucleus in the medulla on way to the cerebellum.

Spinothalamic tracts: These include the anterior and the lateral spinothalamic tracts (Table 3.1). The *anterior spinothalamic* tract lies in the anterior funiculus dorsal to the vestibulospinal tract while the *lateral spinothalamic* tract lies medial to the anterior

Table 3.1: Comparison of anterior and lateral spinothalamic tracts

	Anterior spinothalamic	Lateral spinothalamic
Origin	Centromedian nucleus	Substantia gelatinosa
Crossing	Few segments higher	At once (i.e. at same level)
Termination	Ventral posterolateral nucleus	Ventral posterolateral nucleus
Modalities	Crude touch	Pain
	Pressure	Temperature
Applied importance		Bilateral lesions-cause syringomyelia

spinocerebellar tract. The anterior spinothalamic tract conducts sensations of crude touch and pressure. The lateral spinothalamic tract conducts pain and temperature. Their fibres arise from the posterior horn cells and cross in the anterior white commissure. The pain and temperature fibres cross closer to the central canal and may be involved in *syringomyelia*. In the medulla oblongata the anterior spinothalamic tract joins the medial lemniscus while the lateral spinothalamic tract along with the spinotectal tract constitutes the *spinal lemniscus.* Both spinothalamic tracts terminate in the ventral posterior nuclei of thalamus. The above classical subdivision of the spinothalamic tract into lateral, and anterior is now being rejected.

Spinoreticular and spinotectal tracts: These tracts also conduct pain and temperature sensations. These tracts and terminate in the brainstem reticular formation, peri-aqueductal grey matter and the superior colliculus. Ascending fibres from the reticular formation end in the intralaminar thalamic nuclei, which project widely to the cerebral cortex to bring alertness.

Spino-olivary tract: It conducts proprioceptive impulses. Its fibres originate from deeper laminae of the opposite posterior horn and ascend to the dorsal and medial accessory olivary nuclei. A *dorsal spino-olivary* tract ascends in the posterior funiculus and ends in the inferior olivary nucleus.

Descending Tracts

Corticospinal tracts: These two tracts, *lateral* (crossed) and *anterior* (uncrossed), are also called the pyramidal tracts. Their fibres mainly originate in the motor area of the cerebral cortex. The tract also contains fibres descending from the premotor and somesthetic areas. The fibres descend through the white matter of the cerebrum, crus cerebri, ventral pons and finally the pyramid of the medulla oblongata. In the lower medulla, about 85% fibres cross in the *pyramidal (motor) decussation.* The crossed fibres descend in the lateral funiculus of the spinal cord as the lateral corticospinal tract, which lies deep to the posterior spinocerebellar tract. The uncrossed fibres (15%) descend as the ventral corticospinal tract beside the anterior median fissure. The corticospinal fibres terminate in relation with the interneurons in the laminae IV to VII. Through these interneurons they influence the motor neurons in the anterior horn (lamina IX) on the side opposite to their origin in the motor cortex. The corticospinal fibres along with their cells of origin form the *upper motor neuron* while the anterior horn neurons, which ultimately terminate in relation with the fibres of the striated muscles constitute the *lower motor neuron.*

Rubrospinal tract: This tract lies in the lateral funiculus anterior to the lateral corticospinal tract. Its fibres originate from the red nucleus of the midbrain and immediately crossover to the opposite side. The fibres descend through pons, medulla and the spinal cord to ultimately influence the anterior horn motor neurons. The tract is rudimentary in man and ends at the C3 level. Both, the corticospinal and the rubrospinal fibres influence the more laterally placed anterior horn cells that control distally placed limb muscles. Both are facilitatory to the flexors and inhibitory to the extensors and are important, particularly, for the skilled and precise movements of the fingers.

Vestibulospinal tract: The vestibulospinal tract lies in the anterior funiculus of the spinal cord. Its fibres originate in the lateral vestibular nucleus (Deiter's nucleus) in the medulla. They terminate in synaptic contacts with the anterior horn motor neurons, innervating extensor muscles. The vestibulospinal tract serves to maintain posture and balance by facilitating quick movements in reaction to sudden changes in body position (e.g. falling).

Reticulospinal tract: The reticulospinal fibres originate in several nuclei of the reticular formation of the midbrain, pons and medulla. The fibres, largely ipsilateral, occupy the ventral funiculus and the ventral half of the lateral funiculus. The fibres influence the motor neurons and control motor activities that do not require constant conscious efforts. They also influence autonomic neurons.

Olivospinal tract of Helweg: It occupies a small triangular area immediately lateral to the issuing ventral nerve roots. The tract is confined to the cervical levels and terminates in relation with the anterior horn cells.

Tectospinal tract: The tectospinal tract, present only in the upper cervical regions originates in the superior colliculus, crosses to the opposite side and descends through the brainstem close to the mid line. In the spinal cord, it lies in the ventral funiculus, adjacent to the ventral end of the anterior median fissure. This tract causes head turning in response to sudden visual or auditory stimuli.

APPLIED ANATOMY OF SPINAL CORD

1. **Poliomyelitis:** Polio (poliomyelitis) is a highly infectious viral disease. The poliovirus invades the nervous system and can cause irreversible paralysis in a matter of hours. Polio is spread through person-to-person contact is a preventable viral disease which destroys the motor neurons in the anterior horn of the spinal cord leading to paralysis and atrophy of the muscles (lower motor neuron paralysis).

2. **Syringomyelia:** In this disease, there is a destruction of the central portion of the spinal cord and widening of the central canal beginning usually in the cervical region. The second order neuron fibres conducting pain and temperature, which cross midline in the vicinity of the central canal are affected. A bilateral loss of pain and temperature senses in the area of the skin supplied by the affected cord segments results.

3. **Anterior spinal artery syndrome:** The anterior spinal artery supplies the ventral two-thirds of the spinal cord including the anterolateral funiculi and ventral grey horns. An obstruction in the artery (thrombosis) results in a bilateral loss of pain and temperature (spinothalamic tracts) and motor disturbances (corticospinal tracts and ventral horn cells) below the level of lesion. Dorsal column senses (touch, vibration and position) are not affected.

4. **Dorsal column syndrome:** In a dorsal column lesion, there is loss of vibration and position senses, muscular incoordination (ataxic gait) and astereognosis (inability to recognize objects by feeling only). Dorsal column lesions are found in tabes dorsalis (tertiary stage of syphilis) and vitamin B_{12} deficiency (subacute combined degeneration).

5. **Progressive lateral sclerosis:** It is a hereditary degenerative disease of anterior horn neurons. The patient gradually becomes weaker and dies within 3–10 years.

6. **Amyotrophic lateral sclerosis:** It is a bilateral degenerative disease involving corticospinal fibres, ventral horn cells and motor cranial nerve nuclei. Signs of both upper and lower motor neuron lesions are found.
7. **Familial spastic paraplegia:** The pyramidal tracts undergo a dying-back process. There is upper motor neuron paralysis. It refers to a group of inherited disorders that are characterized by progressive weakness and spasticity (stiffness) of the legs.
8. **Friedreich's ataxia:** It is a hereditary, degenerative disease of the cerebellum and posterolateral portions of the spinal cord.
9. **Spinal injuries:** Commonest sites of spinal injuries are the lower cervical regions and the thoracolumbar junction.

Levels of lesions and associated symptoms are presented in Table 3.2.

Table 3.2: Effects of total transection of spinal cord	
Level of spinal segment	*Symptoms*
Above C4	Respiratory failure (phrenic and intercostal nerves)
C5	Quadriplegia (paralysis of all four limbs)
C6	Paraplegia (both lower limbs paralysed)
	Upper limbs abducted (unopposed deltoid)
	Forearm flexed and supinated (unopposed biceps)
C7	Paraplegia loss of flexion at wrist, extension of fingers
C8	Paraplegia with fingers extended (flexors paralysed)
T1	Paraplegia, paralysis of small muscles of hand and **Horner's syndrome**
Rest of thoracic segments	Paraplegia and paralysis of trunk
L1–L2	Loss of hip flexion
L2–L3	Loss of hip adduction
L3–L4	Loss of hip extension
L4	Loss of dorsi-flexion of foot
L5	Loss of great toe extension
S1–S5	Loss of knee flexion, urinary and rectal incontinence

Brainstem

- What is Brainstem?
  - Development
- Components of Brainstem
- Gross features of Brainstem
  - Appearance from front
- Appearance from back
- Appearance from sides
- Cranial Nerve Nuclei in Brainstem
- Tracts in Brainstem
- Clinical Significance

WHAT IS BRAINSTEM?

The brainstem is the central trunk of the mammalian brain, consisting of the medulla oblongata, pons, and midbrain, and continuing downwards to form the spinal cord. It is the most inferior portion of the brain, adjoining and structurally continuous with the brain and spinal cord. The brainstem gives rise to cranial nerves III through XII and provides the main motor and sensory innervation to the face and neck via the cranial nerves. Though small, it is an extremely important part of the brain, as the nerve connections of the motor and sensory systems from the main part of the brain that communicate with the peripheral nervous system pass through the brainstem. This includes the corticospinal tract (motor), the posterior column-medial lemniscus pathway (fine touch, vibration sensation, and proprioception) and the spinothalamic tract (pain, temperature, itch, and crude touch). The brainstem also plays an important role in the regulation of cardiac and respiratory functions. It regulates the central nervous system (CNS) and is pivotal in maintaining consciousness and regulating the sleep cycle. The brainstem acts as a vehicle for sensory information.

Development

The adult human brainstem emerges from two of the three primary vesicles formed of the neural tube. The mesencephalon is the second of the three primary vesicles, and does not further differentiate into a secondary vesicle. This will become the midbrain (Fig. 4.1). The third primary vesicle, the rhombencephalon (hindbrain) will further differentiate into two secondary vesicles, the metencephalon and the myelencephalon. The metencephalon will

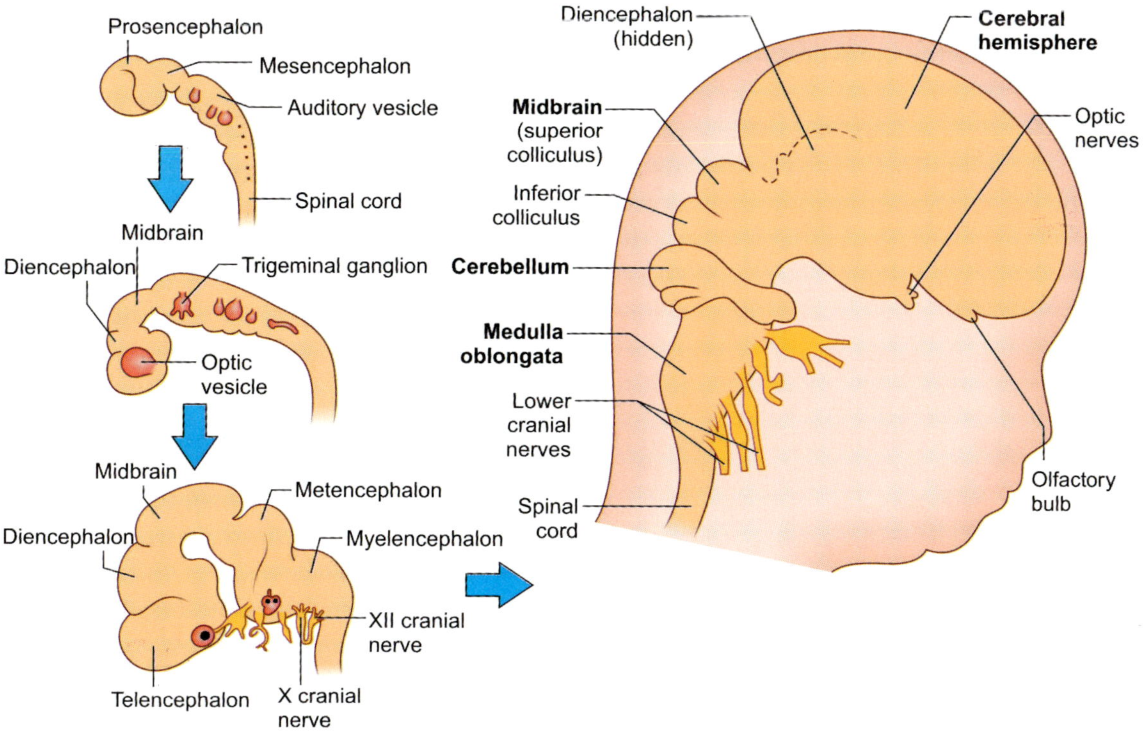

Prosencephalon

Mesencephalon

Auditory vesicle

Spinal cord

Midbrain

Diencephalon

Trigeminal ganglion

Optic vesicle

Midbrain

Diencephalon

Metencephalon

Myelencephalon

XII cranial nerve

Telencephalon

X cranial nerve

Diencephalon (hidden)

Cerebral hemisphere

Midbrain (superior colliculus)

Optic nerves

Inferior colliculus

Cerebellum

Medulla oblongata

Lower cranial nerves

Spinal cord

Olfactory bulb

Fig. 4.1: Development of brainstem components

become the cerebellum and the pons. The more caudal myelencephalon will become the medulla oblongata.

COMPONENTS OF BRAINSTEM

The *three* components of the brainstem are the midbrain, pons, and medulla oblongata of the hindbrain (Fig. 4.2). Sometimes the diencephalon, the caudal part of the forebrain, is also

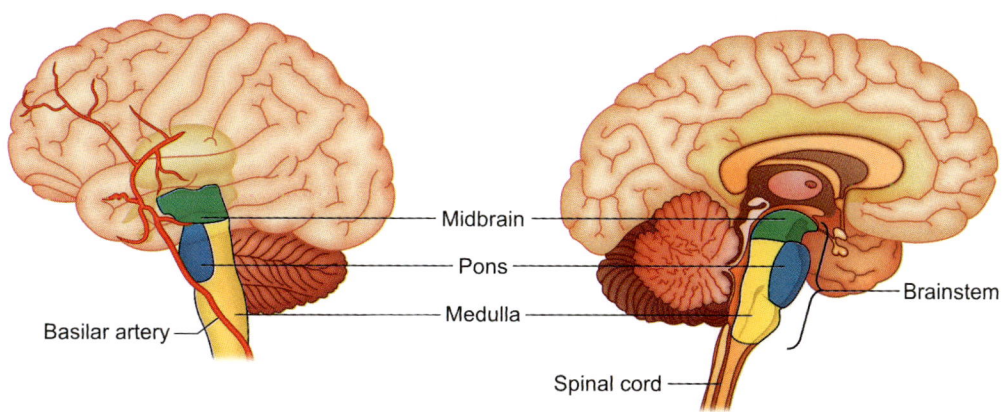

Midbrain

Pons

Medulla

Brainstem

Basilar artery

Spinal cord

Fig. 4.2: Structures of the brainstem are depicted in the diagram, including the midbrain, pons, and medulla

included. Motor and sensory neurons travel through the **brainstem** allowing for the relay of signals between the brain and the spinal cord.

GROSS FEATURES OF BRAINSTEM

The lateral and posterior surfaces of the brainstem are largely hidden from view in an intact brain by the cerebral hemispheres and cerebellum. Hence, the brainstem can be exposed from all aspects by the removal of both these structures. The cut surfaces of the white matter bundles, which connect the brainstem with detached portions, present a massive bundle—the *internal capsule* at the rostral end.

Appearance from Front

The front surface (actually facing inferiorly) shows the emergence of cranial nerves III to XII (all cranial nerves except I (olfactory) and II (optic) both of which are parts of the brain and **do not** emerge from the brainstem (Fig. 4.3A).

Appearance from Back

From behind, the components of the brainstem can be seen after removal of cerebellum, which is connected on each side to each brainstem component—by three white matter bundles called **cerebellar peduncles**. These peduncles from rostral to caudal side are: *superior* (brachium conjunctivum), *middle* (brachium pontis), and *inferior* (restiform body). The midbrain (mesencephalon) consists, on the posterior aspect, of four rounded swellings: two *superior* and two *inferior colliculi*. These four swellings are also called collectively as **corpora quadrigemina** (Fig. 4.3B). The midbrain is associated functionally with vision, hearing, motor control, sleep and wake cycles, alertness, and temperature regulation.

The pons lies between the medulla oblongata and the midbrain. It contains tracts that carry signals from the cerebrum to the medulla and to the cerebellum. It also has tracts that carry

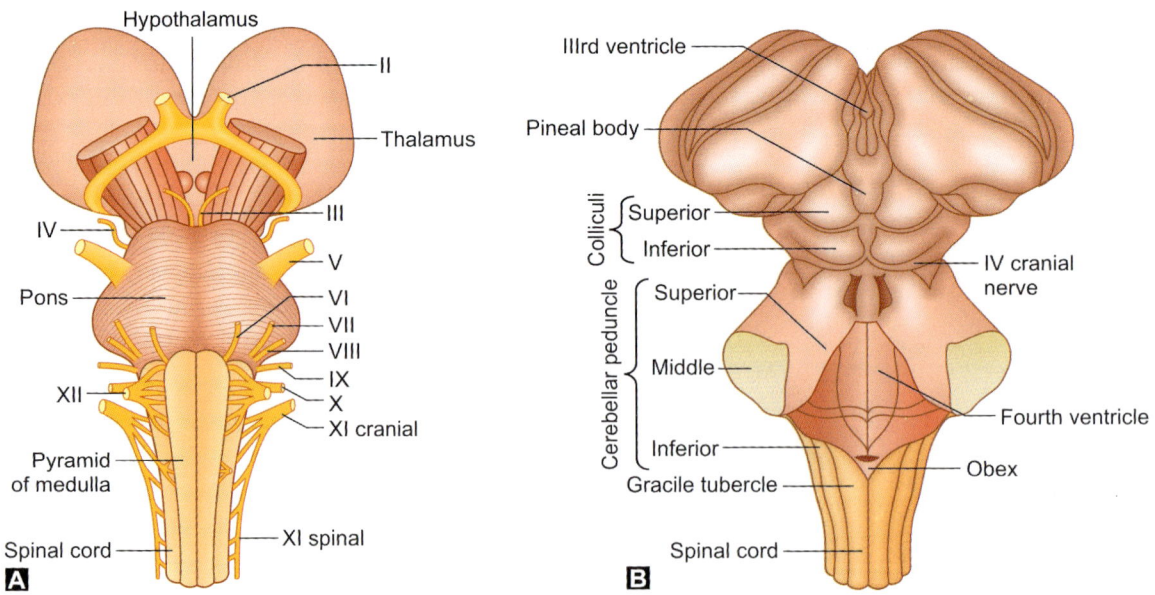

Fig. 4.3: Two views of the brainstem: **A.** from the front, **B.** from the behind

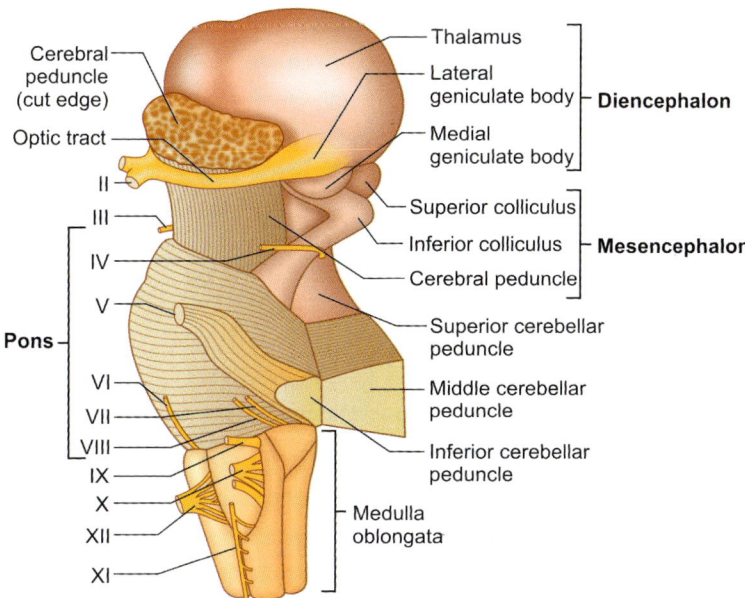

Fig. 4.4: The brainstem from lateral aspect

sensory signals to the thalamus. The medulla oblongata is the lower half of the brainstem continuous with the spinal cord. Its upper part is continuous with the pons. The medulla contains the cardiac, respiratory, vomiting, and vasomotor centres regulating heart rate, breathing, and blood pressure.

Appearance from Sides

The lateral aspect of the brainstem shows the sulci, observed on the surfaces of the spinal cord, which continue upward into the medulla (Fig. 4.4). Above the medulla, only the posterior median sulcus and sulcus limitans are present. The *anterior median sulcus* is partially obliterated in the lower part of medulla oblongata by obliquely crossing pyramidal decussation.

CRANIAL NERVE NUCLEI IN BRAINSTEM

The cell columns identifiable in the grey matter on each side are *four* in number (Fig. 4.5) (*the first two* in basal lamina and the remaining *two* in the alar lamina) as detailed below:
  i. Somatic efferent—supplies striated muscles of the trunk and limbs.
 ii. General visceral efferent—contains preganglionic neurons of the ANS.
iii. General visceral afferent—receives afferents from thoracic and abdominal organs.
iv. General somatic afferent—receives afferents from the body wall.
   In the brainstem, these four columns are fragmented (Fig. 4.6), and not all contribute to each cranial nerve. Their connections are tabulated in Table 4.1.

TRACTS IN BRAINSTEM

There are *three* somatic sensory pathways in the brainstem (Figs 4.7 and 4.8):
  i. Posterior column—**medial lemniscal pathways**—the chief functions of the posterior column are those of *conscious proprioception* and *discriminative touch*. In humans, disturbance of the

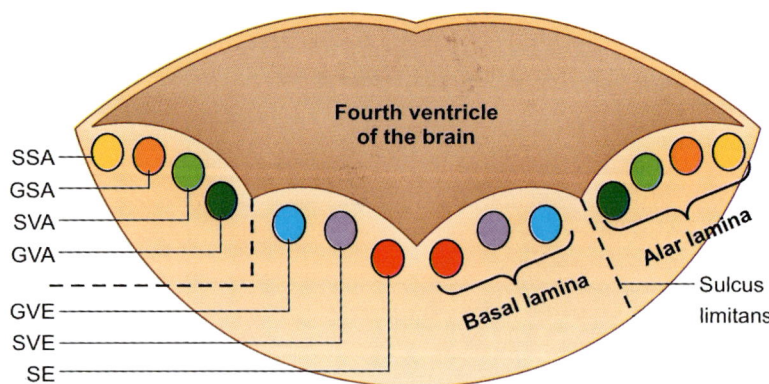

Fig. 4.5: Functional columns in the brainstem are seven in number; four sensory (afferents) in the dorsal or alar lamina; and three motor (efferents) columns in the ventral or basal lamina. These two laminae are separated by sulcus limitans (dotted line). SSA—special somatic afferent, GSA—general somatic afferent, SVA—special visceral afferent, GVA—general visceral afferent, GVE—general visceral efferent, SVE—special visceral efferent, and SE—somatic efferent (sometimes called general somatic efferent)

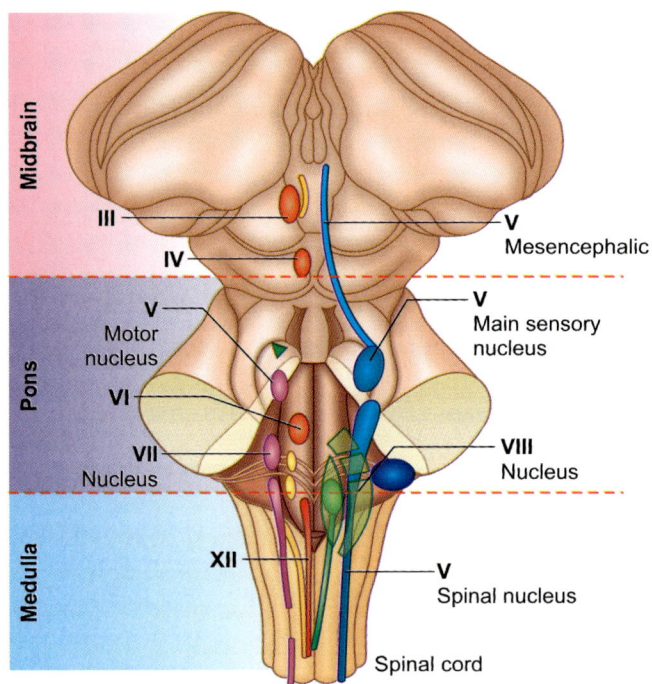

Fig. 4.6: The brainstem: locations of cranial nerves' nuclei in the different parts of brainstem

posterior column function is most often observed in association with demyelinating diseases such as multiple sclerosis—resulting into the classical symptom of **sensory ataxia**—a movement disorder caused by sensory impairment in contrast to *cerebellar ataxia* where a lesion within the motor system is the cause.

ii. Anterolateral **sensory** pathways, which carry peripheral sensations to the brain is referred to as an ascending pathways, or ascending **tracts**. The various sensory modalities each

Table 4.1: Fibers in the seven distinct cell columns in the brainstem

Cell columns	Sensations from/supply to
Special somatic afferent	Sensations from internal ear (balance and hearing)
General somatic afferent	Sensations from skin and mucous membranes, mainly in V nerve territory (oro-naso-facial regions, and dura mater)
Special visceral afferent	Sensations from taste buds located in the endoderm lining the pharyngeal (branchial) arches
General visceral afferent	Sensations from visceral territory of IX and X nerves
General visceral efferent	Cranial parasympathetic (ciliary, pterygopalatine, otic, and submandibular ganglia in the head; and vagal ganglia in thorax and abdomen
Special visceral efferent	To branchial arch musculature of face, jaws, palate, larynx, and pharynx (V, VII, IX, and X nerves)
General somatic efferent	Striated musculature of orbit and tongue (III, IV, VI, and XII)

follow specific pathways through the CNS. The anterolateral pathways comprise the **lateral spinothalamic tracts** serving pain and temperature, and the **anterior spinothalamic tracts** serving touch. The anterior and lateral spinothalamic tracts merge in the brainstem as **spinal lemniscus**. Travelling up the brainstem, the tract moves dorsally.

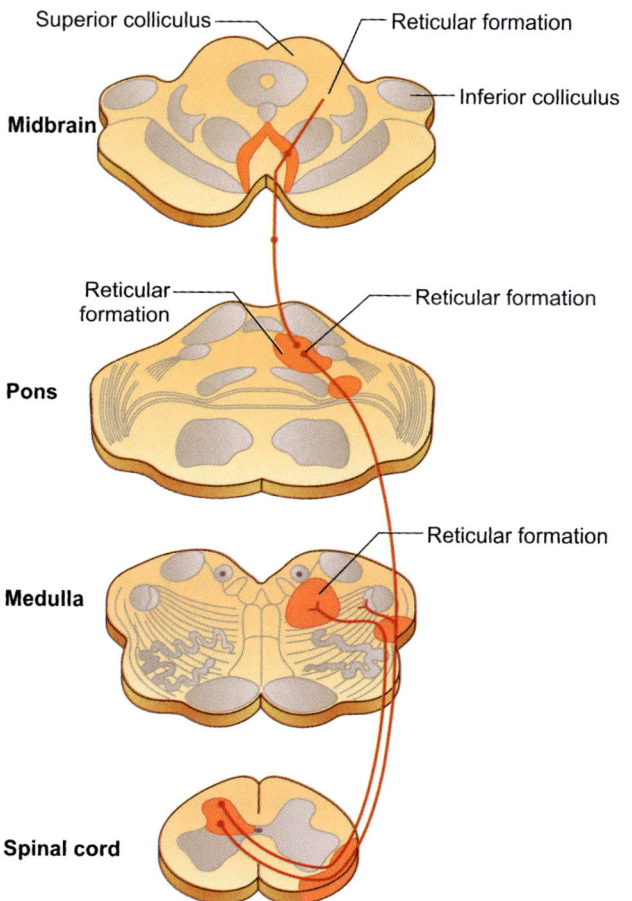

Fig. 4.7: The spinoreticular tract course in the different parts of brainstem

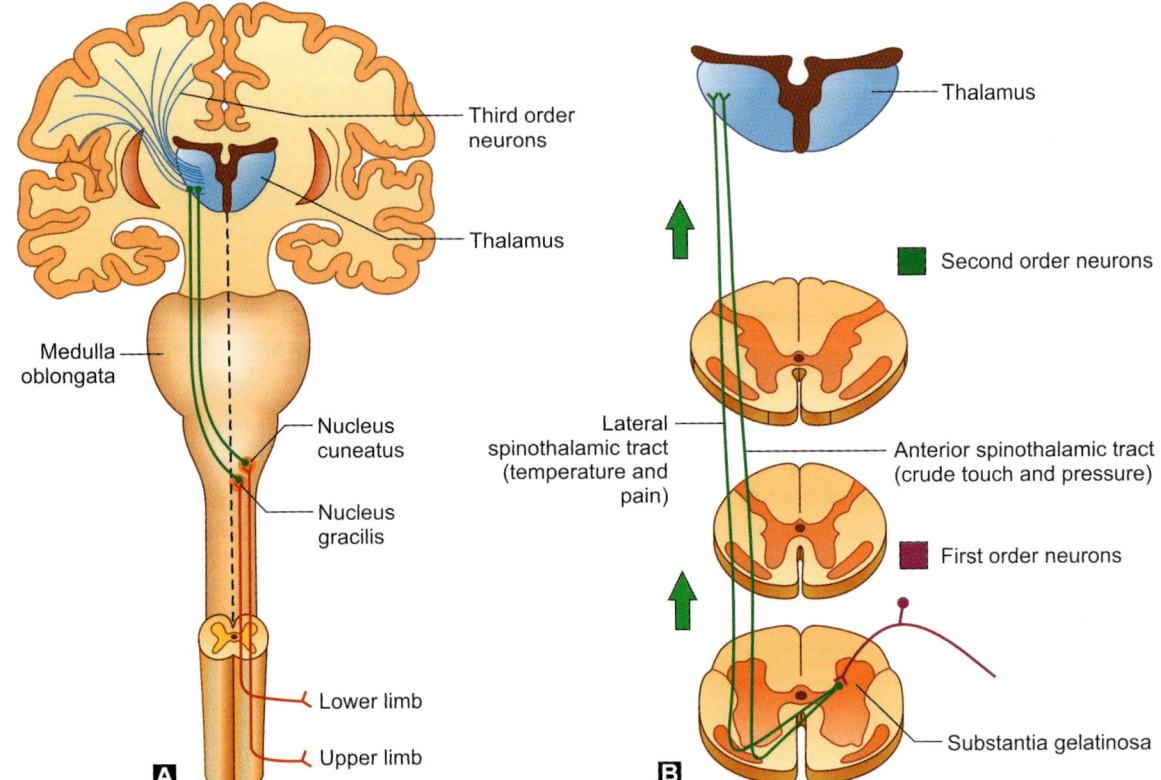

Fig. 4.8: Diagrams of two sensory pathways: **A.** dorsal column or medial lemniscal pathway conveying proprioceptive sense and discriminative touch, **B.** shows course of both spinothalamic tracts: an anterior spinothalamic tract carrying impulses of light touch; and a lateral spinothalamic tract that conveys impulses of pain and temperature sense

CLINICAL SIGNIFICANCE

A **brainstem stroke syndrome** falls under the broader category of stroke syndromes, or specific symptoms caused by vascular injury to an area of brain (e.g. the lacunar syndromes). As the brainstem contains numerous cranial nuclei and white matter tracts, a stroke in this area can have a number of unique symptoms depending on the particular blood vessel that was injured and the group of cranial nerves and tracts that are no longer perfused. Symptoms of a brainstem stroke frequently include sudden vertigo and ataxia, with or without weakness. Brainstem stroke can also cause diplopia, slurred speech and decreased level of consciousness. A more serious outcome is **locked-in syndrome**. The specific lesions in different components of the brainstem are described in subsequent chapters.

Brainstem 1
Medulla Oblongata

- Development of Medulla
- External Features
  - Ventral aspect
  - Dorsal aspect
  - Lateral aspect
- Internal Structure
  - TS of medulla at lower part—pyramidal (motor) decussation
  - TS of medulla at middle part—sensory decussation
  - TS of medulla at mid-olivary level
- Functional Cell Columns in Brainstem
  - Nuclei and their Fibre-bundles
- Clinical Significance of Blood Supply to Medulla Oblongata
  - Occlusion of main arteries supplying medulla
  - Lateral medullary syndrome or Wallenberg syndrome
  - Medial medullary syndrome or inferior alternating hemiplegia

DEVELOPMENT OF MEDULLA

The medulla oblongata, the pons and the cerebellum develop from the rhombencephalon. At first, this part of the neural tube presents features similar to the developing spinal cord. With the formation of pontine flexure, its cavity expands to form the fourth ventricle. The roof plate gets greatly stretched to form the non-nervous ependymal roof of the ventricle. The lateral walls, with the *basal* and *alar plates* separated by the sulcus limitans, form the floor of the ventricle *(fossa rhomboidea)*. The dorsal edges of the alar plate form the *rhombic lip*. Between fourth and fifth weeks (intrauterine life), local resorptions in the roof plate form the apertures of the ventricle.

EXTERNAL FEATURES

The *medulla oblongata* or the *bulb* is the caudal most part of the brainstem. It is pyriform in shape and extends from the lower border of pons to the level of upper border of the first cervical vertebra wider above, the medulla narrows inferiorly to become continuous with the spinal cord. Above, the medulla continues into the pons. It is about 3 cm long and 2 cm broad, in its widest part. Its lower half (closed part) is traversed by the *central canal*. In the upper half (the open part), the central canal moves dorsally and expands to form the cavity of the *fourth ventricle.*

The lower part of medulla oblongata continues, inferiorly into the spinal cord. The cavity of the fourth ventricle lies dorsal to the pons and upper medulla. Posteriorly, the fourth ventricle extends into the white core of the cerebellum.

Ventral Aspect

This aspect of the medulla is separated from the basilar part of the occipital bone. It presents the following features (Fig. 5.1).

* Pyramids are two surface elevations, one on each side, located between the anterior median fissure and the anterolateral sulcus. Each pyramid contains the motor fibres from the cerebral cortex (corticospinal) of the same side.

* The VI cranial (abducens) nerve fibres emerge between the slightly constricted upper end of the medulla and the pons.

* The lower end the pyramid tapers into the anterior funiculus of the spinal cord.

* When traced downwards, approximately 70% fibres leave medullary pyramid in successive bundles and decussate in the anterior median fissure—to form the motor or pyramidal decussation. Having crossed the median plane, these fibres down as the **lateral corticospinal tract** in the lateral white funiculus (Fig. 5.2). The remaining fibres (those in the lateral part of the pyramid) *do not cross the midline*; some pass down as **anterior corticospinal tract** into the anterior funiculus of the same side of the spinal cord, while others deviate backwards and laterally to merge with the lateral corticospinal fibres of the same side.

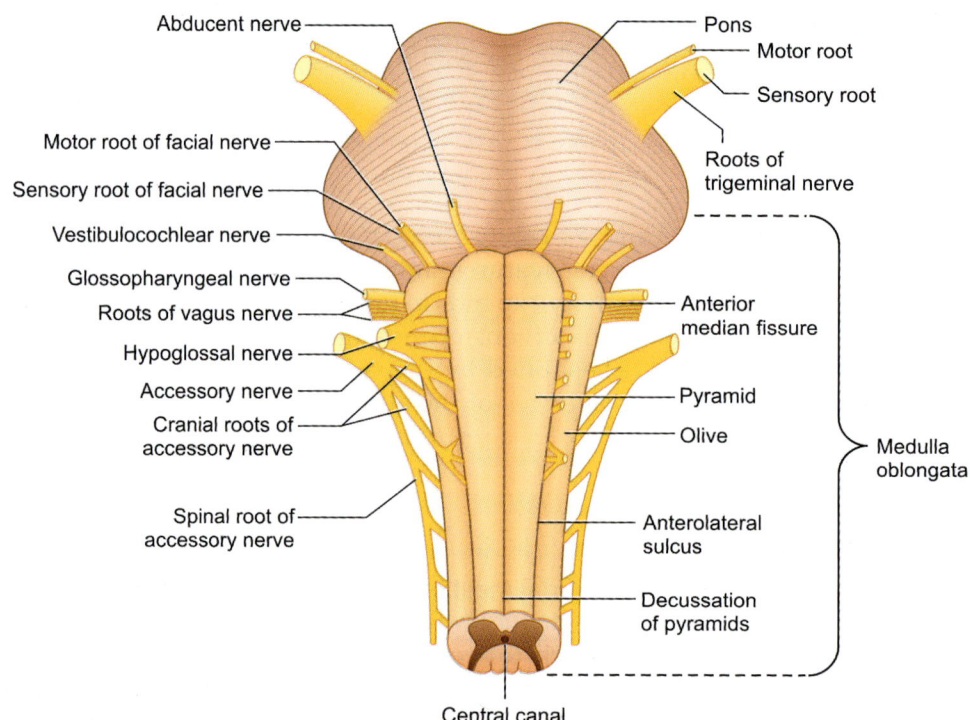

Fig. 5.1: Ventral aspect of the pons and medulla oblongata

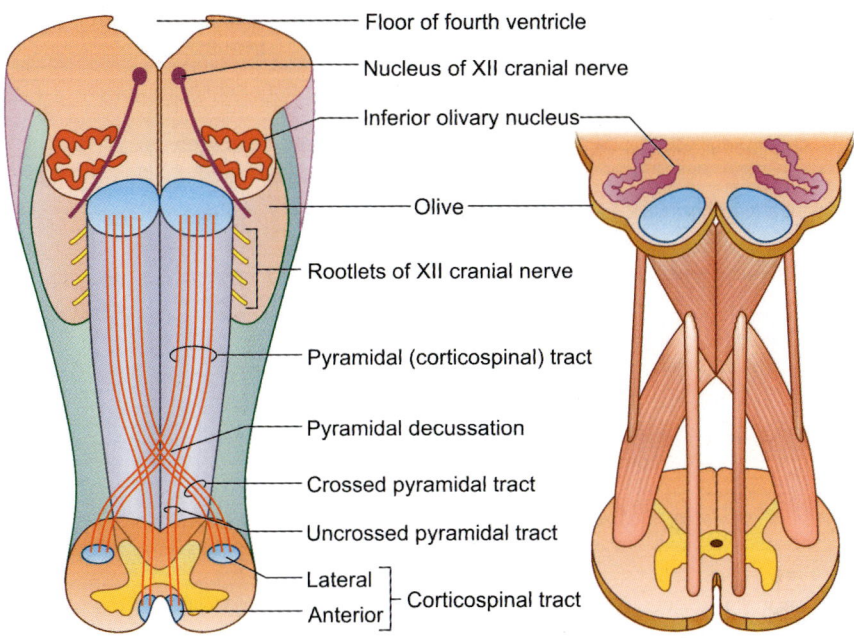

Fig. 5.2: Corticospinal tracts—pyramidal decussation

Dorsal Aspect

Posteriorly the medulla is received into the notch between the two cerebellar hemispheres.

Lower Part

It shows the following:
- *The posterior median sulcus,* which continues inferiorly into the spinal cord.
- *The fasciculi gracilis* and *cuneatus* lie on either side of the posterior median sulcus. They ascend from the spinal cord to end in the nuclei gracilis and cuneatus respectively.
- *The gracile* and *cuneate tubercles* are produced by the nuclei of the same name.
- *The tuberculum cinereum,* produced by the spinal tract and spinal nucleus of trigeminal nerve.

Upper Part

It shows the following (Fig. 5.3):
- It forms the lower half of the floor of fourth ventricle (rhomboid fossa) and presents a *median sulcus.*
- On either side of the median sulcus lie the *hypoglossal* and *vagal triangles* and the *inferior vestibular area* overlying the corresponding vestibular nuclei.
- The *medullary striae,* emerging from the median sulcus course laterally (Fig. 5.3) across the floor of fourth ventricle on their way to the cerebellum.

Lateral Aspect

It is limited in front by the anterolateral sulcus, and behind by the posterolateral sulcus. In the upper part, the lateral surface of the medulla has a prominent oval mass called the olive (Fig. 5.4).

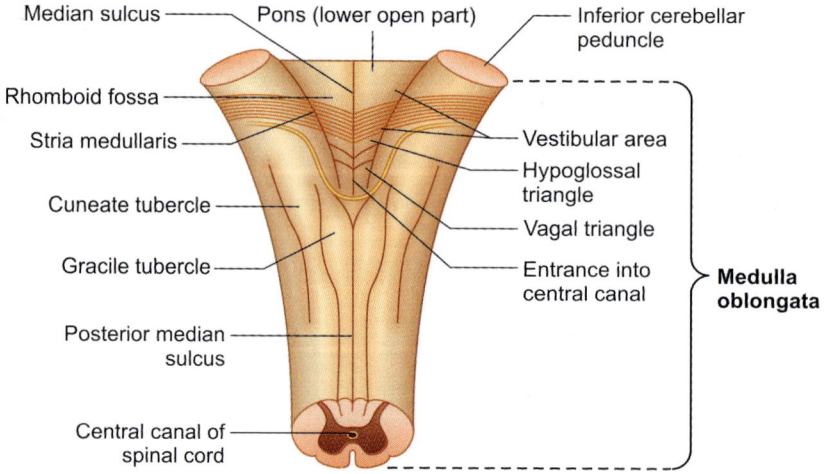

Fig. 5.3: Dorsal aspect of the medulla oblongata

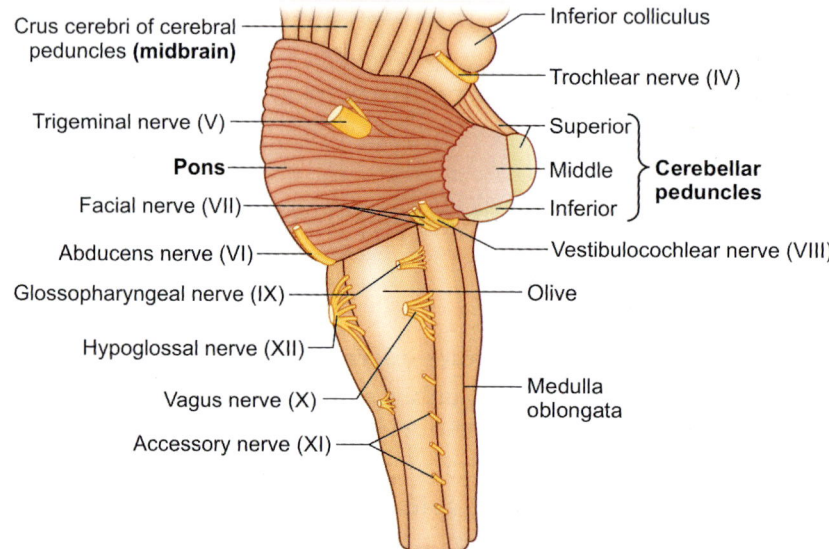

Fig. 5.4: Lateral aspect of the pons and medulla oblongata, shows an oval mass—olive between the anterolateral sulcus (with rootlets of XII cranial nerve in front; and posterolateral sulcus (with rootlets of IX, X, and XI cranial nerves) behind

INTERNAL STRUCTURE

The internal structure of the medulla oblongata is studied, conventionally, by cross-sections cut at following levels from below upwards:

TS of Medulla at Lower Part—Pyramidal (motor) Decussation

The section resembles a spinal cord section except the following differences (Fig. 5.5):
1. Dorsal extensions from the central grey matter pass into the fasciculi gracilis and cuneatus to form their nuclei.

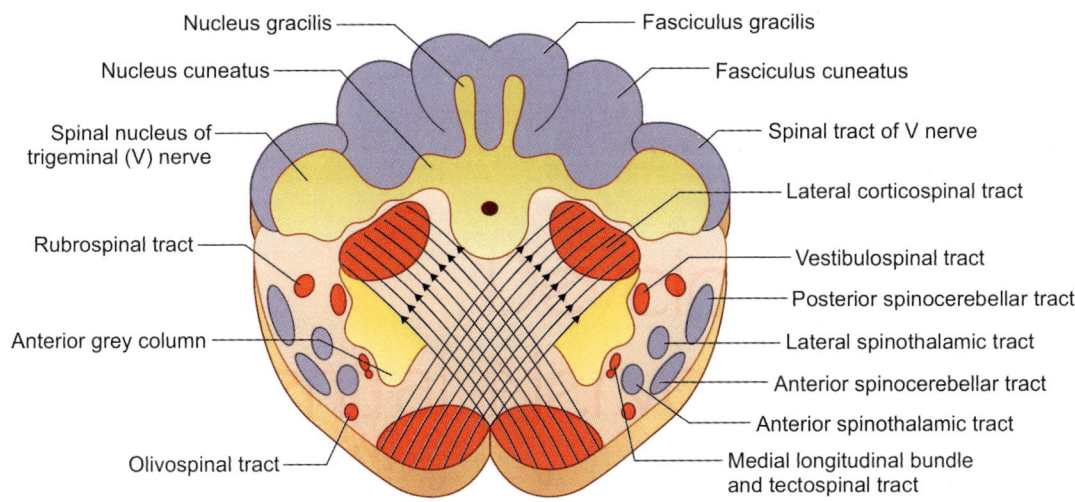

Fig. 5.5: Transverse section through medulla at the level of pyramidal decussation

2. The apex of the posterior grey horn is occupied by the *spinal nucleus of trigeminal nerve*. The fibres of *spinal tract of trigeminal nerve* cap over the nucleus.
3. The anterior median fissure is interrupted by the crossing pyramidal fibres—the *pyramidal decussation. The pyramids* form elongated elevations on either side of the anterior median fissure. Each is produced by the corticospinal fibres, most of which (about 85%) crossover in the pyramidal decussation to the opposite side and descend as the lateral corticospinal tract. The remaining fibres descend in the same half (ipsilateral) of the spinal cord as the anterior corticospinal tract (uncrossed pyramidal fibres).
4. The crossing pyramidal fibres severe the anterior grey horns, which lodge the supraspinal nucleus of first cervical nerve medially, and the *spinal nucleus of accessory nerve* dorsolaterally.

TS of Medulla at Middle Part—Sensory Decussation

The section at this level presents with the following features (Fig. 5.6):
1. *The nuclei gracilis* and *cuneatus* become more pronounced, give rise to the *internal arcuate fibres* and get severed from the central grey matter. These nuclei are *second order neurons* conducting discriminative touch, position and vibration sensations.
2. The internal arcuate fibres course ventrally and medially to decussate with the fibres of the opposite side in the *sensory (lemniscal) decussation.* After crossing over, the fibres ascend in the *medial lemniscus,* on either side of midline. In the decussation the gracile fibres cross ventral to the cuneate fibres.
3. Immediately lateral to the cuneate nucleus lies the *accessory cuneate nucleus* (not shown in the figure). It receives sensory fibres from the fasciculus cuneatus, derived from cervical segments and gives rise to the *posterior external arcuate fibres.* It relays proprioceptive impulses from the upper limb to the cerebellum, through the inferior cerebellar peduncle.
4. Ventrolateral to the cuneate nucleus lies the *nucleus of the spinal tract of trigeminal nerve,* capped by the fibres of the same tract.
5. The central grey matter has the *nuclei of hypoglossal* and *vagus nerves* and *the nucleus of tractus solitarius,* on either side, from ventral to dorsal.

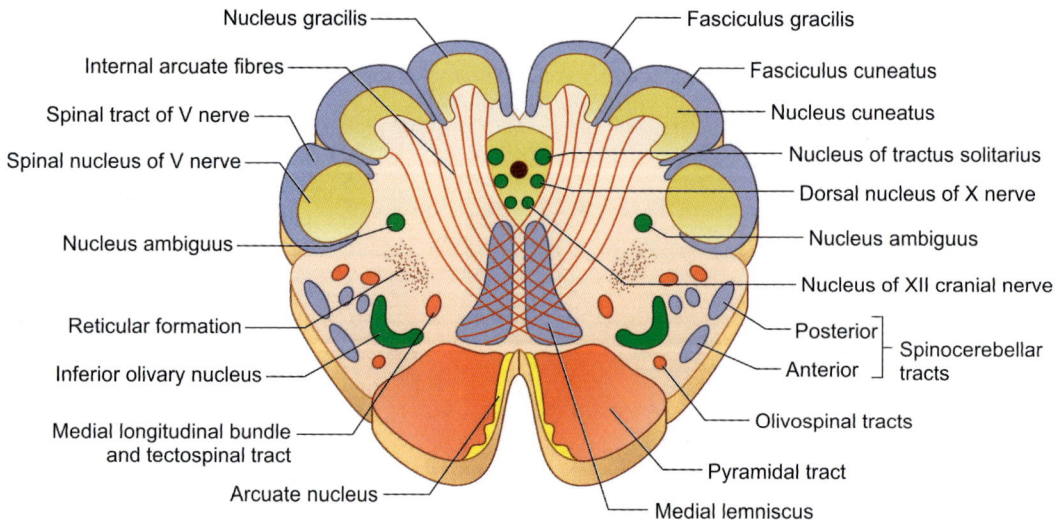

Fig. 5.6: Transverse section through medulla at the level of sensory decussation

6. The *medial longitudinal fasciculus* lies ventral to the hypoglossal nucleus.
7. The *pyramids,* made up of corticospinal and of corticonuclear fibres, lie on either side of the anterior median fissure. Dorsal to them lie the *medial lemniscus* and more laterally the *medial accessory olivary nucleus.*
8. The region between the pyramid and the spinal nucleus of trigeminal nerve presents (i) the *spinocerebellar tracts* superficially, (ii) the *spinothalamic tracts* deep to (i), and (iii) the *rubrospinal, olivospinal, vestibulospinal* and *tectospinal tracts* more deeply, within the *reticular formation.*

TS of Medulla at Mid-olivary Level

The section at this level presents with the following features (Fig. 5.7):

1. The central grey matter is spread over the floor of fourth ventricle. It contains, from medial to lateral, the *hypoglossal nucleus, nucleus intercalatus, dorsal nucleus of vagus* and the *vestibular nuclei.* Ventral to the last named are the *solitary nucleus* and *tract.*
2. Close to the midline, from dorsal to ventral, lie the *medial longitudinal bundle, tectospinal tract, medial lemniscus* and the *pyramid.* Ventromedial to the last named is the *arcuate nucleus.*
3. Laterally, from dorsal to ventral, lie the following structures:
   i. The *inferior cerebellar peduncle* with the *spinal tract of the trigeminal nerve* and its *nucleus* lying ventromedial to it.
   ii. The *anterior spinocerebellar tract in* the floor of the posterolateral sulcus with the *lateral spinothalamic tract (spinal lemniscus)* lying deep to it.
   iii. The *inferior olivary nucleus* (a prominent feature of all sections through the upper half of medulla oblongata) lies deep to the olive. It presents a crumpled bag-like appearance, with its mouth directed medially. Close to the inferior olivary nucleus lie the *medial* and *dorsal accessory olivary nuclei.* Dorsal to the *inferior olivary nuclear complex* lies the *reticular formation.* It has the *nucleus ambiguus* in its ventrolateral part.

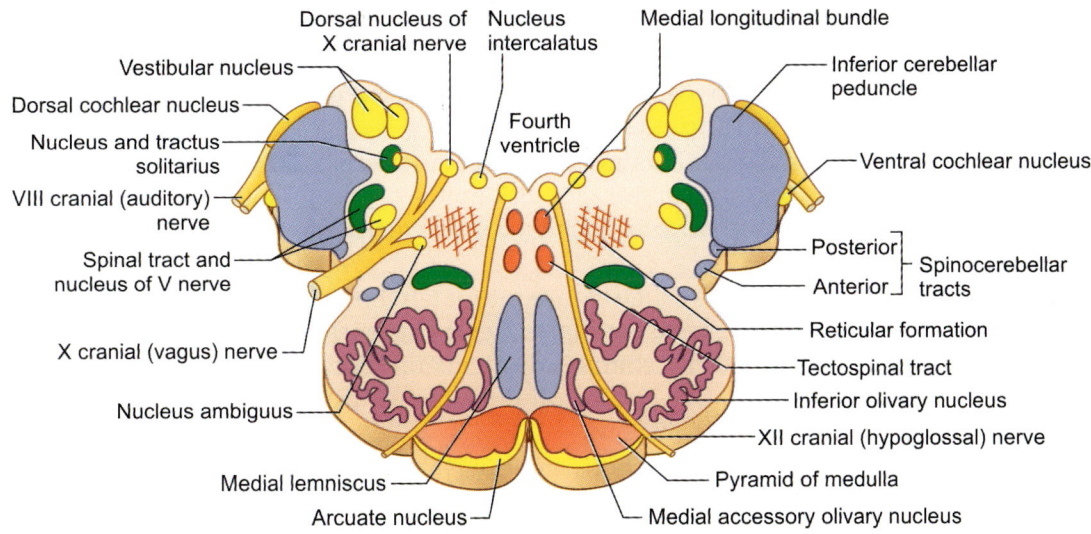

Fig. 5.7: Transverse section through medulla at mid-olivary level

FUNCTIONAL CELL COLUMNS IN BRAINSTEM

In the alar plate develop the four afferent (sensory), and in the basal plate the three efferent (motor) nerve cell columns (Fig. 5.8). These (functional) cell columns give rise to the nuclei associated with the cranial nerves. Some of these nuclei migrate and change their positions (*neurobiotaxis*). The olivary and arcuate nuclei are derived from the rhombic lip.

Nuclei and their Fibre-bundles

The medulla contains several nuclei with many fibre-bundles, listed below:

1. The *hypoglossal nucleus* is the somatic motor nucleus for muscles of tongue. It is situated under the hypoglossal triangle and is ventrally related to the medial longitudinal fasciculus. The fibres arising from this nucleus pass ventrolaterally between the olivary nuclei and the medial lemniscus to emerge through the anterolateral sulcus, lateral to the pyramid. A

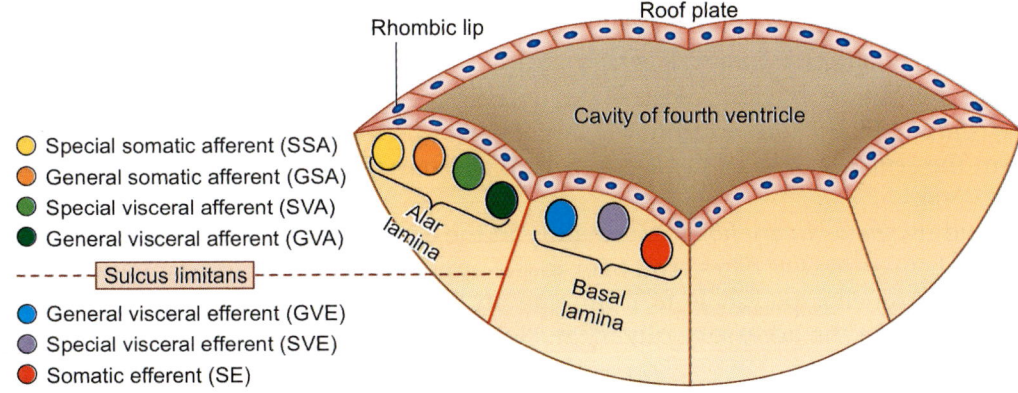

Fig. 5.8: The functional cell columns in the alar and basal plates. The nuclei derived from them are shown on the left side. SSA—Special somatic afferent, GSA—General somatic afferent, SVA—Special visceral afferent, GVA—General visceral afferent, GVE—General visceral efferent, SVE—Special visceral efferent, SE—Somatic efferent

small lesion in this region results in the paralysis involving muscles of the tongue on the same side but the muscles of the body on the opposite side *(alternating hemiplegia).*

2. The *nucleus intercalatus* lies between the hypoglossal and the dorsal vagal nuclei. Gustatory and visceral connections are attributed to it.

3. The *dorsal nucleus of vagus* provides general visceral efferent fibres to the vagus nerve, which are inhibitory to the cardiac muscles and motor to the smooth muscles and glands of the digestive and respiratory tracts (bronchoconstrictor). They also relax the pyloric and ileocaecal sphincters.

4. The *nucleus solitarius* and *tractus solitarius* are intimately related to its tract. Its rostral part is concerned with the sense of taste (special visceral afferent) carried by the VII, IX, and X cranial nerves. The tract is mainly composed of general visceral afferent fibres (IX and X cranial nerves) from the digestive and respiratory tracts, the aortic sinus and the carotid body. The fibres terminate in its nucleus.

5. The *vestibular nuclei* are *four* in number: superior, lateral (Deiter's), medial and inferior. The superior vestibular nucleus lies in the pons. Other nuclei lie in the medulla. They receive fibres from the vestibular nerve and project them to the cerebellum. Efferent fibers are received back from the cerebellum. The vestibular nuclei (mainly from Deiter's nucleus) give rise to the vestibulospinal tract, and contribute liberally to the medial longitudinal fasciculus and mediate the control of posture and muscle tone.

6. *Nucleus* and *spinal tract of trigeminal nerve* carry pain and temperature fibres from the face (and other regions of the trigeminal area) carried by all the three divisions of the trigeminal nerve. They pass to the pons in its sensory root and descend to form spinal tract of trigeminal which is seen in the lower pons, the medulla oblongata and the upper two cervical segments of the spinal cord. The fibres terminate in the *nucleus of V nerve* (second order neurons). Efferent fibres from the nucleus crossover and ascend as the *trigeminal lemniscus* on the opposite side.

7. The *nucleus ambiguus* made up of large motor neurons, lies deeply in the reticular formation. Fibres from this special visceral efferent nucleus pass in the IX, X and XI cranial nerves for the supply of muscles of larynx, pharynx and soft palate (striated muscles of branchial origin). The *inferior salivatory nucleus* that gives preganglionic parasympathetic secretomotor fibres for the parotid gland is located near the rostral tip of the nucleus ambiguus. These fibres travel in the glossopharyngeal nerve.

8. The *inferior olivary* and *accessory olivary nuclei.*
   The inferior olivary nucleus receives:
   - Descending fibres derived from the motor cortex, lentiform nucleus and the red nucleus form the *central tegmental fasciculus,* which surrounds the olivary nucleus and form its *amiculum.*
   - Ascending *spino-olivary fibres* end mainly in the accessory olivary nuclei.
   - Efferent *olivocerebellar fibres* crossover to the opposite cerebellar hemisphere through the inferior cerebellar peduncle to terminate on the Purkinje cells as climbing fibres. The efferents from the accessory olivary nuclei form the *parolivocerebellar tract* that follows the same course.
   - Other olivary efferents descend to the spinal cord as the *olivospinal tract.* The olivary nuclei are associated with the coordination of skilled movements.

9. The *arcuate nucleus* is considered to be formed by the displaced nuclei pontis. Most of its efferents *(anterior external arcuate fibres)* course laterally and dorsally over the surface of the

medulla and pass to the cerebellum through the inferior cerebellar peduncle. Other efferent fibres course internally and emerge through the median sulcus as the *stria medullares*.

10. The *inferior cerebellar peduncle* connects the medulla oblongata and spinal cord. It contains both *afferent* and *efferent* fibres coming to and leaving away the cerebellum respectively as follows.

11. The *medullary reticular formation* includes a network of fibres and a number of scattered nuclei, lying in the region dorsal to the olivary nuclei. The nuclei of reticular formation may be divided into *lateral, medial* and *median (rapheal)* groups. The *lateral parvocellular (small-celled) reticular nuclei* are included in a *superficial ventrolateral area*, which is involved, in the cardiovascular, respiratory, vasoreceptor and chemoreceptor reflexes. The principal projections to the area are from the nucleus of tractus solitarius. A mixed expiratory-inspiratory centre lies in this area. The *medial* group of *gigantocellular medullary* nuclei contribute to the reticulospinal tract. These fibres are concerned with posture and stereotyped movements of the limbs. *Medullary raphe pallidus* and *obscures* of *median* group nuclei mediate the central sympathetic control of cardiovascular functions.

CLINICAL SIGNIFICANCE OF BLOOD SUPPLY TO MEDULLA OBLONGATA

Occlusion of Main Arteries Supplying Medulla

The arteries supplying the medulla with *three* territories—called **'areas of Flechsig'** are shown in Fig. 5.9. The involved arteries are summarised in Table 5.1

The commonest of the brainstem strokes—is the occlusion of blood supply through the posterior inferior cerebellar artery (PICA occlusion).

Manifestation: At the level of dorsolateral medulla and cerebellum (Figs 5.10 and 5.11).

Vascular lesions like hemorrhages into the brainstem have serious consequences because of the presence of nuclei that control the vital functions of *respiration* and *circulation*. Two main clinical conditions are encountered in daily practice. The symptoms and signs listed in Table 5.2 are collectively referred as the **lateral medullary** or **Wallenberg syndrome**—caused by different arteries involved (Fig. 5.10).

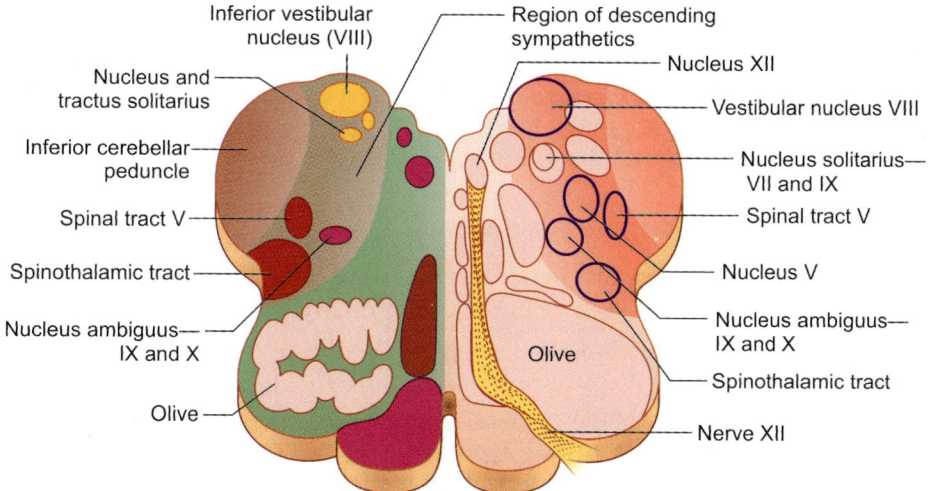

Fig. 5.9: Schematic transverse section through medulla at the level of olive shows structures likely to get involved in occlusion of posterior inferior cerebellar artery (PICA). For lesions see Table 5.2

Table 5.1: Areas supplied by the four arteries supplying the medulla oblongata

Artery	Diagram	Area(s) supplied
1. Anterior spinal artery 2. Posterior spinal artery	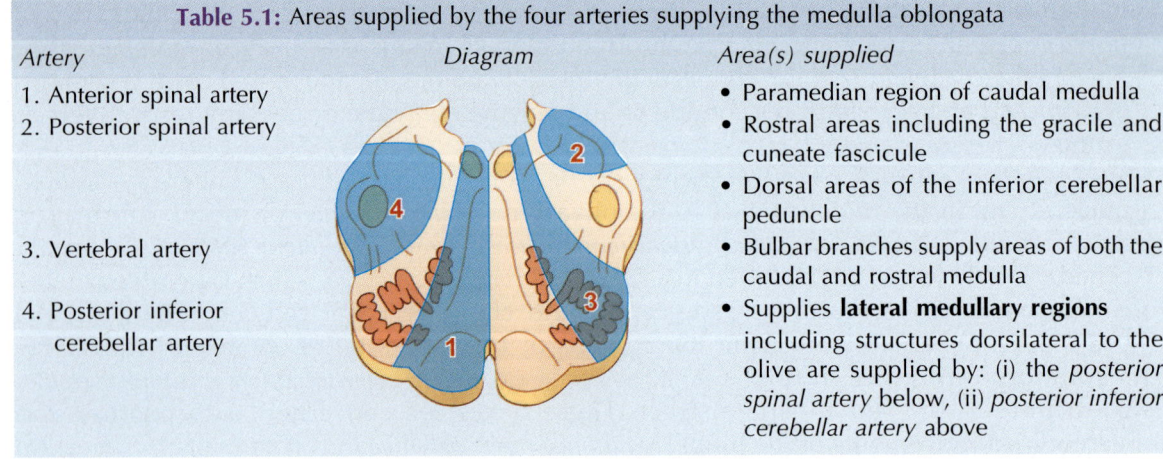	• Paramedian region of caudal medulla • Rostral areas including the gracile and cuneate fascicule • Dorsal areas of the inferior cerebellar peduncle
3. Vertebral artery		• Bulbar branches supply areas of both the caudal and rostral medulla
4. Posterior inferior cerebellar artery		• Supplies **lateral medullary regions** including structures dorsilateral to the olive are supplied by: (i) the *posterior spinal artery* below, (ii) *posterior inferior cerebellar artery* above

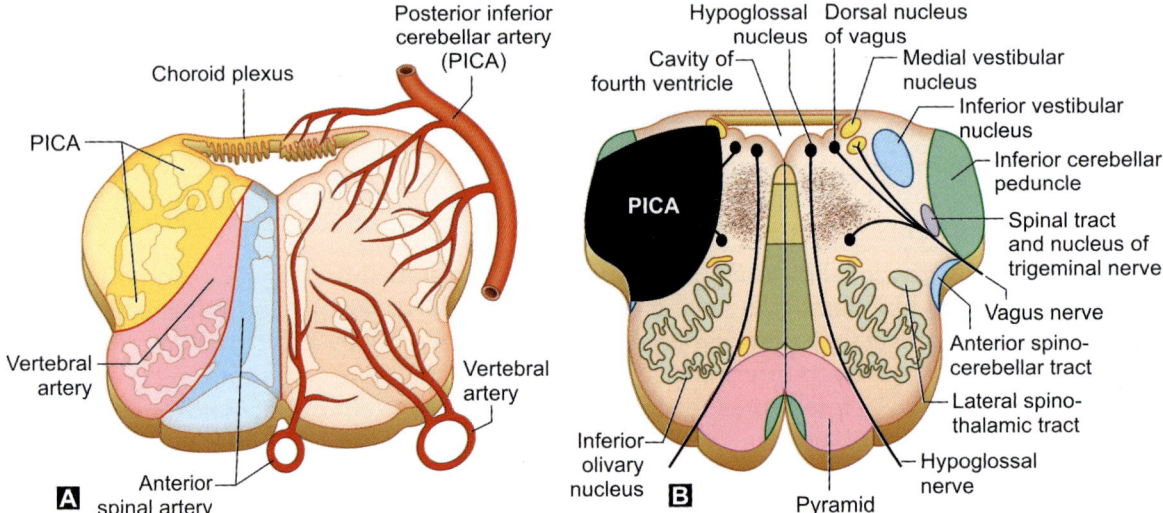

Fig. 5.10: A. Each half of the medulla is supplied by three arteries. Occlusion of individual arteries involves different structures and the symptoms, therefore differ; **B.** shows a section near the pontomedullary portion. PICA—the posterior inferior cerebellar artery territory (shown in black) affects several structure listed in Table 5.2 produce lesions in lateral medullary or Wallenberg syndrome

1. Lateral Medullary Syndrome or Wallenberg Syndrome

Occlusion of the lateral medullary arteries (e.g. posterior inferior cerebellar artery (PICA) and medullary branches of either the PICA or of the vertebral artery) produces the *lateral medullary syndrome of Wallenberg* (Fig. 5.10). The parts involved with the results produced are given below:

  i. **Spinal nucleus and tract of V nerve**—ipsilateral loss of pain and temperature over the area supplied by the V cranial nerve.
 ii. **Lateral spinothalamic tract in spinal lemniscus**—absence of pain and temperature on opposite side of the body. The touch sensation is further reduced rather than abolished.
iii. **Nucleus ambiguus**—there is difficulty in swallowing and phonation due to paralysis of ipsilateral muscles of soft palate, pharynx, and larynx.

Table 5.2: Lesions produced due to areas occluded by PICA supplying the medulla oblongata

Areas affected due to PICA occlusion	Lesion(s) produced
Spinal nucleus CN V	• Ipsilateral sensory loss of face—pain and temperature· Ipsilateral facial pain
Inferior cerebellar peduncle– Ipsilateral cerebellum	• Ipsilateral ATAXIA—arm and leg • Ipsilateral Gait Ataxia
Vestibular nucleus	• Ipsilateral nystagmus • Ipsilateral nausea and vomiting • Ipsilateral vertigo
Nucleus ambiguus	• Ipsilateral hoarseness • Ipsilateral dysphagia
Descending sympathetic fibres	• Ipsilateral Horner's syndrome
Spinothalamic tract	• Contralateral hemisensory loss—pain and temperature

Prognosis is generally quite good with full or near full recovery

iv. **Reticular formation** (involving sympathetic fibers)—lesions in the pathway from hypothalamus—intermediate cell columns cause Horner's syndrome characterised by: (a) small pupil size, (b) slight ptosis, (c) slight enophthalmos, and (d) anhydrosis of face with warm and dry skin.

 If lesion is extensive—the base of inferior cerebellar peduncle and vestibular nuclei get involved producing severe dizziness, ipsilateral cerebellar ataxia, and nystagmus.

2. Medial Medullary Syndrome or Inferior Alternating Hemiplegia

Occlusion of the medial medullary arteries (Fig. 5.11) would cause: (i) **ipsilateral paralysis of the tongue** (due to damaged hypoglossal nuclei—XII cranial nerve), (ii) **contralateral paralysis of the arm and leg** (crossed pyramidal fibres damage), and (iii) **contralateral impairment of touch and sense of position** (medial lemniscus damage). The medial medullary regions (listed above—such as the pyramid, medial lemniscus, and the hypoglossal nucleus are supplied by: (i) the *anterior spinal artery* below, and (ii) direct medullary branches of vertebral artery above.

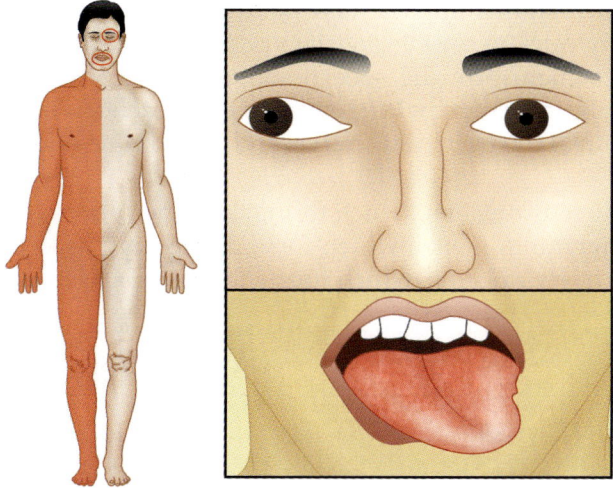
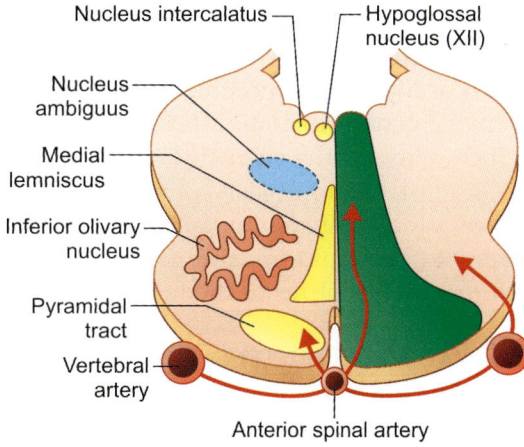

Fig. 5.11: Medial medullary syndrome in medulla affecting the anterior spinal artery and branches from the vertebral artery

Brainstem 2
Pons

DEVELOPMENT OF PONS

During embryonic development, the metencephalon develops from the rhombencephalon and gives rise to two structures: the pons and the cerebellum. The alar plate produces sensory neuroblasts, which will give rise to the solitary nucleus and its special visceral afferent (SVA) column; the cochlear and vestibular nuclei, which form the special somatic afferent (SSA) fibres of the vestibulocochlear nerve, the spinal and principal trigeminal nerve nuclei, which form the general somatic afferent (GSA) column of the trigeminal nerve, and the pontine nuclei which relays to the cerebellum.

Basal plate neuroblasts give rise to the abducens nucleus, which forms the general somatic efferent (GSE) fibers; the facial and motor trigeminal nuclei, which form the special visceral efferent (SVE) column, and the superior salivatory nucleus, which forms the general visceral efferent (GVE) fibres of the facial nerve.

CRANIAL NERVE NUCLEI IN PONS

A number of cranial nerve nuclei are present in the pons:
- *Mid-pons*
  - The 'chief' or 'pontine' nucleus of the trigeminal nerve sensory nucleus (V)
  - The motor nucleus for the trigeminal nerve (V)

- *Lower-pons*
  - Abducens nucleus (VI)
  - Facial nerve nucleus (VII)
  - Vestibulocochlear nuclei (vestibular nuclei and cochlear nuclei) (VIII)

Functions

The functions of these four cranial nerves (V–VIII) include regulation of respiration, controls involuntary actions, sensory roles in hearing, equilibrium, and taste, and in facial sensations such as touch and pain, as well as motor roles in eye movement, facial expressions, chewing, swallowing, and the secretion of saliva and tears. As part of the brainstem, the pons also impacts several automatic functions necessary for life. A section of the lower pons stimulates and controls the intensity of breathing, and a section of the upper pons decreases the depth and frequency of breaths (Table 6.1). The pons has also been associated with the control of sleep cycles.

The pons contains nuclei that relay signals from the forebrain to the cerebellum, along with nuclei that deal primarily with sleep, respiration, swallowing, bladder control, hearing, equilibrium, taste, eye movement, facial expressions, facial sensation, and posture.

Within the pons is the pneumotaxic centre consisting of the subparabrachial and the medial parabrachial nuclei. This centre regulates the change from inhalation to exhalation. The pons is implicated in sleep paralysis, and may also play a role in generating dreams.

EXTERNAL FEATURES OF PONS

The pons is also called the pons cerebelli or **pons Varolii** ('bridge of Varolius'), after the Italian anatomist and surgeon Costanzo Varolio (1543–75). This region of the brainstem includes neural pathways and tracts that conduct signals from the brain down to the cerebellum and medulla, and tracts that carry the sensory signals up into the thalamus.

The pons is involved in the control of breathing, communication between different parts of the brain, and sensations such as hearing, taste, and balance. The pons in humans measures about 2.5 cm (0.98 in) in length. Most of it appears as a broad anterior bulge rostral to the medulla. Posteriorly, it consists mainly of two pairs of thick stalks called middle cerebellar peduncles. They connect the cerebellum to the pons (middle cerebellar peduncle) and midbrain (superior cerebellar peduncle). There are many important nerves that originate in the pons. The **trigeminal nerve** is responsible for feeling in the face. It also controls the muscles that are

Table 6.1: Components and functions of the pons		
Subdivision	Component(s)	Function(s)
Grey matter	Nuclei associated with cranial nerves V, VI, VII, and VIII (in part)	Relay sensory information and issue somatic motor commands
	Apneustic and pneumotaxic centres	Adjust activities of the respiratory rhythmicity centres in the medulla oblongata
	Relay centres	Relay sensory and motor information to the cerebellum
White matter	Ascending tracts	Carry sensory information from the nucleus cuneatus and nucleus gracilis to the thalamus
	Descending tracts	Carry motor commands from higher centres to motor nuclei of cranial or spinal nerves

responsible for biting, chewing, and swallowing. The **abducens nerve** allows the eyes to look from side to side. The **facial nerve** controls facial expressions, and the **vestibulocochlear nerve** allows sound to move from the ear to the brain. All of these nerves start within the pons.

The *pons* is the bulging bridge lying in front of the cerebellum (Fig. 6.1). Transversely running fibres mark its surface. On each side these fibres converge into a thick rounded bundle called the *middle cerebellar peduncle.*

Its ventral aspect presents the *basilar groove* in the midline and laterally, on either side, provides attachments to the roots of the trigeminal nerve. In the midline it shows the groove for basilar artery. More laterally it provides attachments to the two roots, larger sensory and smaller motor, of the *trigeminal nerve* (V cranial nerve). The motor root lies ventromedial to the sensory root (Fig. 6.2). Beyond the attachment of the trigeminal nerve, the pons continues

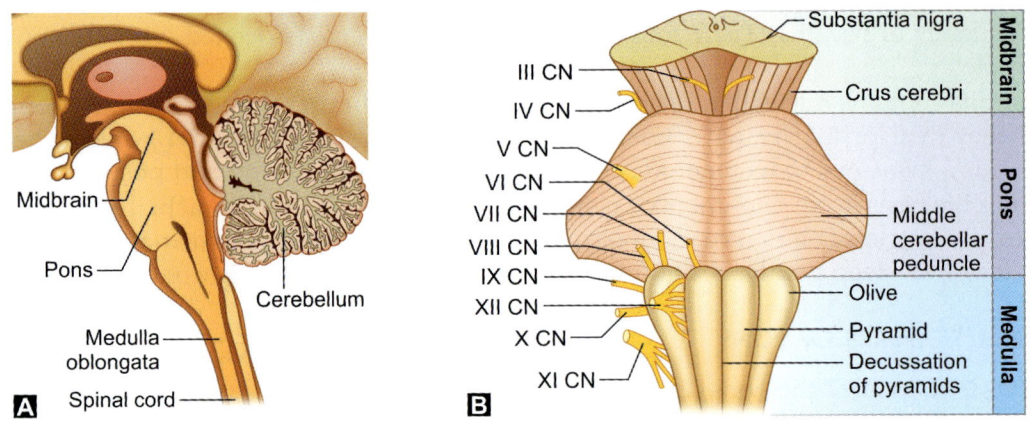

Fig. 6.1A and B: Sagittal section of brainstem shows the three main components. On the right is shown the ventral surface of pons and medulla with cranial nerves attached to each part of brainstem

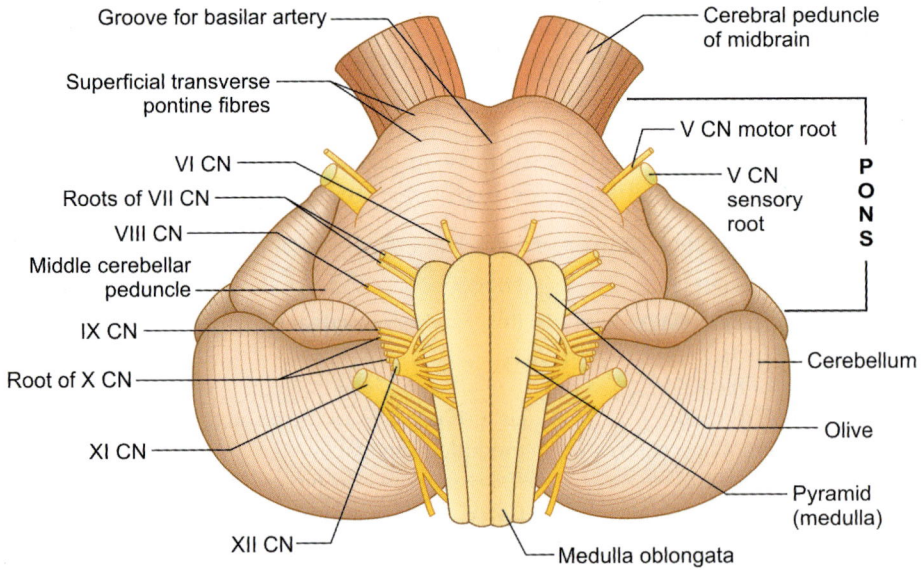

Fig. 6.2: External gross features of brainstem show the emergence of cranial nerves on pons (V, VI, VII, and VIII); and on medulla (IX, X, XI, and XII)

as the *middle cerebellar peduncle* into the cerebellar hemisphere. The *abducens* (VI cranial), *facial* (VII cranial) and the *vestibulocochlear* (VIII cranial nerves) emerge at the lower border of pons. The dorsal surface of the pons forms the upper half of the floor of fourth ventricle. The pons consists of a larger ventral *(basilar)* part and a smaller dorsal *(tegmental)* part.

INTERNAL STRUCTURE OF THE PONS

Ventral or Basilar Part of Pons

Its ventral aspect presents the *basilar groove* in the midline and laterally, on either side, provides attachments to the roots of the trigeminal nerve.
The *basilar* part consists of:
1. Transverse oriented *pontocerebellar fibres.*
2. Longitudinal oriented **descending tracts** *(corticospinal, corticonuclear and corticopontine).*
3. Scattered masses of grey matter called the *nuclei pontis.*
   The corticospinal fibres pass downwards into the medulla to form the pyramids. The corticonuclear fibres end in the cranial nerve (motor) nuclei. The corticopontine fibres end in the nuclei pontis that in turn give rise to transversely oriented pontocerebellar fibres. These fibres crossover to the opposite side and enter the cerebellar hemisphere via the *middle cerebellar peduncle.*

Dorsal or Tegmental Part of Pons

The pontine tegmentum consists of the following:

Long Ascending Fibres

These fibres pass through the pons into the midbrain and are found at both the pontine levels. These include the following:
  i. The medial lemniscus forms a curved and rather coronally oriented band in which the cuneate fibres are medial and the gracile fibres are lateral.
  ii. and iii. The trigeminal and spinal lemnisci lie more laterally.
  iv. The anterior spinocerebellar tract lies dorsolateral to (ii) and (iii). At the upper pontine level this tract enters the *superior cerebellar peduncle to* reach the cerebellum. The superior *medullary velum* stretches between the peduncles of the two sides (Fig. 6.3).
  v. *Other longitudinal fibre bundles:* These are lying more dorsally, close to the midline and include the *medial longitudinal* fasciculus and the tectospinal tract.

TS through Lower Pons

Transversely Disposed Fibres

Intersecting the ascending fibres of medial lemniscus are the transversely running fibres of the *trapezoid body* in the caudal pons (Fig. 6.4). These fibres, derived from the cochlear nuclei, crossover to the opposite side and ascend up as the *lateral lemniscus*, with or without relay in the *nuclei of the trapezoid body* or the *superior olivary nucleus.* Many cochlear fibres do not cross but join the ipsilateral lateral lemniscus.

Pontine Reticular Formation

It forms the central core in each half of the tegmentum at all pontine levels. It is made up of nerve cell groups intermingled with mainly longitudinally oriented nerve fibres. The *locus*

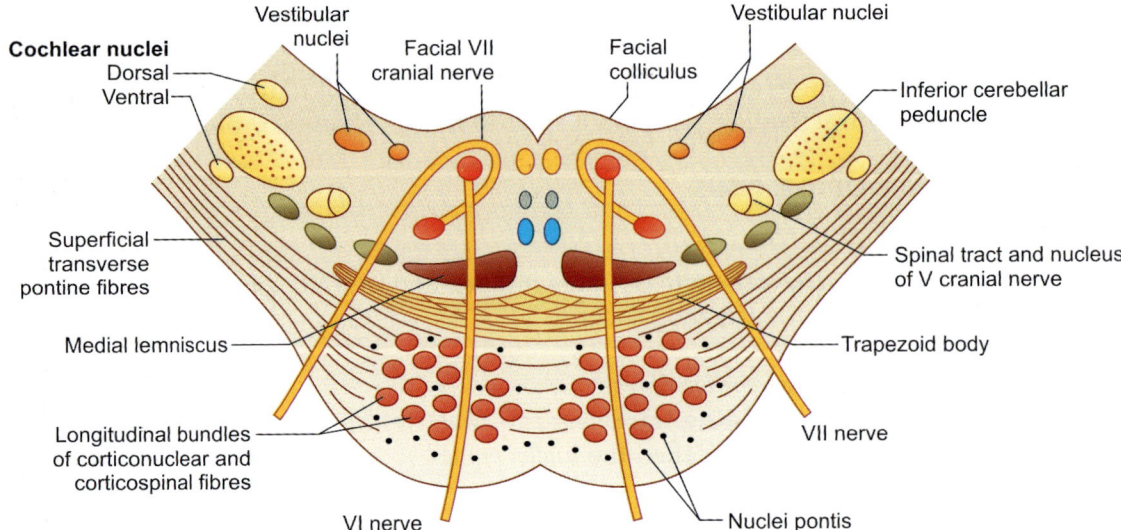

Fig. 6.3: Transverse section of lower pons at the level of facial colliculus (*Courtesy:* Nafis Ahmad Faruqi)

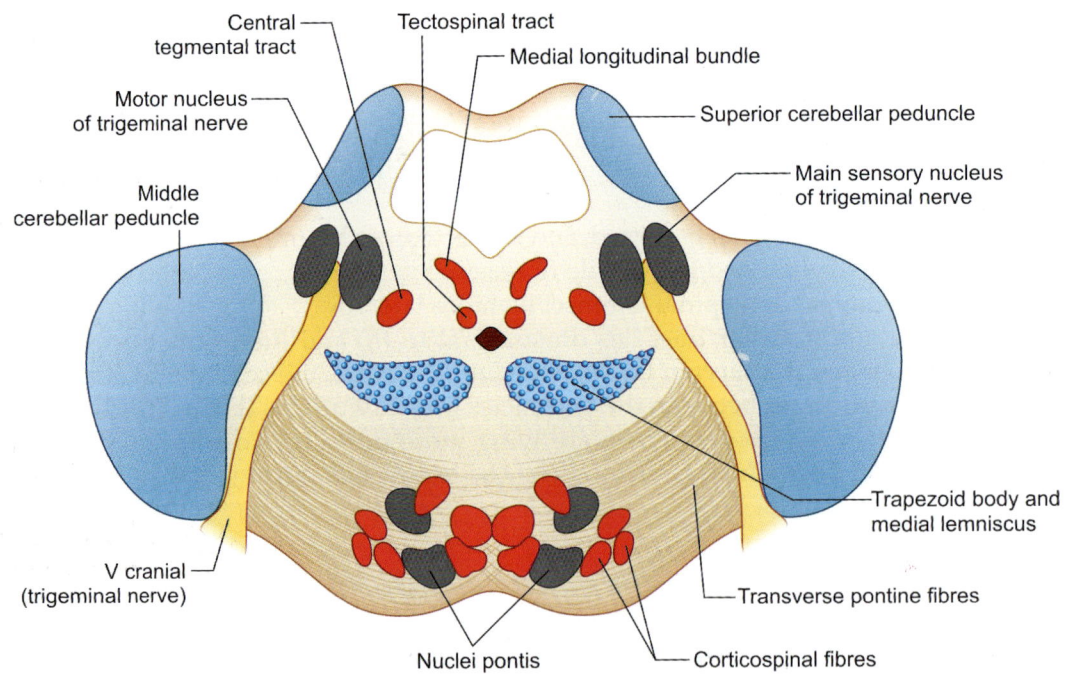

Fig. 6.4: Transverse section of middle pons at the level of main sensory nucleus of trigeminal nerve

coeruleus (an attention centre) and a higher *pneumotaxic centre* lie in the lateral pontine reticular formation. Through the reticular formation also descend the rubrospinal tract, central tegmental tract and the *descending central sympathetic fibres*. In the ventrolateral part of the reticular formation of the lower pons lie the *superior olivary* and the *trapezoid nuclei*.

Nuclei of Cranial Nerves

Nuclei in the lower (caudal) pons: At the caudal pontine levels (Fig. 6.6) are found the nuclei of V (spinal nucleus and tract), VI, VII (facial) and the VIII (cochlear and vestibular) cranial nerves. The *nuclei of the vestibulocochlear nerve* and the *spinal nucleus of the V* are closely related to the inferior cerebellar peduncle. The *cochlear nuclei* lie lateral to the peduncle while the *vestibular nuclei* and the spinal nucleus and tract of V nerve lie to its medial side. The *facial nucleus* lies in the ventrolateral part of the pontine tegmentum dorsal to the dorsal nucleus of the trapezoid body. The fibres of the VII nerve course in a dorsomedial direction to reach the medial side of the abducens nucleus and wind round its dorsal aspect. The fibres then pass ventrolaterally and downwards to the lower border of pons, where they emerge. The *abducens nucleus* lies close to the midline, dorsolateral to the medial longitudinal bundle and deep to the facial colliculus (found in the floor of the fourth ventricle). Its fibres pass ventrolaterally and downwards and emerge at the lower border of pons. The *superior salivatory* (for submandibular and sublingual salivary glands) and *lacrimal nuclei* lie medial to the facial nucleus.

TS through Upper Pons

Nuclei in the upper (cranial) pons: These include the motor and the *principal sensory* nuclei of the *trigeminal nerve* and *the nucleus of the lateral lemniscus.* A transverse section through the upper part of pons (Fig. 6.2) shows the trigeminal motor nucleus under the lateral part of the floor of fourth ventricle. Fibres from the nucleus pass into the motor trigeminal root to supply (mainly) the muscles of mastication. The *principal (superior) sensory nucleus* of the trigeminal nerve lies lateral to the trigeminal motor nucleus. The principal sensory nucleus receives touch, pressure, position and vibration senses from the face area. Fibres from the nucleus crossover and join the medial side of the opposite medial lemniscus. Along the dorsolateral edge of the medial lemniscus lie the trigeminal, the spinal and the lateral lemnisci. The nucleus of the lateral lemniscus lies medial to its fibres. It is a relay station in the auditory pathway.

ARTERIAL SUPPLY OF PONS

The pons is supplied by branches from the basilar artery. There are direct *pontine branches* as well as those derived from the *anterior inferior* and the *superior cerebellar arteries.* The arteries are often classified into *paramedian, short circumferential* and *long circumferential* depending upon whether they enter the pons close to the midline on the ventral aspect, further laterally or elsewhere on the dorsolateral aspect. Occlusion of paramedian arteries involves the corticospinal tract, the medial lemniscus and the nucleus of the VI cranial nerve. Infarcts related to the circumferential arteries usually include parts of the cerebellar peduncles, lateral spinothalamic tract and the nuclei of the cranial nerves V, VII and VIII.

APPLIED ANATOMY AND CLINICAL SIGNIFICANCE OF PONS

1. **Central pontine myelinolysis:** It is a demyelination disease that causes difficulty with sense of balance, walking, sense of touch, swallowing and speaking. In a clinical setting, it is often associated with transplant or rapid correction of blood sodium. Undiagnosed, it can lead to death or locked-in syndrome.
2. **Astrocytoma of pons:** Occurring in childhood, it is the commonest brainstem tumour. Signs of ipsilateral cranial nerve paralysis and contralateral hemiparesis are found.
3. **Pontine haemorrhage:** Paralysis (quadriplegia), pyrexia and pin-point pupil are the cardinal signs of extensive pontine haemorrhage.

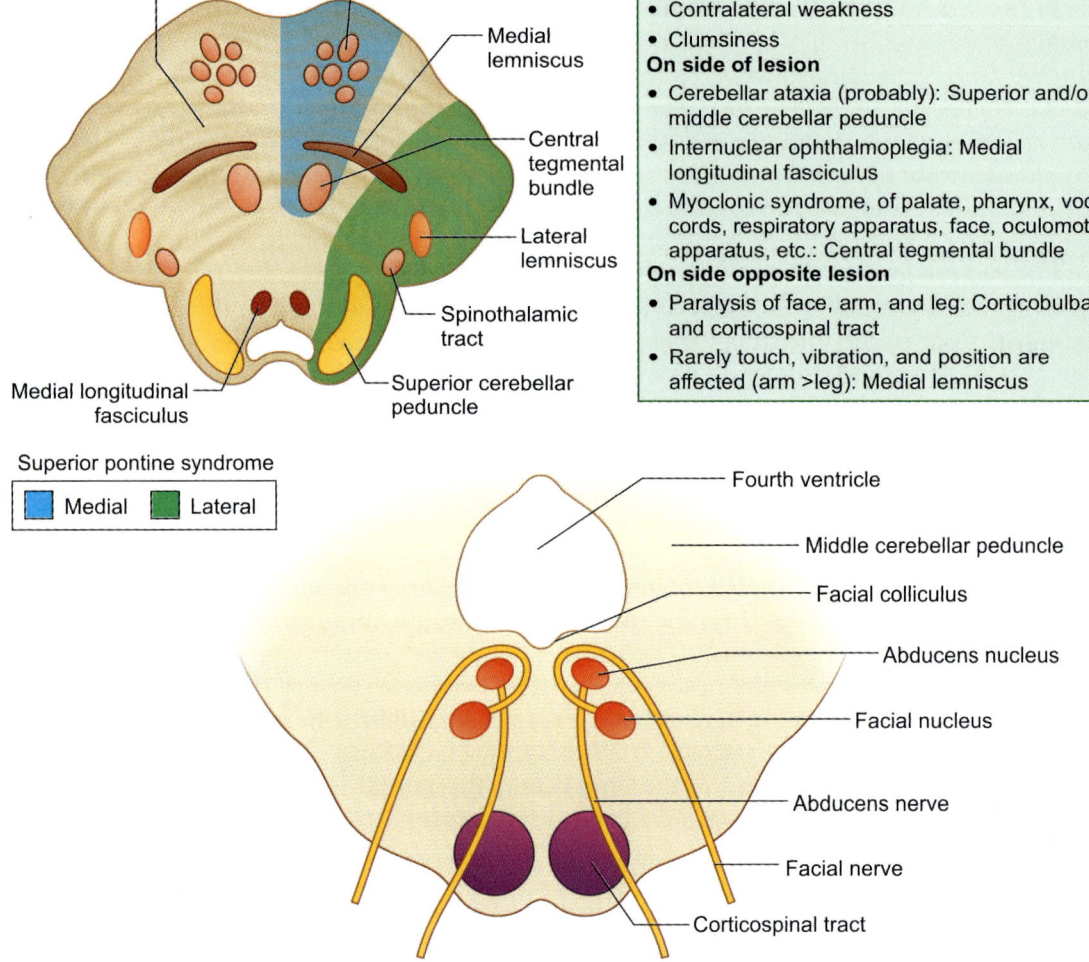

Common symptoms
- Contralateral weakness
- Clumsiness

On side of lesion
- Cerebellar ataxia (probably): Superior and/or middle cerebellar peduncle
- Internuclear ophthalmoplegia: Medial longitudinal fasciculus
- Myoclonic syndrome, of palate, pharynx, vocal cords, respiratory apparatus, face, oculomotor apparatus, etc.: Central tegmental bundle

On side opposite lesion
- Paralysis of face, arm, and leg: Corticobulbar and corticospinal tract
- Rarely touch, vibration, and position are affected (arm >leg): Medial lemniscus

Superior pontine syndrome

■ Medial ■ Lateral

Fig. 6.5: Medial pontine syndrome: Axial section of the brainstem (pons) at the level of the facial colliculus. Somatic motor fibres of the facial nerve (CNVII) are shown going around the abducens nucleus (CNVI)

4. **Medial pontine syndrome (Millard-Gubler syndrome):** There is internal strabismus (VI cranial nerve) and paralysis of muscles of the face (VII cranial nerve) on the same side and paralysis of the muscles (corticospinal tract) and impairment of touch and position senses (medial lemniscus) on the opposite side of the body (contralateral hemiplegia). This syndrome is also called 'medial inferior pontine syndrome' (Fig. 6.5); and has many similarities to medial medullary syndrome, because it is located higher up the brainstem in the pons, it affects a different set of cranial nuclei. Medial pontine syndrome results from occlusion of paramedian branches of the basilar artery.

5. **Lateral Pontine syndrome or Marie-Foix syndrome:** It includes the impairment of pain and temperature on the opposite side (lateral spinothalamic tract) and impairment of facial sensations (V cranial nerve), vertigo, nystagmus and deafness (VIII cranial nerve), facial paralysis (VII cranial nerve) and cerebellar ataxia (middle cerebellar peduncle) on the same side.

A **lateral pontine syndrome** (Fig. 6.6) is a lesion which is similar to the lateral medullary syndrome, but because it occurs in the pons, it also involves the cranial nerve nuclei of the pons.

Damage to the following areas produces symptoms (from medial to lateral):

Structure affected	Presentation
Corticospinal tract	Contralateral spastic hemiparesis, or unilateral paresis, is weakness of one entire side of the body (hemi—means 'half'). Hemiplegia is, in its most severe form, complete paralysis of half of the body. Hemiparesis and hemiplegia can be caused by different medical conditions, including congenital causes, trauma, tumours, or stroke.
Medial lemniscus	Contralateral PCML (aka DCML) pathway loss (tactile, vibration, and stereognosis)
Abducens nerve	Strabismus (ipsilateral lateral rectus muscle paralysis—the affected eye looks down and towards the nose). Abducens nerve lesion localizes the lesion to inferior pons.
Lateral spinothalamic tract	Contralateral loss of pain and temperature from the trunk and extremities.
Facial nucleus and facial nerve (CN VII)	1. Ipsilateral paralysis of the upper and lower face (lower motor neuron lesion). 2. Ipsilateral loss of lacrimation and reduced salivation. 3. Ipsilateral loss of taste from the anterior two-thirds of the tongue. 4. Loss of corneal reflex (efferent limb).
Spinal trigeminal nucleus and tract	Ipsilateral loss of pain and temperature sensation from the face (facial hemianaesthesia)
Vestibular nuclei and intra-axial nerve fibres	Nystagmus, nausea, vomiting, and vertigo
Cochlear nuclei and intra-axial nerve fibres	Hearing loss-ipsilateral central deafness
Middle and inferior cerebellar peduncle	Ipsilateral limb and gait ataxia
Descending sympathetic tract	Ipsilateral Horner's syndrome (ptosis, miosis, and anhydrosis)

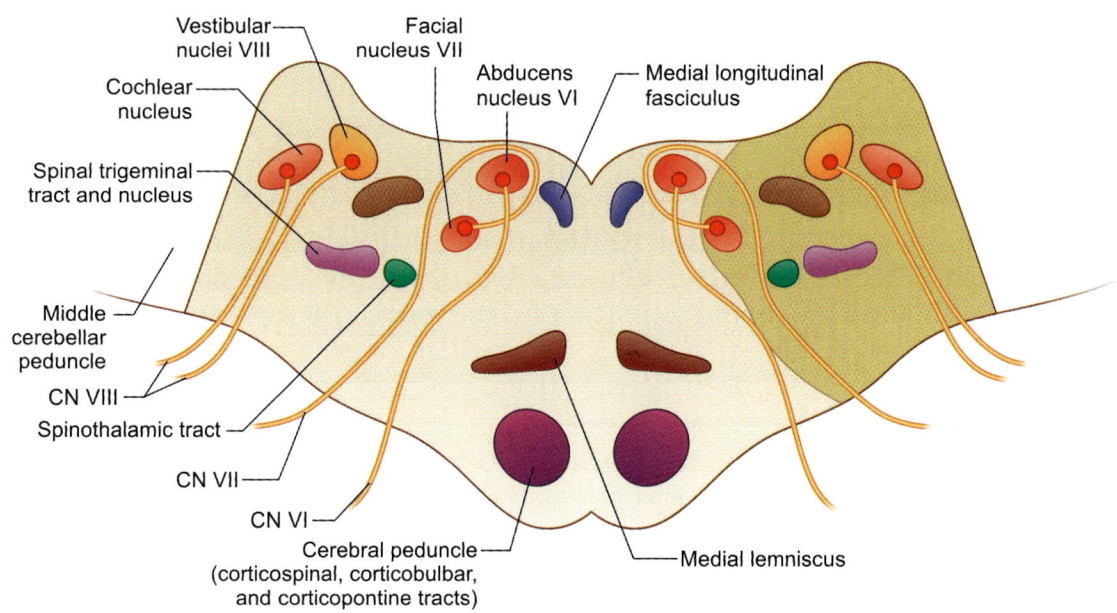

Fig. 6.6: Structures affected in lateral pontine syndrome

Rhombencephalon 1
Cerebellum and Cerebellar Cortex

GENERAL FEATURES

The cerebellum (little or small brain) is the second largest part of the brain. Despite its abundant sensory inputs it is essentially a motor part of the brain. It is transversely fissured, ovoid in form and weighs about 150 g (1/10th of total brain weight). It occupies the posterior cranial fossa and lies under the tentorium cerebelli posterior to the medulla and the pons. It consists of two *hemispheres* joined by a median portion called the **vermis**. The *superior vermis* (Fig. 7.1), not demarcated from the hemispheres, forms a median ridge sloping downwards and posteriorly and also on either side to merge with the gently concave superior surface of the hemisphere.

The inferior surfaces of the two *hemispheres* are convex and are separated by a median depression called the *vallecula*. The *inferior vermis* (Fig. 7.2) projects from the floor of the vallecula. In front, a wide *anterior cerebellar notch* accommodates the medulla and the pons. Three pairs of cerebellar peduncles (superior, middle and inferior) enter the cerebellum through the anterior cerebellar notch. The *posterior cerebellar notch* is narrow and accommodates the falx cerebelli.

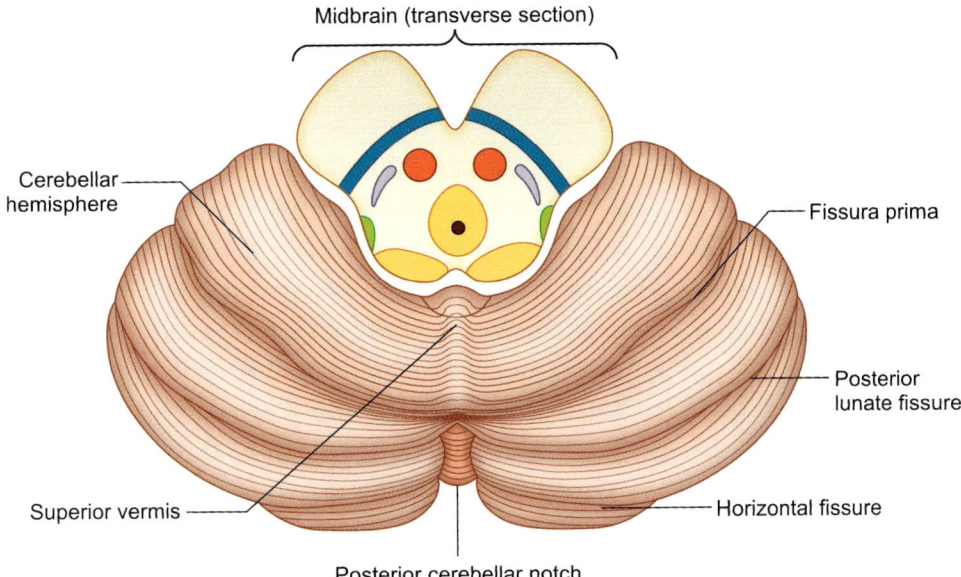

Fig. 7.1: Superior surface of the cerebellum

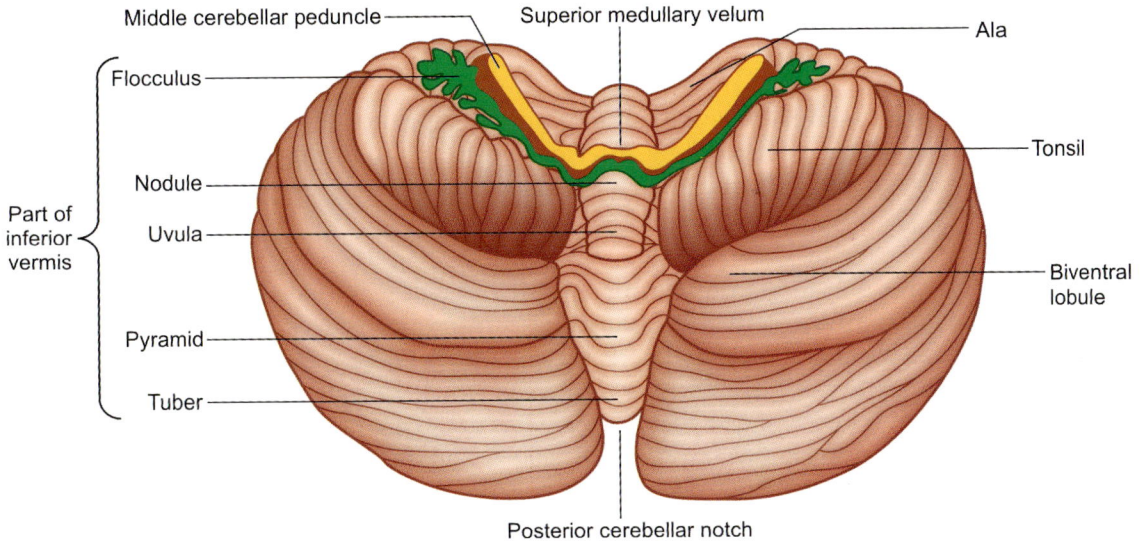

Fig. 7.2: Inferior surface of the cerebellum

MORPHOLOGICAL SUBDIVISIONS

Numerous closely set, almost parallel fissures cut through the surfaces of the cerebellum, separating its *folia*. The *horizontal fissure* running along the lateral and posterior margins is the most conspicuous (Fig. 7.3). It separates the superior and inferior surfaces of cerebellum. Two other fissures are of particular interest.

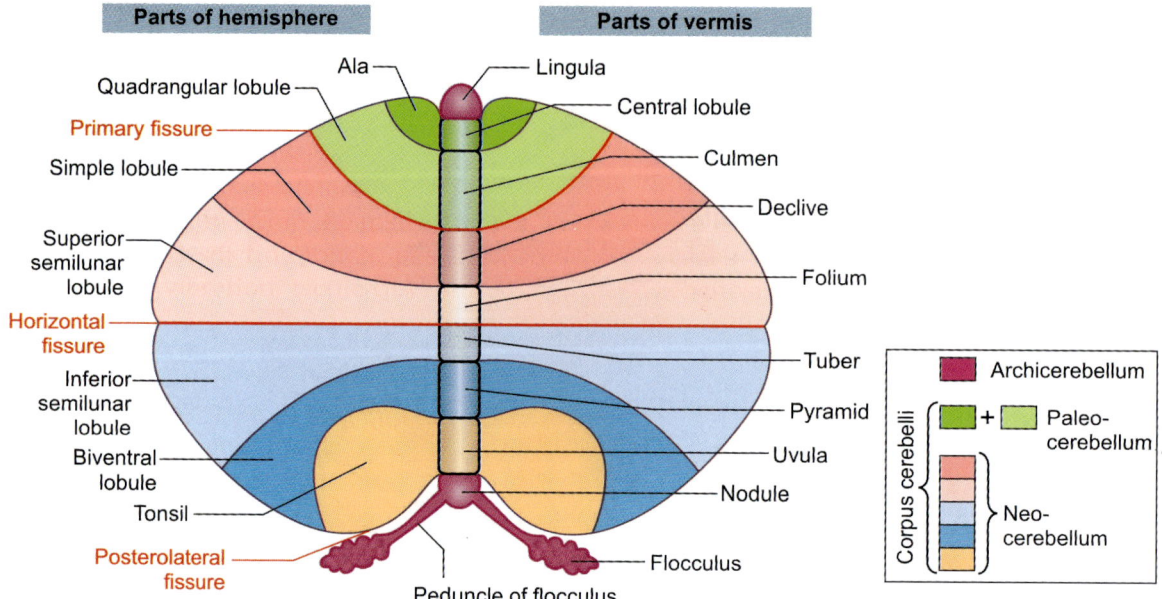

Fig. 7.3: Morphological and functional subdivisions of the cerebellum (*Courtesy:* Nafis Ahmad Faruqi)

Posterolateral fissure: It cuts through the anterior part of inferior surface of cerebellum and demarcates the *flocculonodular lobe* from the rest of cerebellum, which constitutes the *corpus cerebelli.*

Fissura prima: It is a V-shaped fissure running on the superior surface of cerebellum. It cuts the superior vermis at the junction of its anterior two-thirds with the posterior one-third and divides the corpus cerebelli into the anterior and posterior *lobes.*

Superior Surface

Several other fissures subdivide the vermis and hemispheres into *lobules.* The lobes, lobules and fissures, are present on both the superior and inferior surfaces of the cerebellum. The cerebellum has been assumed to be unrolled and laid out flat (Fig. 7.3). The parts of the *superior vermis,* from before backwards are, the *lingula, central lobule, culmen, declive* and the *folium.* The corresponding superior hemispheric parts (lingula has none) are the *ala,* the *anterior* and *posterior quadrangular lobules* and the *superior semilunar lobule.* The declive together with the posterior quadrangular lobule constitute the simple *lobule.*

Inferior Surface

The parts of the *inferior vermis,* from before backwards are, the *nodule, uvula, pyramid* and the *tuber vermis.* The corresponding inferior hemispheric lobules are the *flocculus* (and *paraflocculus*), the *tonsil,* the *biventral lobule* and corresponding to the tuber, the *gracile* and inferior *semilunar lobules.* The lobules on the inferior surface of the cerebellum are also shown in Fig. 7.3. Note the tonsil occupying the anteromedial portion of the inferior surface of the hemisphere. In conditions of raised intracranial pressure the tonsils tend to herniate downwards through the foramen magnum. This compresses the medulla and may cause quadriplegia and respiratory arrest.

FUNCTIONAL SUBDIVISIONS

Flocculonodular Lobe

The **flocculonodular lobe** (vestibulocerebellum) is a **lobe** of the cerebellum consisting of the nodule and the flocculus. The two flocculi are connected to the midline structure called the nodule by thin pedicles (Fig. 7.3). It is placed on the anteroinferior surface of cerebellum. This region of the cerebellum, as suggestive of its name, has important connections to the vestibular nuclei and uses information about head movement to influence eye movement. This lobe is also involved in the maintenance of balance equilibrium and muscle tone.

Corpus Cerebelli

Besides the flocculonodular lobe, the remaining part of cerebellum (of the two lateral portions of the cerebellum) is called *corpus cerebelli* which is subdivided longitudinally into *three* zones based on the projections of fibres to deep cerebellar nuclei. It is separated from the flocculonodular lobe by the posterolateral fissure. The corpus cerebelli is subdivided by the primary fissure into an **anterior lobe** (in front of the fissure), and a **middle lobe** (behind the fissure).

Vermal or **median zone**	Pair of paravermal or **intermediate zone**	Pair of hemisphere or **lateral zones**
Nucleus fastigii	Nucleus interpositus	Nucleus dentatus
Movements of trunk and extensor muscle tone	Movements of proximal limb muscles	Coordination of distal limb muscles for skillful prehensile act
Through vestibule-spinal and reticulospinal tracts	Through rubrospinal tract	Through dentatorubrothalamocortical pathways and descending corticospinal and rubrospinal tracts

The following functional subdivisions of the cerebellum are described.

Vestibulocerebellum (archicerebellum)

It comprises of the flocculonodular lobe and the vestibulocerebellar mossy fibres. The outgoing fibres relay in the nucleus fastigii and pass back to the vestibular nuclei and the reticular formation. From here, vestibulospinal and reticulospinal fibres descend and mediate the movements necessary for maintaining body equilibrium. The vestibulocerebellum also regulates the vestibuloocular reflex, to adjust eye positions in response to head movements.

Spinocerebellum (paleocerebellum)

It comprises of, essentially, the anterior lobe of the cerebellum, lobulus simplex and the pyramid. Its *afferents* include: the *posterior* and *anterior spinocerebellar tracts*, the *cuneocerebellar* and the *trigeminocerebellar tracts.* These tracts bring both proprioceptive and exteroceptive impulses to the cerebellum. The outgoing fibres, from this part of the cerebellum also, relay in the nucleus fastigii and project to the vestibular nuclei (especially the lateral vestibular nucleus). Other fibres terminate in the reticular nuclei. These regions are concerned with the maintenance of *posture* and *muscle tone* and *coordination* of muscles during *stereotyped movements* such as those required in locomotion. Lesions of the anterior lobe usually induce hypotonia.

Neo- or Ponto-cerebellum

It is the largest subdivision of the cerebellum and comprises of the folium, uvula and tuberal parts of the vermis and the entire hemisphere. It receives afferents from all cortical regions (through the corticopontocerebellar fibres) and from the inferior olivary nucleus. The outgoing fibres relay in the dentate, emboliform and the globose nuclei. Efferents from these, project to the motor and premotor cortical regions through the dentatorubrothalamic pathways. These projections regulate skilled movements (based on learning experience) and speech. It is noteworthy that each half of the body is represented in the ipsilateral cerebellar hemisphere. The vermal region mainly controls the trunk, head and neck movements.

DEVELOPMENT OF CEREBELLUM

There are three distinct segments in the developing brain: The prosencephalon, mesencephalon, and rhombencephalon. The rhombencephalon is the most caudal (toward the tail) segment of the embryonic brain; it is from this segment that the cerebellum develops. Along the embryonic rhombencephalic segment develop eight swellings, called *rhombomeres*. The cerebellum arises from two rhombomeres located in the alar plate of the neural tube, a structure that eventually forms the brain and spinal cord. The specific rhombomeres from which the cerebellum forms are: rhombomere 1 (Rh 1) caudally (near the tail) and the 'isthmus' rostrally (near the front). Two primary regions are thought to give rise to the neurons that make up the cerebellum. The **first region** is the ventricular zone in the roof of the fourth ventricle. This area produces Purkinje cells and deep cerebellar nuclear neurons. The **second germinal zone** is the site for the birth of cells in the cerebellum, and is known as the *rhombic lip*, neurons then move by human embryonic week 27 to the *external granular layer*. This layer of cells—found on the exterior of the cerebellum—produces the granule neurons. The granule neurons migrate from this exterior layer to form an inner layer known as the *internal granule layer*. The external granular layer ceases to exist in the mature cerebellum, leaving only granule cells in the internal granule layer. The cerebellar white matter may be a third germinal zone in the cerebellum.

Cerebellum develops from the superior (pontine) rhombic lip. Two rounded swellings are formed in the 6th week of gestation. These join across the midline to form a dumb-bell shaped mass (Fig. 7.4). Transverse grooves, followed by fissures appear on its surfaces. The *posterolateral fissure* appears first. It demarcates the *flocculonodular lobe*. The flocculus and nodule are developed from the **rhombic lip**, and are therefore recognisable **as** separate portions before any of the other cerebellar lobules. The groove produced by the bending over of the **rhombic lip** is here known **as** the floccular fissure; when the two lateral walls fuse, the right and left floccular fissures join **in** the middle line and their central part becomes the post-nodular fissure. The *fissura prima* is the second fissure to be formed (3rd month). It demarcates the anterior lobe. Soon thereafter, the fissura secunda and the prepyramidal fissures are formed. More fissures follow to give the cerebellum its characteristic appearance.

GROSS INTERNAL STRUCTURE

Grey Matter—Intracerebellar Nuclei

The cerebellum has an outer layer of grey matter (cortex) and a white core. Sheets of white matter extend from the white core into the lobes. Four *intracerebellar nuclei* lie on either side within the white core (Fig. 7.5). From lateral to medial side these are: the nuclei *dentatus, emboliformis, globosus* and *fastigii*. The *dentate nucleus* is the largest and consists of an irregularly folded lamina of grey matter. It has a *hilum* directed anteromedially. The *nucleus emboliformis* partially covers its hilum. The *globose nucleus,* lying caudal and medial to emboliform nucleus, is continuous with *nucleus fastigii,* which lies close to the roof of the fourth ventricle. The globose and emboliform nuclei together constitute the *nucleus interpositus.*

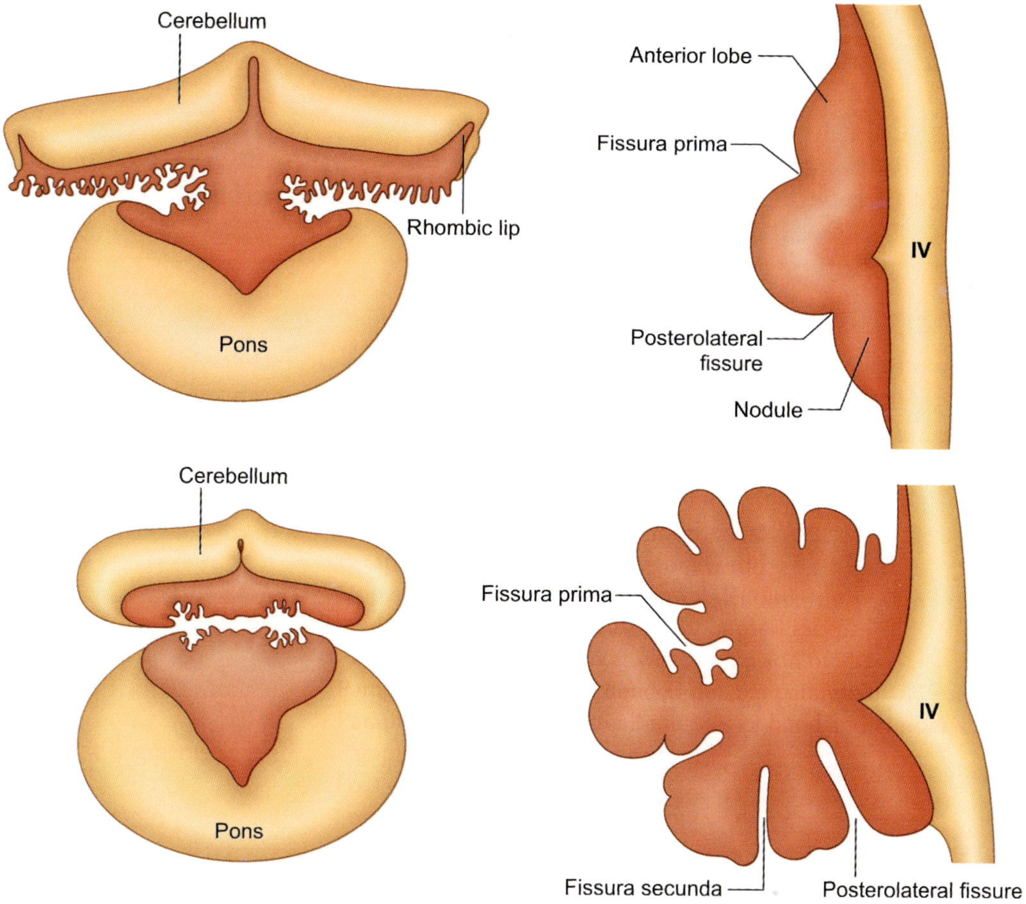

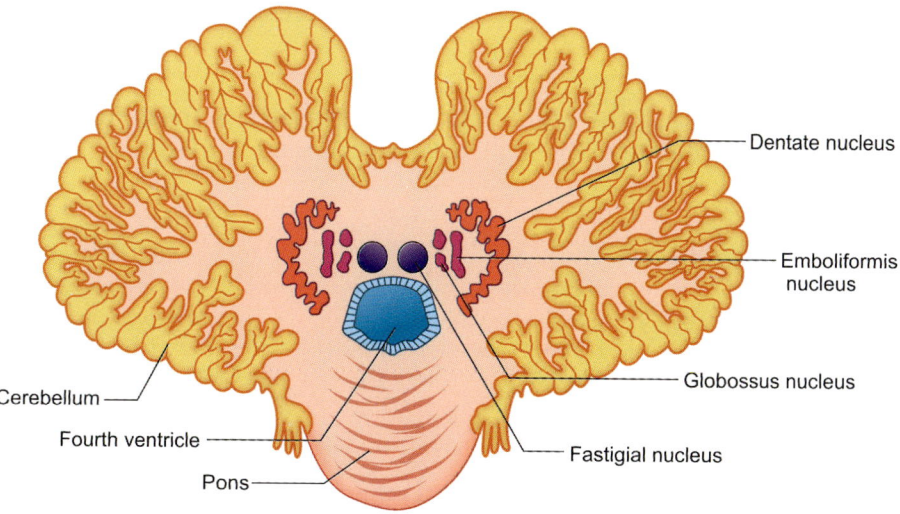

Fig. 7.4: Development of the cerebellum and the appearance of the fissures

Fig. 7.5: Transverse section of the cerebellum at the level of pons and locations of the deep cerebellar nuclei (*Courtesy:* Nafis Ahmad Faruqi)

White Matter—Fibre Tracts

The white matter of the cerebellum consists of:

The Superior Medullary Velum

It is a thin lamina of white matter stretching between the two superior cerebellar peduncles. It forms the upper part of the roof of fourth ventricle. The frenulum veli descends as a thin median ridge on its upper part. The trochlear nerves emerge on either side of the frenulum.

The Inferior Medullary Velum

These are two thin crescentic laminae of white matter lying on either side of the nodule and overlapped by the tonsil of the cerebellum. Narrowing laterally they continue with the peduncle of the flocculus.

The Central White Core of Cerebellum

The white core contains the cerebellar nuclei and extends into the folia of cerebellum. The primary plates and the secondary laminae of white matter, covered by strips of grey matter form a branching pattern called the *arbor vitae cerebelli* seen best in a sagittal section.

Projection Fibres Forming—Cerebellar Peduncles

Three pairs of cerebellar peduncles, the superior, the middle and the inferior, connect the cerebellum to the midbrain, pons and the medulla oblongata respectively. Table 7.1 may be seen for their constituent fibres which are 16 in number; and may be categorized into two subtypes: afferent (Fig. 7.6) and efferent (Fig. 7.7).

Afferent Fibres (Fig. 7.6)

Corticopontocerebellar Fibres

These are derived from all parts of cerebellar cortex, relay in the pontine nuclei and pass through the middle cerebellar peduncle to the opposite cerebellar hemisphere.

Vestibulocerebellar Fibres

From the vestibular nerve and the vestibular nuclei, these fibres pass through the inferior cerebellar peduncle to terminate in the ipsilateral flocculonodular lobe.

Table 7.1: The constituent fibres of the three cerebellar peduncles

Inferior cerebellar peduncle	Middle cerebellar peduncle	Superior cerebellar peduncle
1. Olivocerebellar fibres	1. Pontocerebellar fibres	1. Dentatorubrothalamic fibres
2. Parolivocerebellar fibres	2. Reticulocerebellar fibres	2. Anterior spinocerebellar tract
3. Anterior external arcuate fibres		3. Tectocerebellar fibres, arcuate fibres
4. Posterior external arcuate fibres		4. Rubrocerebellar fibres, arcuate fibres
5. Posterior spinocerebellar tract		5. Trigeminocerebellar fibres
6. Vestibulocerebellar fibres		
7. Reticulocerebellar fibres		
8. Cerebellovestibular fibres		
9. Cerebelloreticular fibres		

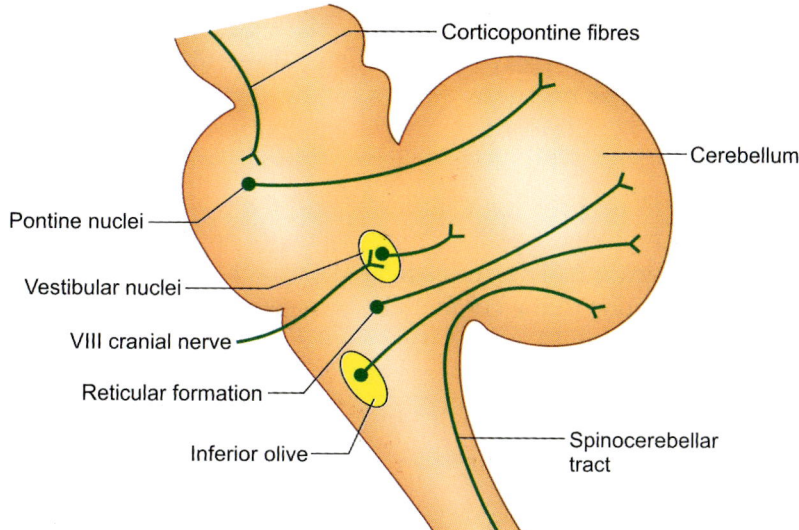

Fig. 7.6: Schematic diagram of the cerebellum to show its afferent fibres

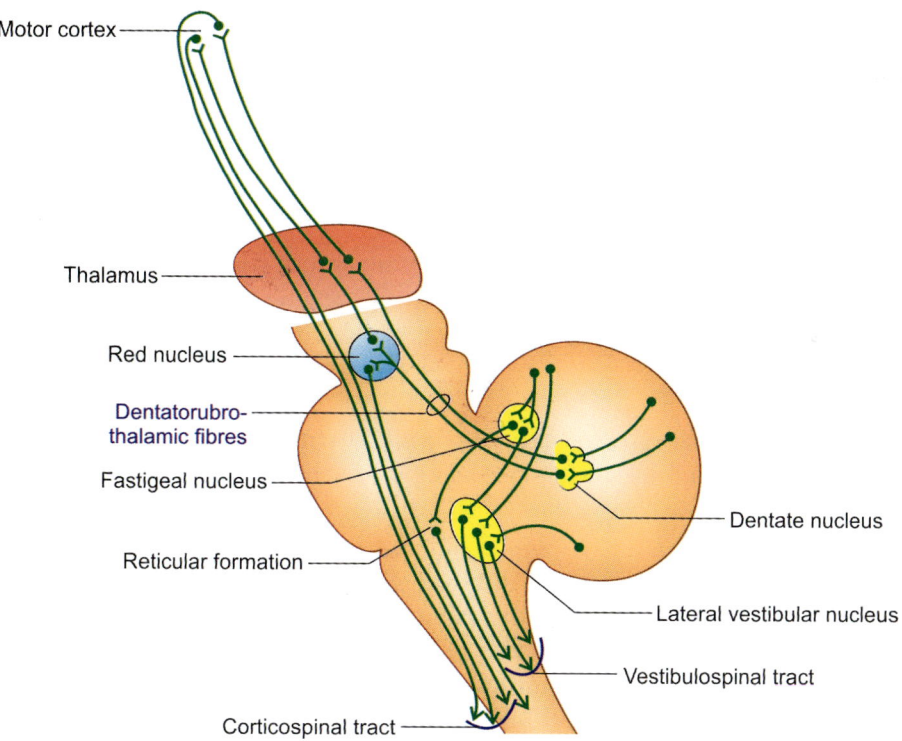

Fig. 7.7: Schematic diagram of the cerebellum to show its efferent fibres

Reticulocerebellar Fibres

From the reticular formation (lateral reticular nucleus) is received the *spinoreticular tract*, which projects bilaterally to the vermis and hemispheres.

Olivocerebellar Fibres

From the inferior olivary and accessory olivary nuclei, these fibres pass through the inferior peduncle to the contralateral hemisphere.

Spinocerebellar Fibres

From the spinal cord, these fibres pass in the anterior and the posterior spinocerebellar and the cuneocerebellar tracts. The spinocerebellar tracts transmit proprioceptive and exteroceptive information from the lower limb. The cuneocerebellar tract conducts similar impulses from the upper limb. The projections to the cerebellum are essentially *ipsilateral.*

Efferent Fibres (Fig. 7.7)

The cerebellar efferents originate in its nuclei and include the following:

Dentatorubrothalamic Fibres

These fibres conducted by the superior cerebellar peduncle, cross the midline in the lower midbrain, and pass through the contralateral red nucleus, with or without relay, to terminate in the thalamus. From the thalamus the impulses are relayed to the motor cortex.

Cerebellovestibular Fibres

From *fastigial nucleus* the cerebellovestibular fibres reach to the vestibular nuclei of both sides. The cerebellar efferents to the vestibular nuclei (lateral vestibular nucleus) are relayed to the anterior horn cells of the spinal cord in the *vestibulospinal* tracts.

Cerebelloreticular Fibres

The efferents to the reticular nuclei are relayed to the spinal cord in the *reticulospinal tract.*

MICROSCOPIC STRUCTURE OF CEREBELLUM

Layers in Cerebellar Cortex

The cerebellar cortex presents the same structure in all its parts (homogeneity of cortex). It consists of (1) the granular layer, (2) the Purkinje cell layer, and (3) the molecular layer (Fig. 7.8).

Granular Layer

This layer contains a large number of small-sized granule cells and a limited number of (large sized) *Golgi cells*. The granule cells send their axons outwards into the molecular layer, where they bifurcate in a typical T-shaped manner. The opposite axonal branches extend along the longitudinal axis of the folium (parallel fibres) to make synaptic contacts with the dendrites of several Purkinje cells. The *Golgi cell* axon ramifies in the granular layer while its dendrites pass out into the molecular layer where they ramify in all the directions.

Purkinje Cell Layer

This layer consists of a single row of large pear-shaped Purkinje cells. Their richly arborising dendrites extend in a plane transverse to the long-axis of the folium. The axon is basal in origin and passes in the white matter to terminate in contact with the cerebellar nuclei.

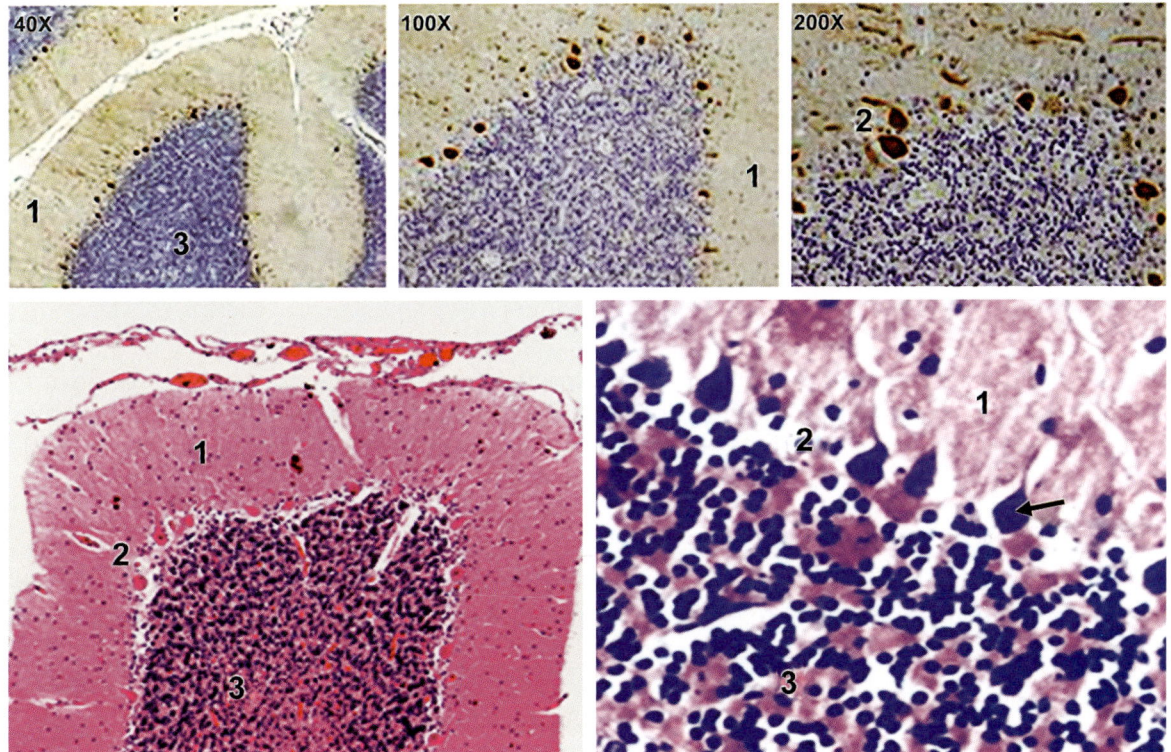

Fig. 7.8: Photomicrographs show three distinct layers in the cerebellar cortex at different magnification: molecular layer (1), Purkinje cell (2) layer in a single row, and granule cell layer (3) characterised by numerous small-sized neurons. The photomicrograph at the lower right corner depicts typical flask-shaped Purkinje neurons (arrow) at higher magnification

Molecular Layer

This layer contains dendritic branches of the Purkinje and the Golgi cells and an abundance of the axons of granule cells. Two types of interneurons, the superficially located *stellate cells* and deeply placed *basket cells,* are also present.

Connections of the Cerebellar Nuclei

The cerebellar nuclei are connected with motor nuclei in the brainstem and, through the thalamus, with the motor cortex. Purkinje cells of the anterior vermis and the vestibulo-cerebellum affect eye muscles, axial muscles and proximal limb muscles through the vestibular nuclei. The hemispheres influence ipsilateral limb muscles through the dentate and interposed nuclei and their connections with the contralateral motor cortex. The paravermal region and the interposed nuclei, forming the *pars intermedia* are mainly involved in the ipsilateral limb muscle control.

The *efferents* from the *fastigial nucleus* pass through the inferior cerebellar peduncle. Efferents from the other nuclei pass through the superior peduncle to end in the opposite red nucleus and the thalamus.

Cortical Inputs and Outputs

Cortical Inputs

Two types of afferent fibres to the cortex of cerebellum are described, the *climbing fibres* and the *mossy fibres.*

Climbing Fibres

These fibres, originate in the inferior olivary nucleus (hence named *olivocerebellar*), and synapse with the dendrites of a single Purkinje cell (Fig. 7.9).

Mossy Fibres

These are more numerous and arise from a variety of sources. Each *mossy fibre* divides to synapse with the dendrites of a number of granule cells (and axons of Golgi cells) in complex synapses called the *glomeruli* (Fig. 7.10). The axon of a granule cell, in turn, synapses with the dendrites of hundreds of Purkinje cells.

Nature of Neuronal Connections

1. The synapses between the climbing fibres and the Purkinje cells, mossy fibres and the granule cells and between the granule cells and the Purkinje cells are all *excitatory.* The total input to the cortex is, therefore, excitatory.
2. The *Golgi axons* inhibit the granule cells and the *stellate* and the *basket cells* inhibit the Purkinje cells. These cells serve to limit the area of cortical excitation.

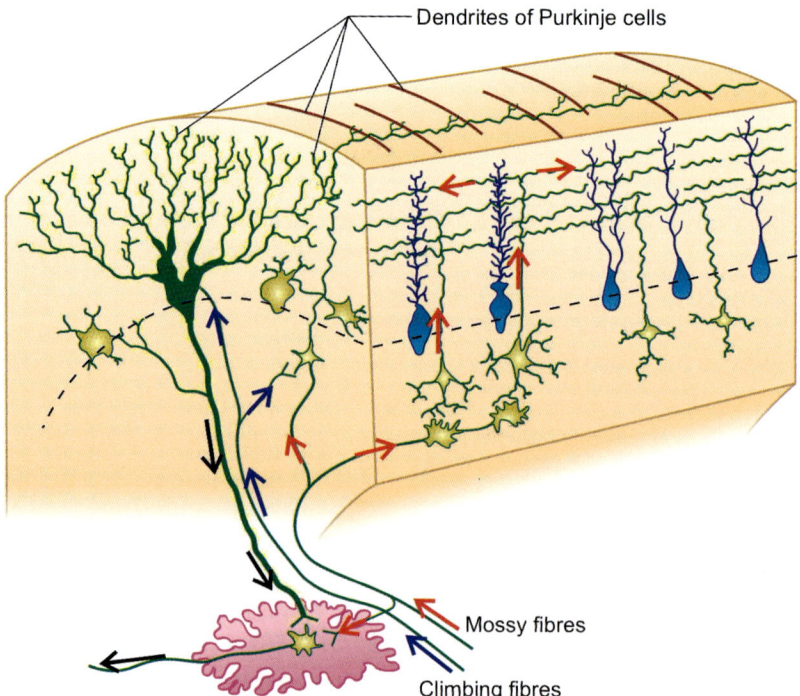

Fig. 7.9: A 3-D transverse section through a cerebellar folium and the climbing and mossy fibres coming to the cerebellum

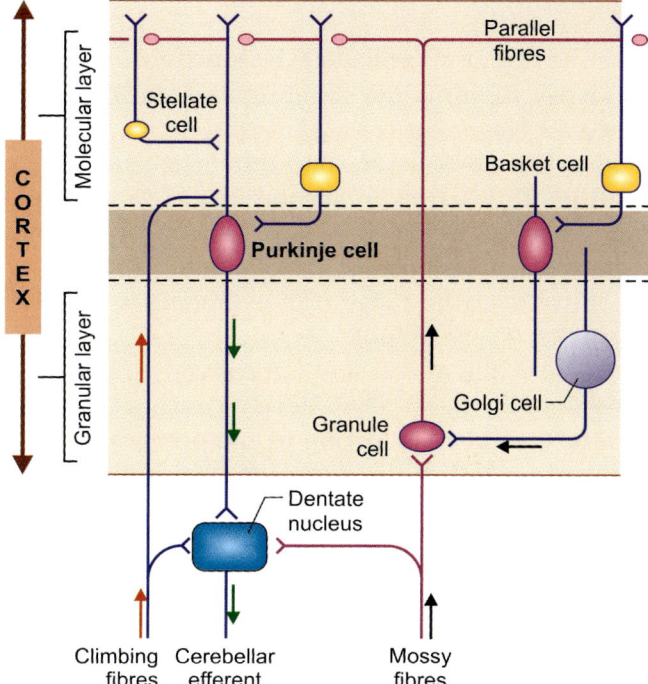

Fig. 7.10: Diagrammatic sketch of cerebellar circuitry

3. The Purkinje cells inhibit the intracerebellar nuclei.
4. Neurons of the deep nuclei are, excitatory. Ascending fibres to the Purkinje cells supply collaterals to these nuclei. These collaterals act as emergency circuits in diseases involving the Purkinje cells.

Cortical Outputs

Purkinje cell axons are the only efferent fibres leaving the cerebellar cortex. They provide afferent fibres to the cerebellar nuclei. The dentate nucleus receives axons from the Purkinje cells in the lateral part of cerebellar hemisphere. The emboliform and globose nuclei receive axons from the paravermal region and the nucleus fastigii receives fibres from the vermian region.

FUNCTIONS OF CEREBELLUM

The cerebellum is necessary for normal movements. Lesions of cerebellum impair movements and motor learning. As already described there are three functional subdivisions of the cerebellum, associated with different functional modalities.
1. The vestibulocerebellum helps in the maintenance of the body equilibrium.
2. The spinocerebellum is concerned with the coordination of muscles during the stereotyped movements such as are required for the control of the posture and locomotion.
3. The pontocerebellum controls skilled movements and speech. The cerebellum coordinates the sequence and force of muscular contraction during postural and voluntary movements of trunk and limbs.
4. Cerebellum is also important for the smooth pursuit movements of the eyeball.

Cerebellar Dysfunction

The following effects may be found in cerebellar dysfunction.

1. **Dysequilibrium:** Tendency to fall while standing and staggering gait (incoordination of limb and axial muscles).
2. **Hypotonia:** Diminution of the muscle tone and inhibited tendon reflexes.
3. **Muscular incoordination:** This results in asynergia, i.e. diminished capacity for smooth, orderly and coordinated action between muscle groups. A complex movement may be carried out as irregular disjointed episodes *(decomposition of movements)*.
4. **Dysmetria:** Loss of control over the range of movements is called dysmetria, in which a patient either 'undershoots' or 'overshoots'.
5. **Tremors:** These are absent while at rest and appear only during a movement, especially towards the end of the movement.
6. **Dysarthria (speech defect):** There is slowing of the onset, slurring and jerk intermittent sound production, due to incoordination of speech muscles.
7. **Nystagmus:** Eyes cannot be fixed on an object. They drift away due to incoordination of eye muscles.

Localisation of Cerebellar Disease

Damage to the vermis and the flocculonodular lobe causes imbalance and trunkal ataxia. There is swaying of the body, staggering gait and tendency to fall backwards. Nystagmus is often present.

Lesions of hemisphere result in hypotonia, tremors and incoordination.

(*Note:* 1. Cerebellar functions cannot be tested in sleep or coma. 2. Cerebellar lesions do not affect memory, mentation consciousness, sensory perception or autonomic functions).

Rhombencephalon 2
Fourth Ventricle and Area Postrema

- Development of Fourth Ventricle
- Boundaries of Fourth Ventricle
  - Angles
  - Lateral boundaries
  - Roof
- Tela Choroidea of Fourth Ventricle
  - Floor (Rhomboid Fossa)
  - Recesses
  - Applied anatomy
- Area Postrema

Inside the brain, there are four cavities, called **ventricles.** The right and left lateral ventricles and the third and **fourth ventricles** compose the *ventricular system.* The fourth ventricle is the cavity of hindbrain. It lies posterior to the upper part of medulla oblongata and pons and anterior to the cerebellum (Fig. 8.1).

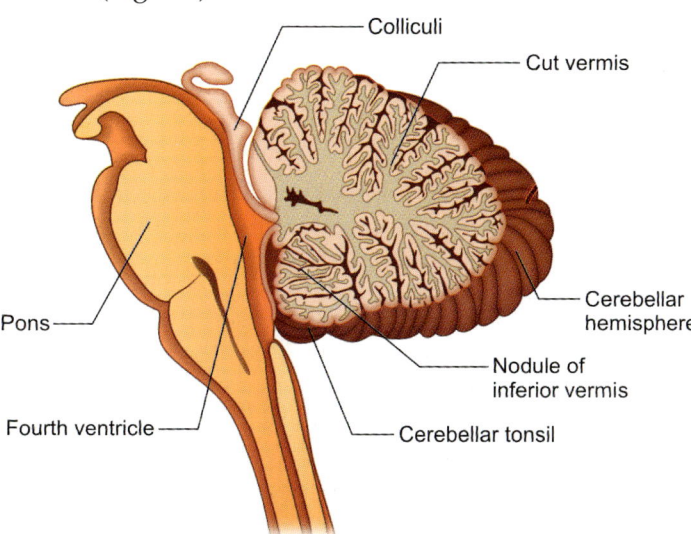

Colliculi

Cut vermis

Pons

Cerebellar hemisphere

Nodule of inferior vermis

Fourth ventricle

Cerebellar tonsil

Fig. 8.1: Location of the tent-like fourth ventricle on the posterior surface of the pons and the upper part of the medulla. It is rhomboid in shape (diamond-shaped)

DEVELOPMENT OF FOURTH VENTRICLE

Much like other portions of the ventricular system inside the brain, the fourth ventricle develops from the area inside the neural tube. During gestation, the ventricles form during the first three months of pregnancy. During this time of development, it is possible for circulation to be blocked by overproduction of cerebrospinal fluid, causing a condition called *hydrocephalus*.

The fourth ventricle is found in the posterior region of the pons and medulla and is rhomboid in shape. Superiorly, it narrows to become continuous with the aqueduct of the midbrain. Inferiorly, it narrows and leads into the central canal of the medulla. This in turn is continuous with the central canal of the spinal cord. The fourth ventricle is widened at the point called the lateral recess.

BOUNDARIES OF FOURTH VENTRICLE

This ventricle has a roof and a floor. The roof is composed of the cerebellum, located at the back of the brain, and the floor is formed by the rhomboid fossa, a depression in the brainstem. Within the floor is the facial colliculus, sulcus limitans, and the obex.

Angles

It has a superior, an inferior, and two lateral angles. The *superior angle* leads through the cerebral aqueduct to communicate with the cavity of third ventricle. The *inferior angle* continues downwards as the central canal in the closed part of medulla oblongata. The *lateral angles* are drawn outwards as the *lateral recesses* which open through the *lateral apertures (foramina of Luschka)* into the subarachnoid space.

Lateral Boundaries

Superolateral—The superior cerebellar peduncles
Inferolateral—From above downward three structures seen are:
  i. Inferior cerebellar peduncles.
 ii. Cuneate tubercles.
iii. Gracile tubercles.

Roof

The roof is *tent-like* and extends into the white core of the cerebellum (Fig. 8.2). This portion presents three recesses of the fourth ventricle: a *median dorsal* and two *lateral dorsal recesses* one on either side. The roof slopes both rostrally and caudally.

Rostral slope of the roof (also called fastigium) is formed by:
  i. Superior cerebellar peduncles.
 ii. Superior medullary velum.

Caudal slope of the roof is formed by:
  i. Inferior medullary velum.
 ii. Tela choroidea of the fourth ventricle.
iii. Tenia: A narrow white ridge attached along the lower part of lateral boundaries.
 iv. Obex: A small fold opposite the inferior angle.

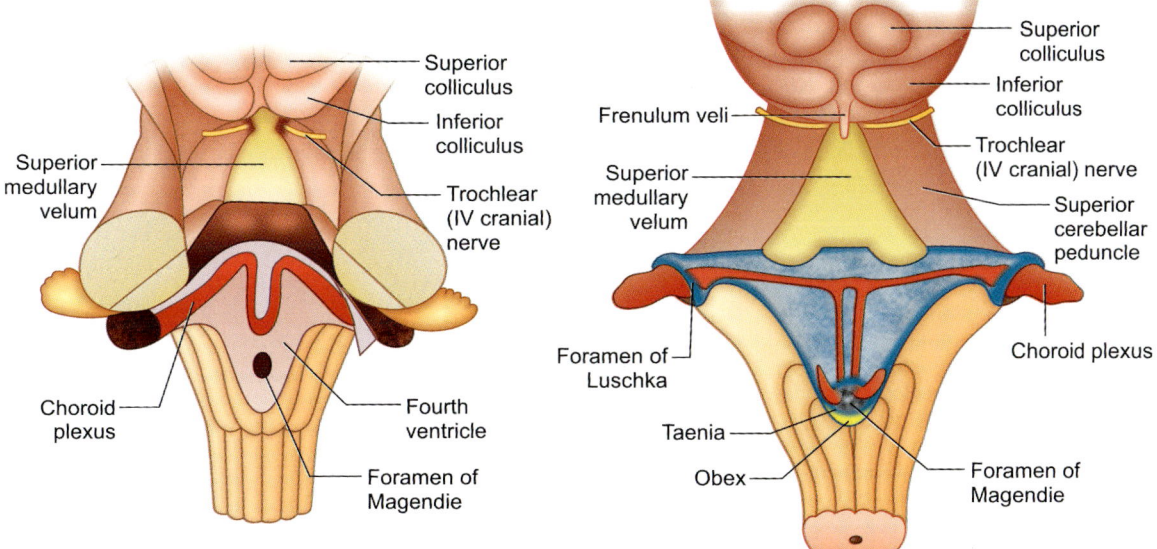

Fig. 8.2: Removal of the cerebellum from the posterior aspect of the brainstem exposes the tent-like roof of the fourth ventricle. The upper portion of roof is formed entirely by the superior medullary velum. The lower portion of the roof is formed by inferior medullary velum, and the tela choroidea (red in the right sketch). At the lateral angles of the ventricle, the roof is widest and is continued on each side into a tubular lateral recess through which choroid plexus escapes into the subarachnoid spaces

TELA CHOROIDEA OF FOURTH VENTRICLE

The tela choroidea is a fold of pia matter containing blood vessels and forming the lower non-nervous part of the roof of fourth ventricle. A median aperture called the foramen of Magendie is present in the lower portion of the ventricle's roof. Through this aperture the fourth ventricle communicates with the subarachnoid space (cerebello-medullary cistern).

The *choroid plexus* is a vascular tuft projecting into the fourth ventricle through lower part of its roof. The plexus is T-shaped with a duplicated vertical limb. It is supplied by the branches of the posterior inferior cerebellar arteries and secretes CSF into the ventricle. Portions of the plexus protrude through the apertures of the ventricle to secrete CSF directly into the subarachnoid space.

Floor (Rhomboid fossa)

The floor of the fourth ventricle is formed by the dorsal surfaces of the upper half of medulla oblongata and the pons. It presents the following features (Figs 8.3 and 8.4).
1. The *median sulcus*, which divides the floor into symmetrical right and left halves.
2. The *medial eminence* is present on either side of the median sulcus. A little above its middle the medial eminence presents a small localised elevation called the *facial colliculus*. It overlies the abducent nucleus and the facial nerve fibres wind round the nucleus. The lower part of the medial eminence constitutes the *hypoglossal triangle*, which overlies the hypoglossal nucleus and the nucleus intercalatus.
3. The *sulcus limitans* forms the lateral limit of the medial eminence. The sulcus presents the *locus ceruleus* in its upper part, the *superior fovea* opposite the facial colliculus and the *inferior fovea* in its lower part. The locus coeruleus is a bluish-grey area overlying a mass of pigmented

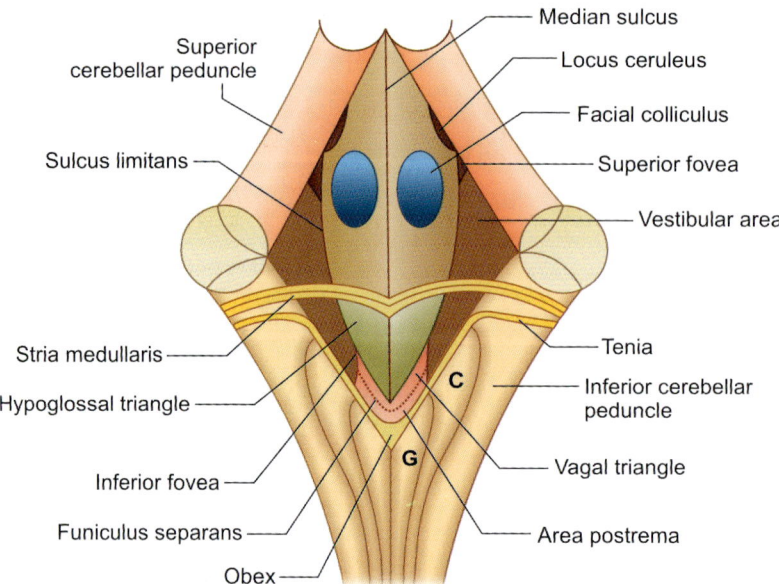

Fig. 8.3: The floor of the fourth ventricle is composed by the posterior surface of the pons and the upper part of the medulla. It is rhomboid in shape (diamond-shaped) and exhibits several features

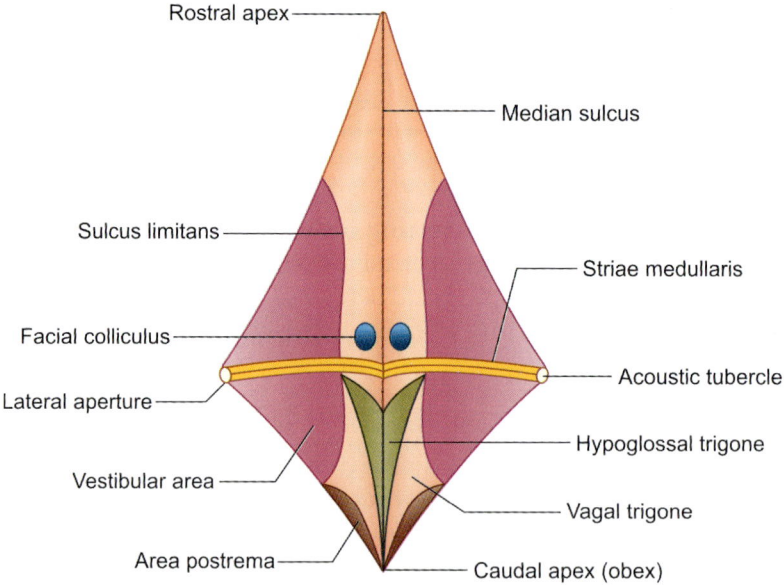

Fig. 8.4: The floor of the fourth ventricle is composed by the posterior surface of the pons and the upper part of the medulla. Notice facial colliculus and area postrema

melanin containing neurons. The neurons are adrenergic, have widespread projections and are active only in awake, attentive animals. They are involved in controlling the level of alertness.

4. The *vagal triangle (ala cineria),* which lies below the inferior fovea and lateral to the hypoglossal triangle, overlies the *dorsal nucleus of vagus nerve. A* thin ridge of ependyma called the *funiculus separans* running across the vagal triangle demarcates the *area postrema* in its lower part. The blood–brain barrier is modified (or absent) over the area postrema. Stimulation of this area by certain drugs (apomorphine, digitalis derivatives) initiates vomiting. The area is accordingly called the *chemoreceptor trigger zone (CTZ).*
5. The *vestibular* area lies lateral to the superior and inferior foveae and extends into the lateral recess. It overlies the *vestibular nuclei* and extending into the lateral recess, overlies the *dorsal cochlear nucleus.*
6. The *stria medullares* are transversely running fibres coursing across the floor of fourth ventricle, about its middle. The fibres are derived from the arcuate nuclei and emerge through the median sulcus. Laterally, the fibres pass to the cerebellum along the inferior cerebellar peduncle.

Recesses

The fourth ventricle presents five recesses, two paired and one unpaired. The paired recesses are *lateral* and *lateral dorsal* recesses. The *median dorsal recess is* unpaired.

The *lateral recesses* extend, on either side, in the form of a narrow curved pouch from about the middle of the fourth ventricle. Each is prolonged between the inferior cerebellar peduncle and the peduncle of flocculus and is open laterally (foramen of Luschka). The choroid plexus protrudes into the subarachnoid space through the foramen. The filaments of the IX and X cranial nerves cross the recess anteriorly.

The median and the two lateral dorsal recesses extend into the white core of cerebellum and are blind. The *median dorsal recess* lies above the nodule. The *lateral dorsal recesses, which* extend further dorsally into the cerebellar core, lie above the inferior medullary velum. Only a thin layer of white matter separates the cavity of the lateral dorsal recess from the intracerebellar nuclei.

The *choroid plexus* in the roof of fourth ventricle secretes cerebrospinal fluid (CSF), which is also secreted by the choroid plexuses in the third and lateral ventricles. A *median aperture (foramen of Magendie)* in the lower part of the roof of fourth ventricle and the two *lateral apertures (foramina of Luschka)* allow the CSF to escape out into the subarachnoid space.

Applied Anatomy

The three apertures of the fourth ventricle (foramina of Luschka and Magendie) permit the CSF secreted in the ventricles of the brain to pass out into the subarachnoid space. Obstruction of the foramina will result in the accumulation of CSF and dilation of the ventricles, giving rise to hydrocephalus.

AREA POSTREMA

The area postrema is a medullary structure in the brain that controls vomiting. Its privileged location in the brain also allows the area postrema to play a vital role in the control of autonomic functions by the central nervous system. It is one of the circumventricular organs, enabling the dual role of being a sensor for circulating chemical messengers in the blood, as well as integrating neural inputs in the brainstem.

The area postrema (Fig. 8.4) is a small protuberance found at the inferoposterior limit of the fourth ventricle. Specialised ependymal cells are found within the area postrema.

These specialised ependymal cells differ slightly from the majority of ependymal cells (ependymocytes), forming a unicellular epithelium lining of the ventricles and central canal.

The area postrema is separated from the vagal triangle by the funiculus separans, a thin semitransparent ridge. The vagal triangle overlies the dorsal vagal nucleus and is situated on the caudal end of the rhomboid fossa or 'floor' of the fourth ventricle.

The area postrema is situated just before the obex, the inferior apex of the caudal ventricular floor. Both the funiculus separans and area postrema have a similar thick ependyma-containing tanycyte covering. Ependyma and tanycytes can participate in transport of neurochemicals into and out of the cerebrospinal fluid from its cells or adjacent neurons, glia or vessels. Ependyma and tanycytes may also participate in chemoreception. The eminence of the area postrema is considered a circumventricular organ because its endothelial cells do not contain tight junctions, which allows for free exchange of molecules between blood and brain tissue. This unique breakdown in the blood–brain barrier is partially compensated for by the presence of a tanycyte barrier.

Brainstem 3
Midbrain

- Development of Midbrain
- External Features of Midbrain
  - From ventral aspect
  - From dorsal aspect
- Internal Structure of Midbrain
  - Crus cerebri
  - Substantia nigra
  - TS at level of inferior colliculus
    - Nucleus of inferior colliculus
    - Trochlear nucleus
    - Trigeminal mesencephalic nucleus
    - Reticular nuclei
    - Superior cerebellar peduncle
    - Trigeminal, medial and spinal lemnisci
  - TS at superior collicular level
    - Red nucleus
    - Oculomotor nucleus
    - Mesencephalic nucleus of trigeminal nerve
    - Superior colliculus
    - Pretectal area
    - Fibre bundles from white matter
- Arterial Supply of Midbrain
- Midbrain Lesions due to Vascular Insufficiency
  - Weber's syndrome (superior alternating hemiplegia)
  - Benedict's (paramedian midbrain) syndrome
  - Claude's syndrome
  - Parinaud's syndrome
- Blockage of Cerebral Aqueduct

DEVELOPMENT OF MIDBRAIN

Midbrain, also called **mesencephalon**, is the region of the **developing** vertebrate brain that is composed of the tectum and tegmentum. The **midbrain** serves important functions in motor movement, particularly movements of the eye, and in auditory and visual processing. A deep furrow, the **rhombencephalic isthmus**, separates the mesencephalon from the rhombencephalon. The mesencephalon has basal efferent (motor) and alar afferent (sensory) plates (Fig. 9.1A). The mesencephalon's alar plates form the anterior and posterior colliculi as relay stations or visual and auditory reflex centres, respectively. Also form red nucleus and substantia nigra (Fig. 9.1B).

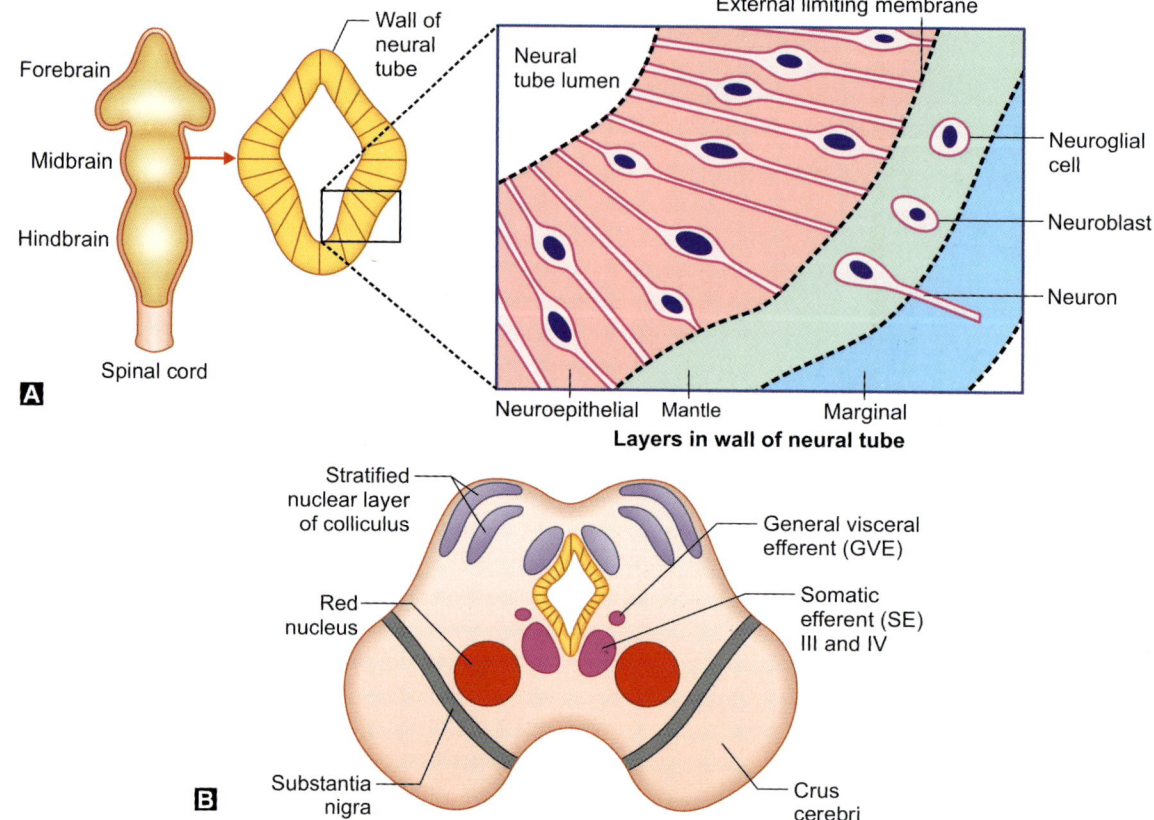

Fig. 9.1: A. The mesencephalon develops from both basal efferent (motor) and alar afferent (sensory) plates, **B.** also during development are formed red nucleus and substantia nigra

Only the two serving the oculomotor (III cranial) nerve arise from the mesencephalic neuroblast; The somatic motor III nerve nucleus (Fig. 9.2) controls the movements of all but the superior oblique and lateral rectus extrinsic ocular muscles. The GVE (general visceral efferent) Edinger-Westphal nucleus supplies parasympathetic pathways to the pupillary constrictor and the ciliary muscles of the eye globe.

EXTERNAL FEATURES OF MIDBRAIN

The midbrain is about 2 cm long, passes through the tentorial notch and connects the hindbrain with the forebrain. It is traversed by the *cerebral aqueduct (of Sylvius)*. The *tectum* (roof), the part of midbrain posterior to the aqueduct, consists of paired superior and inferior colliculi. Anterior to the plane of aqueduct lie the *cerebral peduncles*. Each cerebral peduncle consists of (1) the *crus cerebri* anteriorly, (2) the *substantia nigra* in the middle, and (3) the *tegmentum* posteriorly.

From Ventral Aspect

The *midbrain* on its ventral surface shows *crura cerebri* (singular, *crus cerebri*), which are the masses of white matter that diverge as they pass from the upper border of pons to enter the cerebrum. They enclose the *interpeduncular fossa* whose boundaries and contents are as follows:

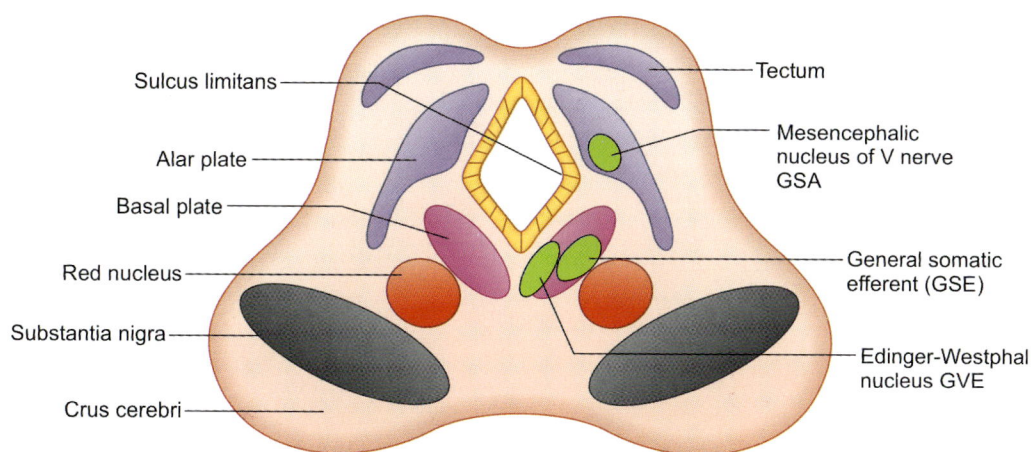

Fig. 9.2: Four cranial nerve nuclei develop during midbrain development: (i) GSA: represented by mesencephalic nucleus of V cranial nerve; (ii) and (iii) GSE: represented by the motor nuclei of III and IV cranial nerves; and (iv) GVE: represented by Edinger-Westphal nucleus, the fibres from which course via the inferior division of III cranial nerve in the orbital cavity

Boundaries

Anteriorly	*Optic chiasma*
On either side	*Optic tract* and *crus cerebri*
Posteriorly	*Upper border of pons*

Contents

Named from before backwards, are constituents of hypothalamus (a part of diencephalon).
- Infundibulum of the hypophysis cerebri
- Tuber cinerium
- Mammillary bodies
- Posterior perforated substance.

The cerebral aqueduct traverses the midbrain and divides it into the *tectum* (dorsally) and the *cerebral peduncles* (ventrally). The periaqueductal grey region of the tegmentum is made up of grey matter (neural tissue with relatively few axons covered in myelin) and surrounds the cerebral aqueduct, a short canal that runs between the third and fourth ventricles of the brain. The periaqueductal grey appears to function primarily in pain suppression, a result of its naturally high concentrations of endorphins.

From Dorsal Aspect

On the dorsal aspect of the midbrain (Fig. 9.3) are seen the 4 colliculi *(corpora quadrigemina)* separated by the *cruciform sulcus*. The tectum (from Latin for 'roof') makes up the rear portion of the midbrain and is formed by two paired rounded swellings, the superior and inferior colliculi. The superior colliculus receives input from the retina and the visual cortex and participates in a variety of visual reflexes, particularly the tracking of objects in the visual field. The inferior colliculus receives both crossed and uncrossed auditory fibres and projects upon the medial geniculate body, the auditory relay nucleus of the thalamus. Between the two superior colliculi lies the *pineal body* and immediately below the inferior colliculi emerge

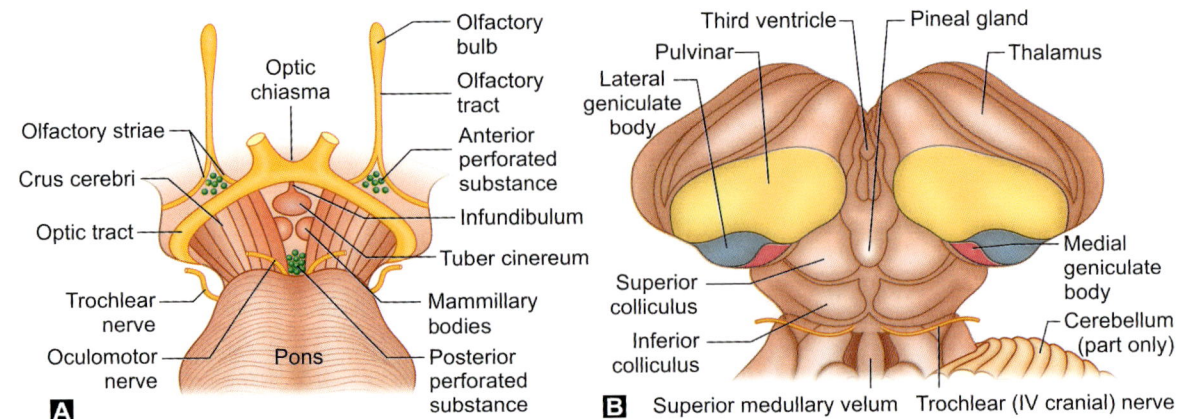

Fig. 9.3: External features of the midbrain seen from the ventral **A.** and dorsal **B.** aspects

the *trochlear nerves* (Fig. 9.3B). Ridges of white matter extending from the lateral side of each colliculus constitute their *brachia*.

The *superior brachium* is a bundle of fibres derived mainly from the optic tract that runs over the posteroinferior surface of the thalamus to reach the superior colliculus. The *inferior brachium* is made up of auditory fibres and extends anterosuperiorly from the inferior colliculus, to the *medial geniculate body* (a part of thalamus).

The tegmentum is located in front of the tectum. It consists of fibre tracts and three regions distinguished by their colour—the red nucleus, the periaqueductal grey, and the substantia nigra. The substantia nigra is a large pigmented cluster of neurons that consists of two parts, the pars reticulata and the pars compacta. Cells of the pars compacta contain the dark pigment melanin; these cells synthesise dopamine and project to either the caudate nucleus or the putamen, both of which are structures of the basal ganglia and are involved in mediating movement and motor coordination.

The red nucleus is a large structure located centrally within the tegmentum that is involved in the coordination of sensorimotor information. Crossed fibres of the superior cerebellar peduncle (the major output system of the cerebellum) surround and partially terminate in the red nucleus. Most crossed ascending fibres of that bundle project to thalamic nuclei, which have access to the primary motor cortex. A smaller number of fibres synapse on large cells in caudal regions of the red nucleus; those give rise to the crossed fibres of the rubrospinal tract, which runs to the spinal cord and is influenced by the motor cortex.

Also within the midbrain are the crus cerebri, tracts made up of neurons that connect the cerebral hemispheres to the cerebellum. The midbrain also contains a portion of the *reticular formation*, a neural network that is involved in arousal and alertness. Cranial nerves in the midbrain that stimulate the muscles controlling eye movement, lens shape, and pupil diameter form the nuclear complex of the oculomotor nerve and the trochlear nucleus.

Each crus is crossed by:

1. The *optic tract* superiorly, where the crus emerges from the cerebrum.

2. The *taenia pontis* (a white ridge) inferiorly, near the upper border of pons.

3 & 4. The *posterior cerebral* and the *superior cerebellar arteries,* also near the upper border of pons.

Laterally the crus is overlapped by the parahippocampal gyrus, is crossed by the trochlear nerve and has the longitudinal *lateral sulcus* under which lie the fibres of the lateral lemniscus. Along the medial aspect of the crus lies the *medial sulcus.* The oculomotor nerve emerges from the medial sulcus.

INTERNAL STRUCTURE OF MIDBRAIN

The crus cerebri and the substantia nigra, present a uniform structure throughout the midbrain. The tegmentum, the central grey matter and the tectum present distinctive features in the upper midbrain (level of the superior colliculus) and the lower midbrain (level of the inferior colliculus).

Crus Cerebri

Each crus cerebri is made up of fibres descending from all parts of the cerebral cortex to the nuclei pontis *(corticopontine fibres)*; and fibre descending from the sensorimotor cortex to the motor nuclei of the cranial nerves *(corticonuclear fibres)* and the spinal cord motor neurons *(corticospinal fibres).* The corticospinal and corticonuclear fibres occupy the intermediate two-thirds of each crus. Of the corticopontine, those arising from the frontal lobe *(frontopontine fibres)* occupy the medial one-sixth, while the fibres from the other lobes *(temporo-, parieto- and occipitopontine) occupy* the lateral one-sixth of the crus cerebri.

Substantia Nigra

It is a curved pigmented lamina of grey matter comprising of melanin containing multipolar neurons. Broader medially than laterally it, extends through the whole midbrain and also extends into the subthalamic region. The substantia nigra has massive reciprocal connections with the basal ganglia and consists of a dorsal *pars compacta* and a ventral *pars reticularis.* The cells in the compact part synthesise dopamine that is carried through their axons into the striatum (putamen and caudate nucleus). Degeneration of these cells causes a deficiency of dopamine in the striatum and produces Parkinson's disease. The reticular part of the substantia nigra has fewer cells some of which are dopaminergic and contain melanin but the majority are GABA-ergic neurons. The latter projects to the ventral anterior and dorsomedial thalamic nuclei. The pars reticularis is continuous superiorly with the internal segment of globus pallidus and is, like-wise, rich in iron.

The cerebral aqueduct, also known as the aqueductus mesencephali, mesencephalic duct, sylvian aqueduct, or aqueduct of Sylvius, is within the mesencephalon (or midbrain), contains cerebrospinal fluid (CSF), and connects the third ventricle in the diencephalon to the fourth ventricle within the region of the mesencephalon and metencephalon, located dorsal to the pons and ventral to the cerebellum.

TS at Inferior Collicular Level

The **grey masses** at this level (Figs 9.4 and 9.5) include the *nucleus of inferior colliculus* in the-tectum, the *nuclei of IV* and *V cranial nerves* in the central grey and the *reticular nuclei* in the tegmentum.

Nucleus of Inferior Colliculus

It is ovoid in form and is covered by a layer of fibres derived from the lateral lemniscus. Many of these fibres terminate in the nucleus and are relayed to the ipsilateral medial geniculate body through the inferior brachium. Other fibres pass to the contralateral medial geniculate

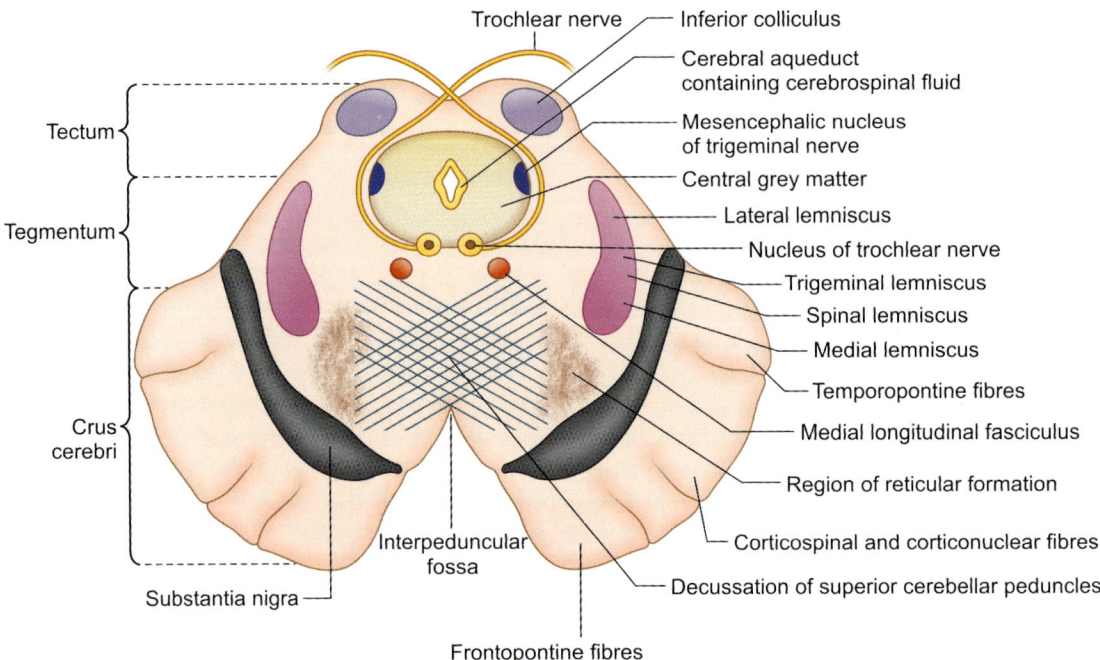

Fig. 9.4: Internal structure of midbrain is seen in a TS at the level of inferior colliculus

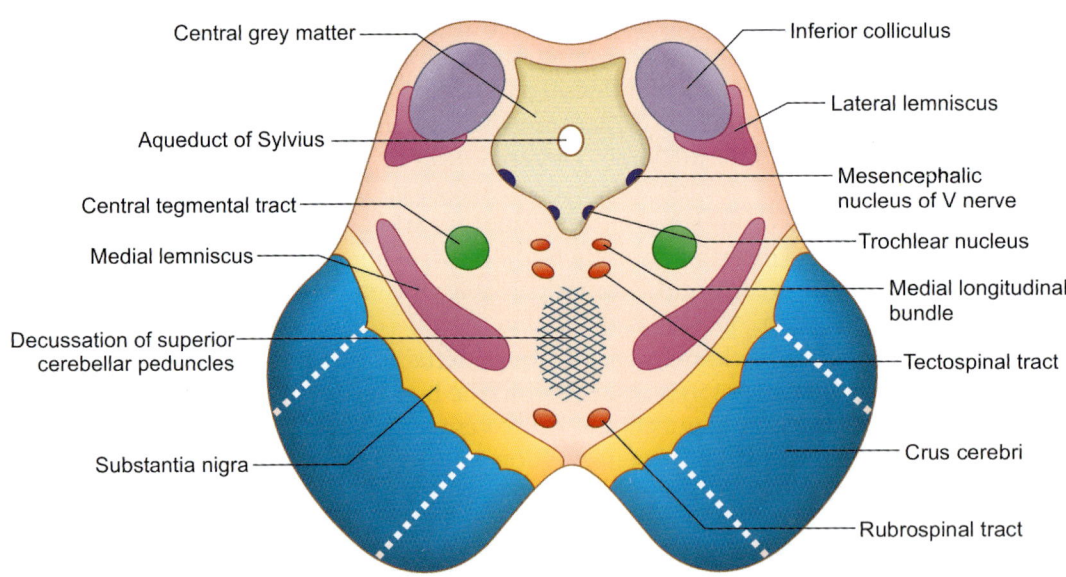

Fig. 9.5: The transverse section of midbrain at the level of inferior colliculus

body, via the *intercollicular commissure*. Projection fibres from the inferior colliculus mediate reflex turning of the eyes and head towards a loud noise *(auditory reflex)*. The impulses pass first to the superior colliculus from which tectotegmental and tectospinal fibres project to the motor cranial nerve nuclei and the spinal motor neurons. The inferior colliculus thus acts as a centre for the auditory reflex. It also helps to localise the source of sound.

Trochlear Nucleus

It lies in the ventral part of the central grey matter, close to the midline and dorsal to the medial longitudinal bundle. Its outgoing fibres pass laterally and dorsally round the central grey matter, turn caudally to decussate in the superior medullary velum and finally emerge on either side of the frenulum veli. The trochlear nerve may have originally supplied muscles of the pineal eye, thus accounting for its dorsal course.

Trigeminal Mesencephalic Nucleus

This nucleus forms a curved lamina of large ovoid unipolar neurons extending through the whole midbrain. It lies laterally in the central grey matter and receives proprioceptive impulses from the masticatory, facial and ocular muscles. The neurons in this nucleus are the only primary sensory somata in the CNS.

Reticular Nuclei

The main reticular nuclei in the midbrain include a laterally placed *pedunculopontine* and medially placed *cuneiform* and *dorsal raphe nuclei.* The latter constitute the mesencephalic pain control centre that sends spinal projections.

 The **white matter** at this level of midbrain has all the tracts of the pontine tegmentum. In addition, it has the decussation of fibres of the superior cerebellar peduncle.

Superior Cerebellar Peduncle

The fibres of superior cerebellar peduncle are essentially derived from the dentate nucleus of cerebellum. They enter the dorsolateral part of the midbrain tegmentum and pass ventromedially to decussate with the fibres of the opposite side. After crossing over, majority of the fibres ascend to the red nucleus and (with or without relay) pass to the ventral lateral nucleus of thalamus. Other fibres descend to terminate in the reticular formation of the pons and medulla oblongata and in the inferior olivary nucleus. The superior cerebellar peduncle also conducts the ventral spinocerebellar tract to the cerebellum.

Trigeminal, Medial and Spinal Lemnisci

These continue upwards from the pons and form a curved band dorsolateral to the substantia nigra. The lateral lemniscus occupies the dorsal edge of this band. Some of its fibres pass into the inferior colliculus to be relayed to the medial geniculate body. Other fibres pass directly to the medial geniculate body through the inferior brachium. The *medial longitudinal fasciculus* lies ventral to the *nucleus of the trochlear nerve* and ventral to it lies the *tectospinal tract.*

TS at Superior Collicular Level

The **grey masses (nuclei)** at this level include the *red nucleus,* the *oculomotor nuclear complex, mesencephalic trigeminal nucleus, superior colliculus* and the *pretectal nucleus* (Figs 9.6 and 9.7).

Red Nucleus

The red nucleus, which is the most prominent feature at this level, is a pinkish ovoid mass of nerve cells (Fig. 9.8). It is about 5 mm in diameter and is situated dorsomedial to the substantia nigra. Its pinkish colour is due to the presence of an iron containing pigment in its multipolar and mostly small sized cells. Larger neurons are few and restricted to its lower levels.

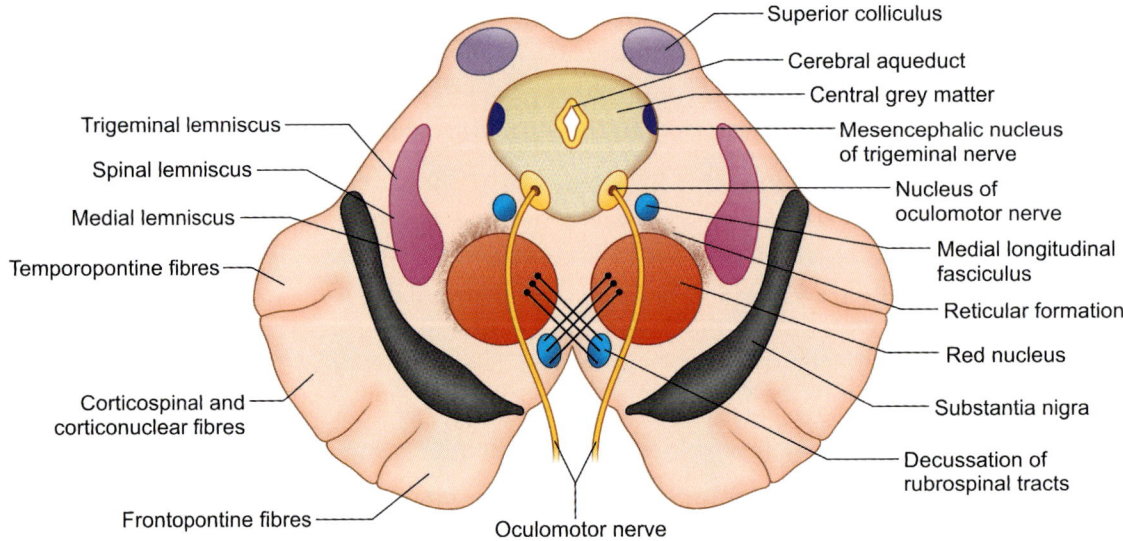

Fig. 9.6: Internal structure of midbrain is seen in a TS at the level of superior colliculus

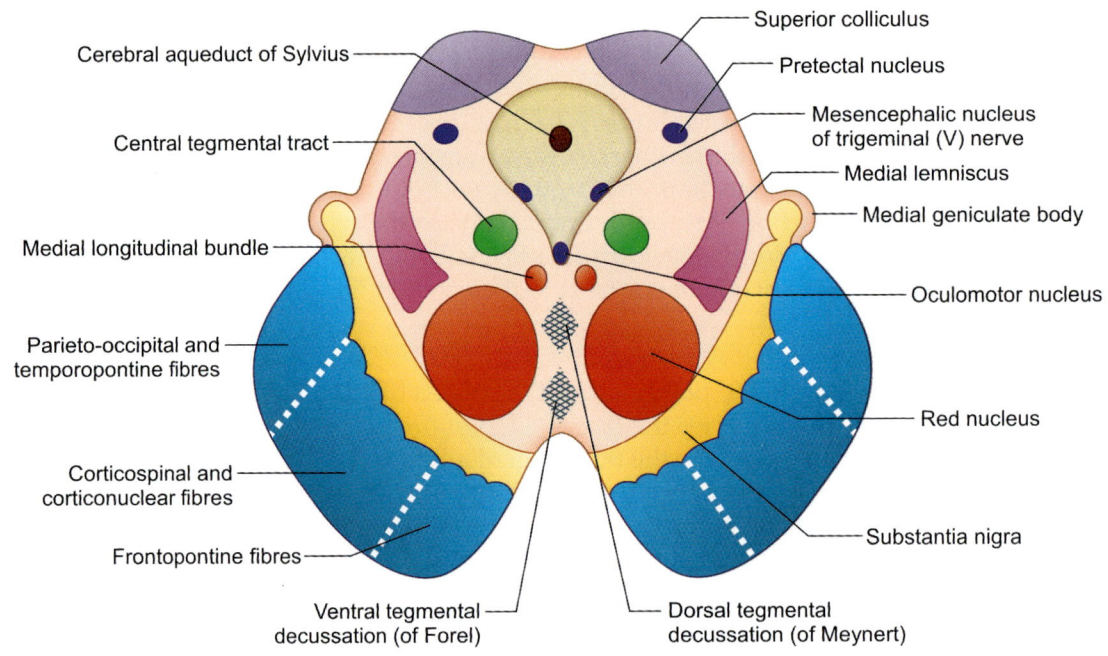

Fig. 9.7: The transverse section of midbrain at the level of superior colliculus

Afferent connections
1. *Corticorubral* fibres from the ipsilateral sensorimotor cortex.
2. *Dentatorubral* fibres from the opposite dentate nucleus.
3. Fibres from the globus pallidus.
4. Fibres from the subthalamic nucleus (Fig. 9.8)

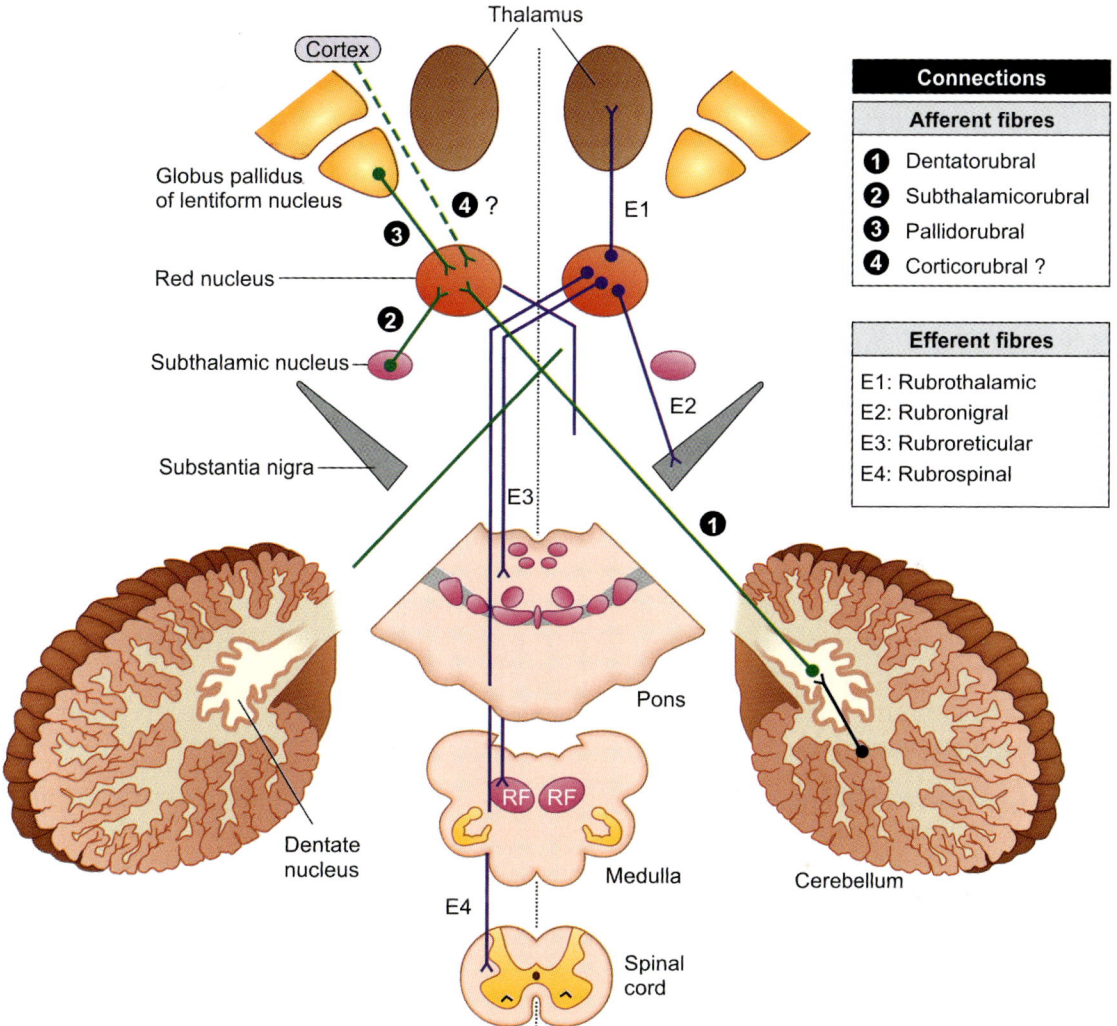

Connections

Afferent fibres
❶ Dentatorubral
❷ Subthalamicorubral
❸ Pallidorubral
❹ Corticorubral ?

Efferent fibres
E1: Rubrothalamic
E2: Rubronigral
E3: Rubroreticular
E4: Rubrospinal

Fig. 9.8: Schematic diagram of connections of the red nucleus: afferents (green line) and efferents (blue lines). Two decussations may be noted in the tegmental area: (i) dorsal tegmental decussation (of Meynert) in blue; and (ii) ventral tegmental decussation (of Forel) in green

Efferent connections
1. *Rubrospinal tract:* These fibres originate from the large neurons in the caudal portion of the red nucleus. The fibres turn medially and decussate in the *ventral tegmental decussation (of Forel).* After crossing over the fibres descend through the brainstem into the lateral funiculus of the spinal cord. The tract is small in man and limited to the upper 2 or 3 cervical segments of the spinal cord.
2. *Rubrothalamic fibres.* These fibres pass to the ventrolateral nucleus of thalamus.
3. Rubronigral fibres to the substantia nigra.
4. *Central tegmental fasciculus.* It constitutes the largest group of efferents from the red nucleus. The fibres project to the inferior olivary nucleus.

Oculomotor Nucleus

The nucleus of oculomotor nerve lies in the ventromedial part of the central grey matter dorsal to medial longitudinal fasciculus. Dorsal to the main nucleus is the *accessory oculomotor nucleus (of Edinger-Westphal)* that is parasympathetic in function and is distributed to the sphincter pupillae and ciliary muscles of the eye. Fibres arising from the oculomotor nuclei pass ventrally, through the red nucleus and the medial part of substantia nigra to emerge through the medial sulcus of crus cerebri.

Mesencephalic Nucleus of Trigeminal Nerve

It occupies the lateral part of central grey matter and presents features already described.

Superior Colliculus

The superior colliculus presents laminar architecture and the following layers, from superficial to deep, are described.
1. The *stratum zonale, which* consists, chiefly, of nerve fibres derived from the occipital cortex (external occipitotectal tract).
2. The *stratum cinereum* (superficial grey layer) forms a crescentic grey lamina and consist of small interneurons.
3. The *stratum opticum* consists of fibres derived from the optic tract. A number of large cells present in this layer send efferent fibres to retina.
4. The *stratum lemnisci* which is subdivided into four layers, i.e. intermediate grey and white, and deep grey and white. The former two are receptive layers, the latter two give efferents.

Afferents to superior colliculus: The superior colliculus receives visual impulses from the retina and occipital cortex; pain, temperature and tactile impulses from the spinal cord and auditory impulses from the inferior colliculus.

Efferents from superior colliculus: Efferents from the superior colliculus pass to the pluvinal, several brainstem nuclei and the spinal cord. Fibres to the pluvinal are relayed to the occipital cortex forming an *extrageniculate retinocortical pathway* for visual orientation and attention. Bulk of the efferent fibres, however, descends in the *tectospinal* and *tectobulbar tracts.*

The *tectospinal* and *tectobulbar fibres* arise from the superior colliculi and sweep ventrally and medially to decussate with the fibres of the opposite side in the *dorsal tegmental decussation (of Meynert).* The tectospinal tract, small in humans, descends ventral to the medial longitudinal fasciculus in the brainstem. In the spinal cord it lies in the anterior funiculus. The tectobulbar tract accompanies the tectospinal tract and terminates in the *pretectal area,* the *accessory oculomotor nuclei* and the *paramedian pontine reticular formation (PPRF).* These regions project to the III, IV and VI cranial nerve nuclei, which supply eye muscles.

Functions of superior colliculus
1. *Fixation of eye on an object:* Signals for fixation originate in the visual areas in the occipital cortex and are relayed through the superior colliculus to the nuclei of nerves controlling eye movements. Damage to the colliculus abolishes the capability of eye fixation to an important highlight in the visual field.
2. *Visual reflex:* Superior colliculus receives visual impulses from the retina (of the two sides) as well as the occipital cortex and under their influence it can bring about reflex turning of the eyes and head towards the source of stimulus and to follow an object moving across the

field of vision. Since auditory as well as general sensory signals also reach the superior colliculus these stimuli too can evoke such a reflex response.

Pretectal Area

It is a poorly defined region of neuronal masses lying at the junction of midbrain and diencephalon and extending caudally to the superior colliculus. It receives fibres from the occipital cortex and the optic tract through the superior brachium and sends efferent fibres to the Edinger-Westphal nucleus of the same as well as of the opposite side. The constriction of pupil in response to light *(pupillary light reflex)* is mediated through this pathway. Because of bilateral connections, pupil constricts on the same *(direct light reflex)* as well as the opposite side *(consensual light reflex)*. The fixation of eye at an object *(fixation reflex)* and adaptation of the eyes for near vision *(accommodation reflex)* are also mediated through the pretectal nucleus. Accommodation includes eye convergence, lens thickening and pupillary constriction.

Fibre Bundle from White Matter

The white matter at the superior collicular level of midbrain consists of a number of longitudinal fibre bundles (Fig. 9.9). These include the *medial* and *dorsal longitudinal fasciculi,* and the *central tegmental fasciculus* described below.

The medial longitudinal fasciculus: It is a heavily myelinated fibre bundle situated close to the midline, immediately ventral to the somatic motor nuclei of the cranial nerves 3, 4, 6 and 12. Cranially the fasciculus extends to the *interstitial nucleus of Cajal,* which lies close to the cranial opening of the cerebral aqueduct. The bundle is connected to the motor ocular nuclei, to the vestibular and reticular nuclei, nucleus of lateral lemniscus, and to the spinal nucleus of

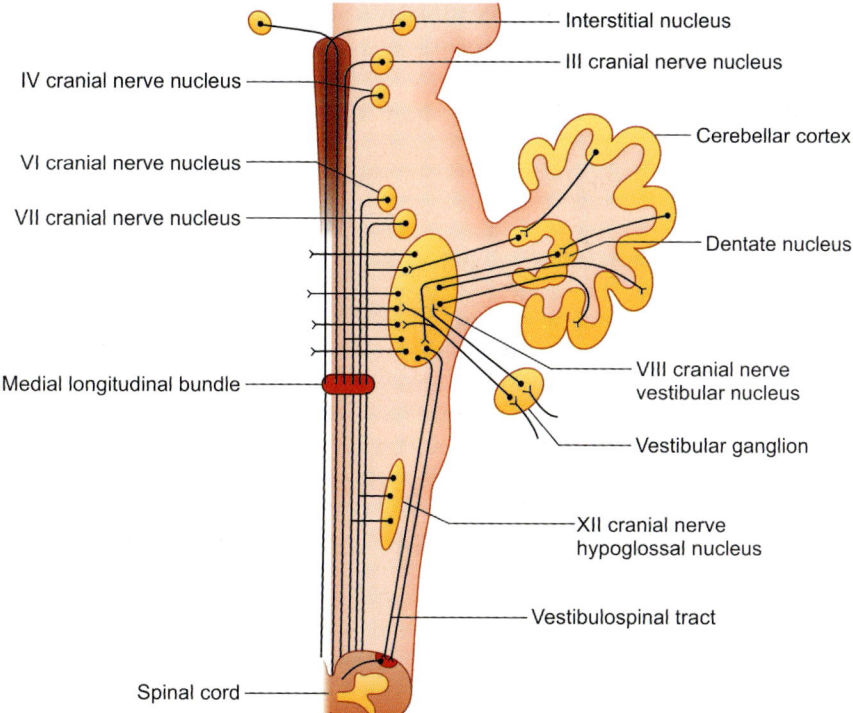

Fig. 9.9: Constituent fibres of the medial longitudinal bundle

the XI nerve. The principal contribution to the bundle is from vestibular nuclei of the same as well as of the opposite side.

The bundle appears to ensure coordinated movements of the eyes and head in response to the stimulation of the vestibulocochlear nerve. Lesions of the bundle are associated with *internuclear ophthalmoplegia.*

Dorsal longitudinal fasciculus (of Schütz): This unmyelinated fasciculus runs in the central grey matter of midbrain, pons and medulla. It consists of fibres descending from the hypothalamus notably from the paraventricular nucleus to the brainstem reticular nuclei, dorsal nucleus of vagus and to the autonomic neurons in the spinal cord. It conducts hypothalamic impulses' to the preganglionic sympathetic and parasympathetic neurons.

Central tegmental fasciculus (of Forel): This fasciculus consists of fibres descending from the motor cortex and the lentiform nucleus. The parvocellular part of red nucleus, contributes heavily to this uncrossed fasciculus as it traverses the nucleus on its way to the inferior olivary nucleus and the brainstem reticular formation.

The *medial lemniscus* (along with the spinal and the trigeminal lemnisci) occupies a more lateral position at this level. It forms a curved band dorsilateral to the red nucleus.

ARTERIAL SUPPLY OF MIDBRAIN

The midbrain is supplied: (i) mainly from basilar system by the posterior cerebral, posterior communicating, and anterior choroidal arteries, and (ii) a lesser extent by from branches of the internal carotid artery.

The vessels from the posterior cerebral artery can be divided into medial and lateral groups. The medial vessels supply the inner parts of the midbrain including the oculomotor nucleus. The lateral vessels supply lateral portions of the crus and the tegmentum.

> **Applied Anatomy of Midbrain**
>
> Vascular lesions involving the medial vessels produce a peculiar type of crossed paralysis involving the oculomotor nerve on the same side and hemiplegia on the opposite side *(Weber's syndrome).*

MIDBRAIN LESIONS DUE TO VASCULAR INSUFFICIENCY

The midbrain syndromes (significant overlap between these three syndromes) (Table 9.1).

Blockage of Cerebral Aqueduct

Blockage or stenosis of the cerebral aqueduct (of Sylvius) is a narrowing of the aqueduct which blocks the flow of cerebrospinal fluid (CSF) in the ventricular system. The narrowing can lead to hydrocephalus, specifically as a common cause of congenital and/or **obstructive** hydrocephalus.

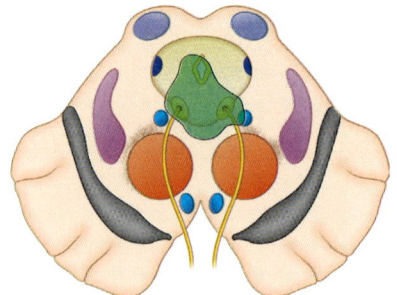

Table 9.1: Midbrain lesions due to vascular insufficiency

Cranial nerve(s)/ Tract(s) involved	Section of midbrain with affected area (in green shaded area) or box in Figure Parinaud's syndrome	Clinical features/remarks
III cranial nerve corticospinal	**Weber's syndrome** 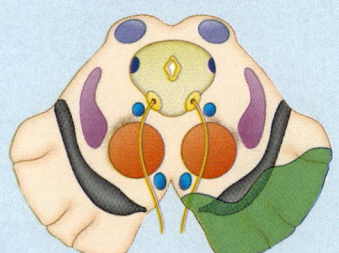	Oculomotor palsy Crossed hemiplegia Condition is also known as superior alternating hemiplegia
III cranial nerve Tegmentum at the level of superior colliculus Affecting 1. Red nucleus 2. Corticospinal tract 3. Brachium conjunctivum	**Benedict's syndrome** 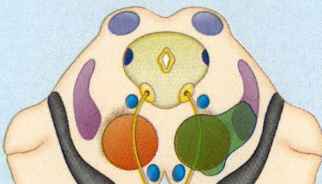	Oculomotor palsy Contralateral cerebellar ataxia Tremors Corticospinal signs Alternative name: Paramedian midbrain syndrome Variant is **Claude's syndrome** presentation almost same: • III nerve palsy • Contralateral hemiplegia • Tremors
III cranial nerve Dorsal midbrain	**Parinaud's syndrome** 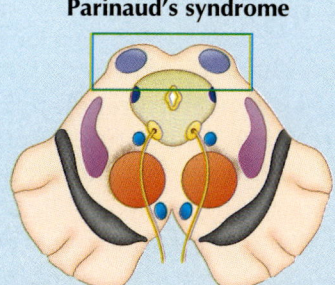	**Supranuclear** mechanism for upward gaze and other structures in periaqueductal grey matter resulting into **paralysis of upward gaze** and **accommodation** with **fixed pupils**

Notice considerable overlap of the affected territories in three syndromes in midbrain vascular lesions

Diencephalon 1
Thalamus, Metathalamus and Epithalamus

INTRODUCTION TO FOREBRAIN

The **forebrain** or **prosencephalon** consists of (Fig. 10.1):

i. The **diencephalon** or **interbrain** or **between brain**—forming the midline rostral most component of the developing brain axis (the future brainstem), about 1.9% of the total brain weight, is a large part of the third ventricle and the structures which surround it.

ii. The **telencephalon** or **endbrain**, consisting of two cerebral hemispheres one on each side constitutes the largest part about 83.0% of the total brain weight.

A curved **forebrain** structure called *hippocampus* is part of the limbic system and is involved in learning and forming new memories. Another **forebrain** structure—*thalamus* processes sensory information for all senses except smell, relaying that information to the cerebral cortex.

DEVELOPMENT OF DIENCEPHALON

The *diencephalon* consists of the thalamus, hypothalamus and epithalamus. The *third ventricle* is the cavity of diencephalon. The *thalamus* above and the *hypothalamus* below form its lateral wall. In its floor lie the *infundibulum* of the hypophysis cerebri, *tuber cinerium* and the *mammillary body*, which are parts of *hypothalamus*. Posteriorly, the third ventricle extends into the stalk of the *pineal body*, which is a part of *epithalamus*. The anterior boundary of the third ventricle is

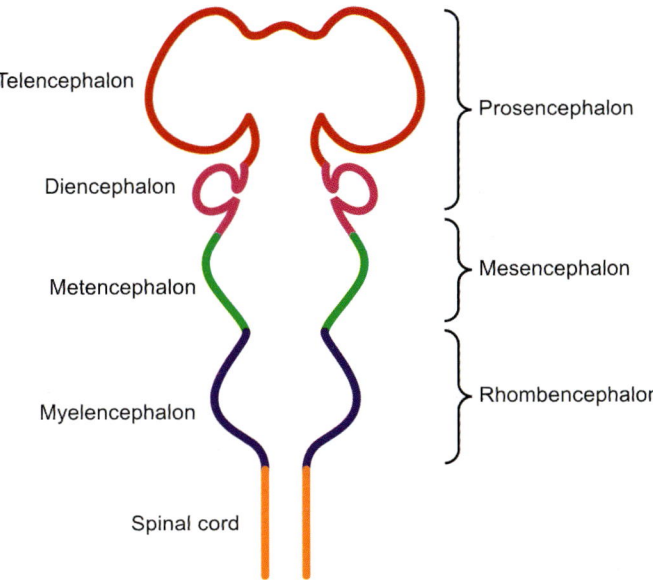

Telencephalon

Diencephalon

Metencephalon

Myelencephalon

Spinal cord

Prosencephalon

Mesencephalon

Rhombencephalon

Fig. 10.1: Diagram depicts the main subdivisions of the embryonic vertebrate brain. These regions will later differentiate into forebrain, midbrain and hindbrain structures

formed by the *lamina terminalis*, a thin sheet of grey matter stretching from the rostrum of corpus callosum to the upper surface of optic chiasma. The third ventricle communicates with the lateral ventricles through the *interventricular foramina* (of Monro). Caudally, it communicates with the fourth ventricle through the *cerebral aqueduct* (of Sylvius).

PARTS AND FUNCTIONS OF DIENCEPHALON

The diencephalon, (*inter-* or *between brain*) lies between the two cerebral hemispheres and encloses the cavity of third ventricle. It is made up of four main components: (i) the **thalamus** (the dorsal thalamus; including lateral and medial geniculate bodies), (ii) the subthalamus (the ventral thalamus), (iii) the **hypothalamus**—an integral part of the **endocrine system**, with the key function of linking the **nervous system** to the **endocrine system** via the **pituitary gland**, and (iv) the epithalamus (pineal body and habenula). Distinct parts of diencephalon (Fig. 10.2) perform numerous vital functions, from regulating wakefulness to controlling the autonomic nervous system.

These parts of the diencephalon are described in separate chapters in this book. This present chapter includes the **dorsal thalamus** including the metathalamus consisting of two geniculate bodies, and epithalamus.

DORSAL THALAMUS

The thalamus is critically involved in a number of functions including relaying sensory and motor signals to the cerebral cortex and regulating consciousness, sleep, and alertness.

The thalami are a pair of large ovoid masses of grey matter lying on either side of the cavity of third ventricle. These account for about 80% of the total diencephalic mass. Each thalamus is 4 cm long and has two ends (poles) and four surfaces.

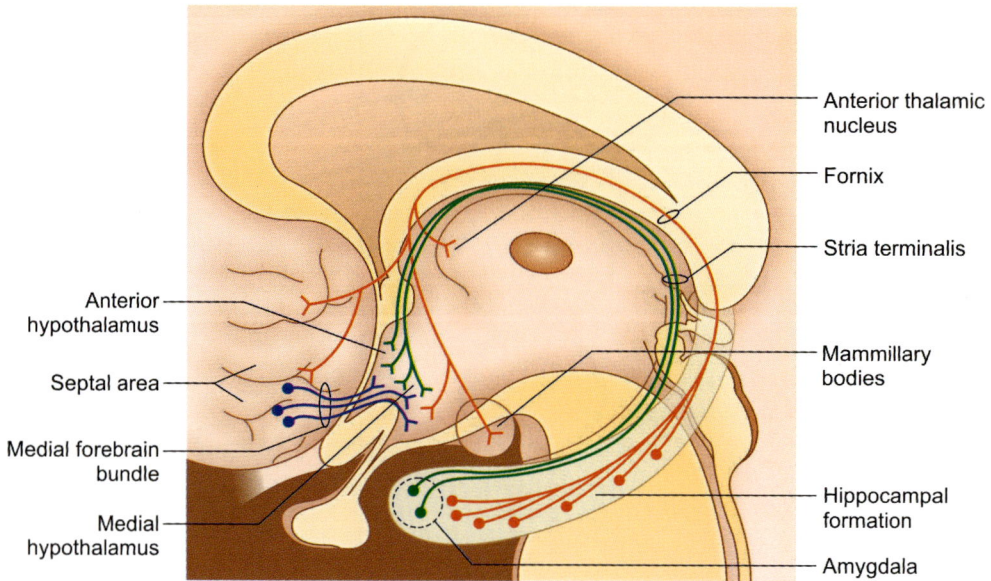

Fig. 10.2: Sagittal section through the diencephalon shows constituents of fornix, hippocampal formation, and other main fibre bundles

The narrow anterior pole of thalamus forms the posterior boundary of the interventricular foramen. The expanded posterior pole called the *pulvinar* is directed dorsolaterally. It lies above and lateral to the superior colliculus.

The superior surface of thalamus is covered by a layer of white matter called the *stratum zonale*. Lateral part of this surface forms the floor of lateral ventricle while its medial part is covered by the fornix. The *taenia thalami,* a ridge of white matter produced by the fibres of the stria medullares thalami runs along the medial edge of this surface.

The medial surface of thalamus forms most of the lateral wall of third ventricle. It is lined by the ventricular ependyma and is joined with the corresponding surface of the opposite thalamus by the *interthalamic adhesion (massa intermedia).*

The lateral surface of thalamus is covered by a layer of white matter called the *external medullary lamina* and is separated from the lentiform nucleus by the posterior limb of internal capsule (Fig. 10.3).

The inferior surface of thalamus rests on the *subthalamus* caudally and the *hypothalamus* rostrally. The rostral parts of the red nucleus, the substantia nigra and the *subthalamic nucleus* occupy the subthalamus.

Parts of Thalamus

The *medullary laminae* of thalamus are layers of myelinated fibres that appear on cross sections of the thalamus. The specific layers are:

- External or *lateral medullary lamina* separating the lateral surface of thalamus from the subthalamus (Chapter 11) and thalamic reticular nucleus covering the lateral surface (Fig. 10.3).
- Internal or *medial medullary lamina*, which is a 'Y'-shaped sheet of white matter, within the substance of the thalamus, which divides the thalamic mass into anterior, medial and lateral parts. The lateral part is the largest out of the three parts. It includes the **pulvinar.**

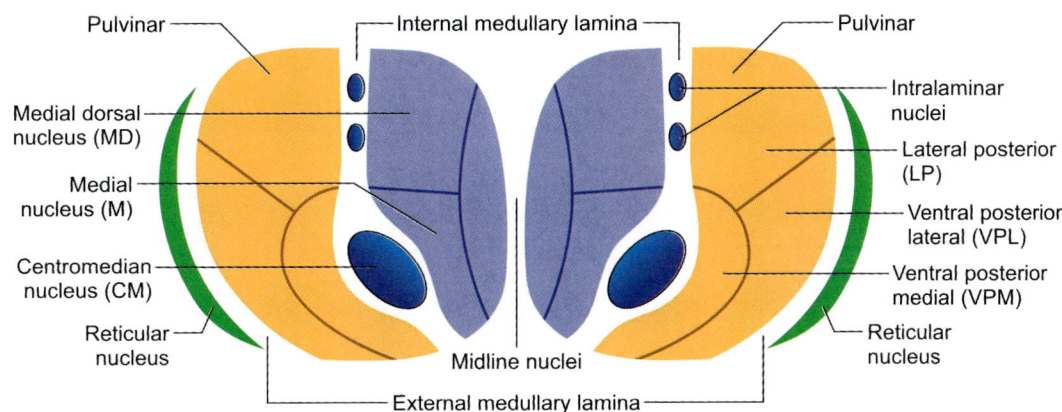

Fig. 10.3: Diagrammatic sketch shows midline, intralaminar, and main nuclei of thalamus. Notice that the reticular nuclei are located outside the external medullary laminae

The lateral part is subdivided into a dorsolateral portion continuous posteriorly with the pulvinar and a ventral portion. Each of these parts contains the corresponding group of the nuclei of thalamus. Nuclei have their specific care also present within the internal medullary lamina *(intralaminar nuclei),* over the lateral surface *(reticular nuclei)* and in the massa intermedia *(midline nuclei).*

Nuclei of Thalamus

The following are the main nuclear groups and their principal constituents.
1. *The anterior group*
   Anteroventral (AV) nucleus
2. *The medial group*
   Mediodorsal (MD) nucleus
3. *Lateral group* (lying in the dorsolateral portion).
   i. Lateral dorsal (LD) nucleus
   ii. Lateral posterior (LP) nucleus
   iii. Pulvinar (PUL)
4. *Ventral group*
   i. Ventral anterior (VA) nucleus
   ii. Ventral lateral (VL) nucleus
   iii. Ventral posterior (VP) nucleus
       a. Ventral posterior lateral (VPL) nucleus
       b. Ventral posterior medial (VPM) nucleus
5. The *medial geniculate bodies*
6. The *lateral geniculate bodies* (earlier included in metathalamus)
7. *Intralaminar nuclei*
   i. Anterior intralaminar nuclei
   ii. Nucleus centrum medianum (CM)
8. *Midline nuclei*
9. **The *reticular nucleus (R)***

With the growth of the cerebral cortex, the mediodorsal nucleus (MD) and the pulvinar have greatly expanded in the human brain.

Connections of Thalamic Nuclei

The thalamus has extensive connections with the cerebral cortex and is the major route for the subcortical impulses on way to the cortex. All cortical connections are reciprocal. The corticothalamic and thalamocortical connections are excitatory at both ends. The indirect route from the cortex through the reticular nucleus is inhibitory and plays a restrictive role. The thalamus is the key structure involved in cognitive and behavioural functions (Table 10.1).

Table 10.1: The thalamic nuclei and their connections

Nuclear groups	Main nuclei	Afferents (tracts from)	Efferents (to)
Anterior	Anteroventral (AV)	Mammillothalamic tract	Cingulate gyrus
Medial	Mediodorsal (MD)	• Primary olfactory area • Amygdaloid body	Prefrontal cortex
Lateral	Lateral dorsal (LD) Lateral posterior (LP)	• Superior colliculus • Cingulate gyrus (post.) • Parietal association area	Bi-directional
	Pulvinar (PLV)	• Association cortices • Retina	Bi-directional Striate area
Ventral	Ventral anterior (VA)	?	?
	Ventral lateral (VL)	• Corpus striatum • Cerebellum • Substantia nigra	• Premotor area • Primary motor area • Frontal lobe
	Ventral posterior medial (VPM)	Trigeminothalamic tract	Somatosensory cortex
	Ventral posterior medial (VPL)	• Medial lemniscus • Spinal lemniscus	Somatosensory cortex
Metathalamic	Medial geniculate body (MGB)	• Lateral lemniscus • Inferior colliculus	Primary acoustic area
	Lateral geniculate body (LGB)	Optic tract	Primary visual area
Intralaminar	Anterior parvocellular group	• Lateral spinothalamic tract • Reticular formation • Superior colliculus	Diffuse cortical projections
	Posterior group centrum medianum	• Corpus striatum • Substantia nigra • Cerebellum	Motor and premotor areas
Midline	Midline nuclei	• Hippocampus • Cingulate gyrus	Bi-directional
Reticular	Reticular nucleus	• All thalamocortical • Corticothalamic	All thalamic nuclei

Anterior Group Nuclei

The anterior nuclei of thalamus form an important link in the following two-way neuronal circuit called **Papez Circuit** from hippocampus to gyrus cinguli and back (Fig. 10.4).

Hippocampus ↔ Fornix Mammillary body ↔ Thalamus (Nucleus AP) ↔ Gyrus cinguli

James Papez (1937) considered this circuit as the principal pathway mediating emotional reactions. Presently, however, the anterior nucleus is considered to be involved in the mediation of attention and encoding of memory. In Korsakoff's psychosis, characterised by loss of recent memory, lesions in the mammillothalamic system are common.

Medial Group Nuclei

The mediodorsal (MD) is the principal nucleus in this group. The nucleus largely projects to the prefrontal cortex, which is the seat of higher mental functions.

Ablation or disease in the nucleus causes changes in personality, motivational drive and intellectual performance. There is indifference to pain. Similar changes are also produced by the ablation of frontal cortex (*prefrontal lobotomy*)—an operation that relieves tension, anxiety, aggression and obsessive thinking.

Lateral Group Nuclei and Pulvinar

These receive subcortical afferents from the superior colliculus and have reciprocal connections with the prefrontal, parietotemporal and occipital association areas (vide infra).

Ventral Group Nuclei

Ventral Anterior Nucleus

Its connections and functions are not known.

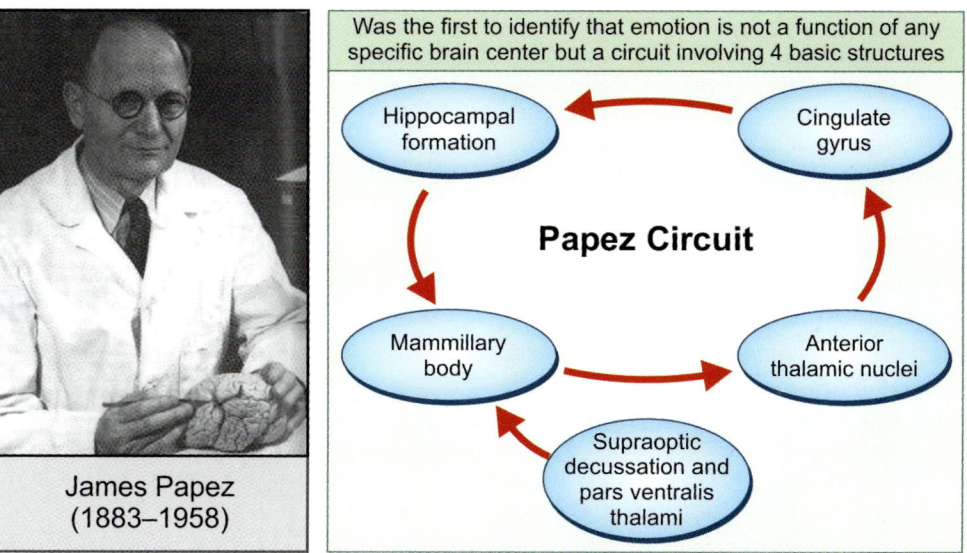

Fig. 10.4: James Papez hypothesised that emotions are not controlled by any specific brain center but a circuit involving four basic structures

Ventral Lateral Nuclear Complex

It has three subdivisions. The *anterior division* receives fibres from the corpus striatum, projects to the premotor and supplementary motor cortices and modulates voluntary movements of the contralateral body. The *posterior division* receives fibres from the deep cerebellar nuclei, has reciprocal connections with the primary motor area and is active during voluntary movements. Its surgical ablation relieves parkinsonian tremors.

The *medial division* receives afferents from the substantia nigra and has diffuse frontal lobe projections.

Ventral Posterior Nuclei (VPL and VPM)

The VPL nucleus of the thalamus receives somatic sensory stimuli from the opposite side of body, carried by the medial lemniscus (touch, pressure vibration and kinesthesis) and the spinal lemniscus (touch, pain and temperature). The trigeminal lemniscus carries all types of somatic sensory impulses from the head region to the VPM nucleus. The VPM also receives taste sensations. Both these nuclei project to the primary somatosensory cortex in the postcentral gyrus (areas 3, 1 and 2) for the conscious appreciation of sensory stimuli.

Intralaminar Nuclei

The intralaminar nuclei consist of anterior group of smaller (parvocellular) nuclei receiving fibres from the lateral spinothalamic tract, reticular formations and the superior colliculus. These nuclei have widespread cortical connections. The posterior group includes the nucleus centrum medianum that receives fibres from the corpus striatum, substantia nigra and the cerebellar nuclei. Efferents pass to the motor and premotor areas. Its damage results in bradykinesia.

Midline Nuclei

These are reciprocally connected with the hippocampal formation and the cingulate gyrus and may play a role in memory and arousal.

Reticular Nucleus

It is a thin curved sheet of large sized cells. It is situated on the lateral aspect of thalamus between the external medullary lamina and the internal capsule. The nucleus is criss-crossed by both thalamocortical and corticothalamic fibres, imparting to it a reticular appearance and providing collateral fibres to the nucleus. Its efferent fibres pass to all the nuclei of thalamus.

Arterial Supply of Thalamus

The following four branches of posterior cerebral artery (Fig. 10.5) supply thalamus
1. Posterior communicating (polar) artery
2. Paramedian thalamic-subthalamic arteries
3. Thalamogeniculate arteries
4. Posterior (medial and lateral) choroidal arteries

1. ***Thalamoperforating arteries:*** Derived from the posteromedial group of central arteries, they supply the anterior and medial parts of thalamus.
2. ***Thalamogeniculate arteries:*** Derived from the posterolateral group of central arteries, they supply the posterolateral part of thalamus.
3. ***Posterior choroidal artery:*** Its branches supply the dorsal part of thalamus.

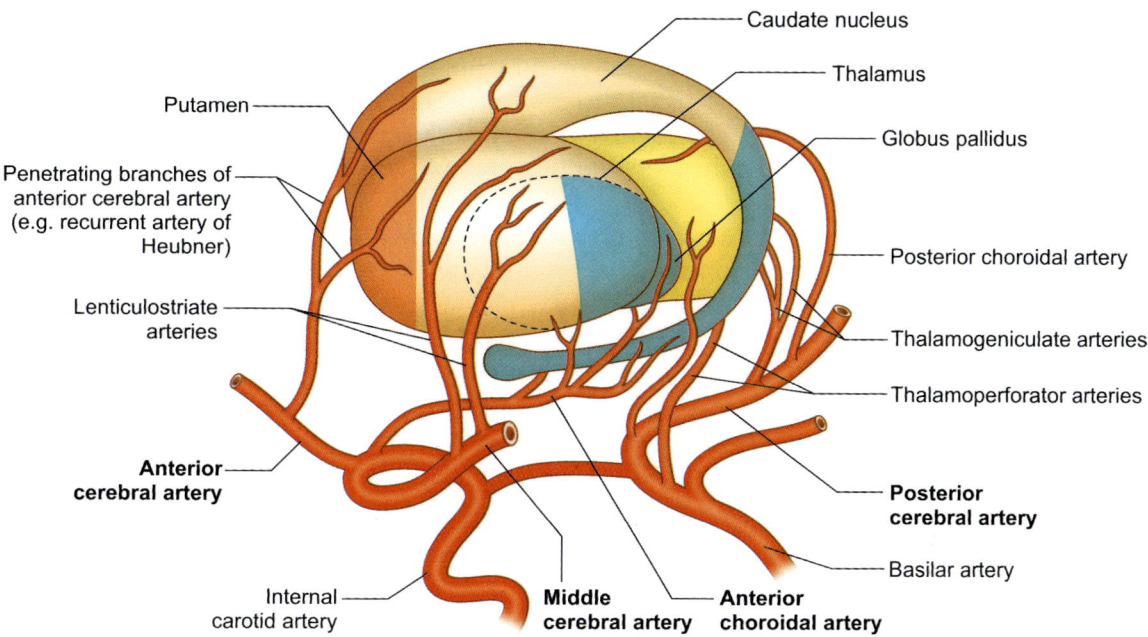

Fig. 10.5: The arteries of thalamus are derived from the posterior cerebral and posterior communicating arteries

Clinical manifestations of thalamic lesions

1. *Disturbances of alertness*

   Sudden bilateral lesions of the thalamus (infarcts) produce somnolence and coma, which are generally transient.
2. *Disturbances of mood and affect*

   There is apathy and lack of drive for motor expression.
3. *Memory disturbances*

   There is loss of recent memory. Storage of new information is affected.
4. *Sensory disturbances*

   a. There is contralateral anaesthesia. The sensory loss is more pronounced on the face and the distal limb.

   b. Thalamic pain.

   It is characterised by excruciating, burning and knife-like pain felt on the side opposite to the infarct. Since the pain from a pinprick is not felt the condition is called *anaesthesia dolorosa* (painful anaesthesia).

METATHALAMUS

The metathalamus consists of two geniculate bodies: Medial and lateral.

Medial Geniculate Body

The medial geniculate body, a relay station on the *auditory pathway*, lies lateral to the superior colliculus. Auditory impulses conducted by the lateral lemniscus ascend to the inferior colliculus and are carried to the medial geniculate body through the inferior brachium with or without relay in the inferior colliculus.

Structurally, it is a mass of nerve cells, which presents a knee-shaped profile in section, and hence its name. Efferent fibres arising from its dorsal aspect constitute the *acoustic radiation*, which passes to the acoustic area 41 in the anterior transverse temporal gyrus. Descending corticogeniculate projections are also described and serve to modulate the centripetal inputs.

Lateral Geniculate Body

The lateral geniculate body (Fig. 10.6) a small ovoid ventral projection from the posterior part of thalamus is a relay station in the *visual pathway*. Anteriorly, it receives the (larger) lateral 'root' (branch) of the optic tract. The medial branch of the tract projecting to the midbrain regions forms the superior brachium. Retinal fibres passing in the medial branch of the optic tract mediate optic reflexes.

Histologically, the lateral geniculate body is made up of six laminae numbered 1 to 6 from the ventral aspect. At the ventral concavity (the *hilum*) the fibres of the optic tract enter. Those from the ipsilateral eye end in the layers 2, 3 and 5 while the crossed fibres from the contralateral eye terminate in the layers 1, 4 and 6. Efferent *geniculocalcarine* (*optic radiation*) fibres emerge dorsally. These pass through the retrolentiform part of internal capsule to terminate in the primary visual area.

The interlaminar zones receive corticothalamic projections from the visual areas and from the superior colliculus.

Applied Significance of Geniculate Bodies

Lesions of the medial geniculate body do not lead to pronounced deafness unless they are bilateral, since both cochlear organs are represented in each lateral lemniscus.

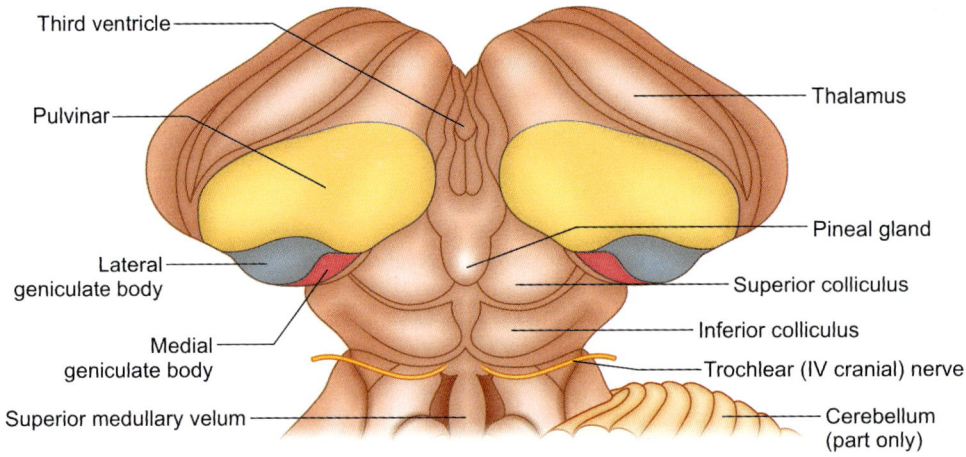

Fig. 10.6: Posterior view of diencephalon and midbrain

EPITHALAMUS

The epithalamus is a posterior segment of the diencephalon (Fig. 10.7). The diencephalon is a part of the forebrain that also contains the thalamus, the hypothalamus and pituitary gland. The epithalamus includes the **habenular complex** comprising: (i) hebenula and their interconnecting fibres the habenular commissure and the stria medullaris thalami, (ii) the pineal gland, and (iii) the posterior commissure.

The epithalamus functions as a connection between the limbic system to other parts of the brain. Some functions of its components include the secretion of melatonin by the pineal gland (involved in circadian rhythms) and regulation of motor pathways and emotions. The epithalamus includes the following structures.

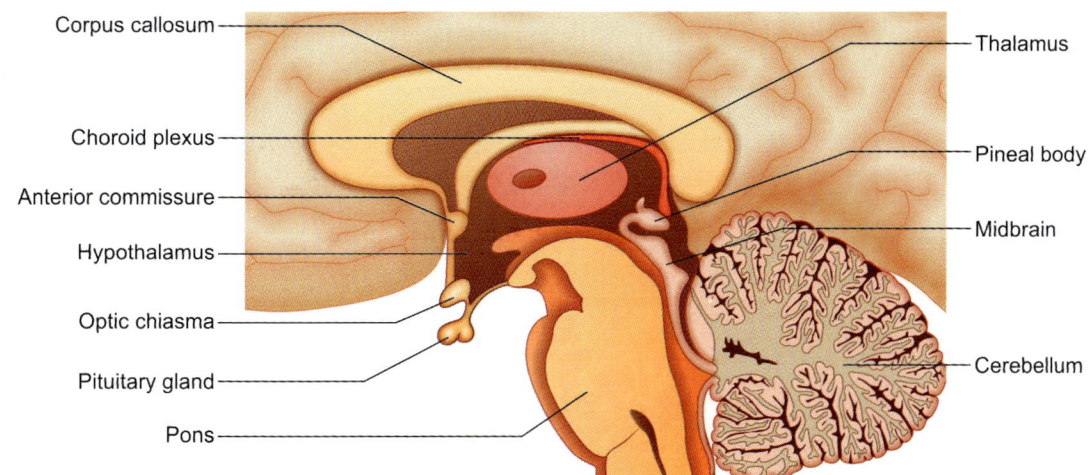

Corpus callosum

Choroid plexus

Anterior commissure

Hypothalamus

Optic chiasma

Pituitary gland

Pons

Thalamus

Pineal body

Midbrain

Cerebellum

Fig. 10.7: Sagittal section of the brain through diencephalon shows the location of the pineal, one of the three structures constituting the epithalamus

Habenular Complex

The habenular complex consists of a pair of the medial and lateral habenular nuclei. Each habenular nucleus is situated under the habenular trigone, a depressed region anterior to the superior colliculus and medial to the pulvinar.

Stria medullaris thalami: Stria medullaris thalami is the principal afferent bundle to the habenular nucleus. Its fibres end in the habenular nucleus of the same side and also crossover to the opposite side in the habenular commissure. The **stria medullaris** is a part of the epithalamus. It is a fiber bundle containing afferent fibers from the septal nuclei, lateral preopticohypothalamic region, and anterior thalamic nuclei to the habenula. It forms a horizontal ridge on the medial surface of the thalamus, and is found on the border between dorsal and medial surfaces of thalamus, superior and lateral to habenular trigone. It projects to the habenular nuclei, from anterior perforated substance and hypothalamus, to habenular trigone, to habenular commissure, to habenular nucleus.

The main outflow from the habenular nucleus (fasciculus retroflexus) passes to the interpeduncular nucleus from where the fibres are relayed to the midbrain reticular formation. Efferent from here control the autonomic centres associated with salivation (superior and inferior salivary nuclei) and those controlling the gastric and intestinal secretions and motility. Motor centres controlling mastication and swallowing are also influenced. Ablation of the habenula produces changes in metabolism, endocrine regulation and thermoregulation.

Pineal Body

The pineal body (gland) or *epiphysis cerebri* is a small (8 mm in length), pear-shaped structure lying below the splenium of corpus callosum and occupying the depression between the two superior colliculi (Fig. 10.8). It is attached to the posterior part of the roof of diencephalon by a short *pineal stalk*.

Microscopic Structure

The pineal body consists in humans of a lobular parenchyma of *pinealocytes* surrounded by connective tissue spaces. The gland's surface is covered by a pial capsule (Fig. 10.9). Four

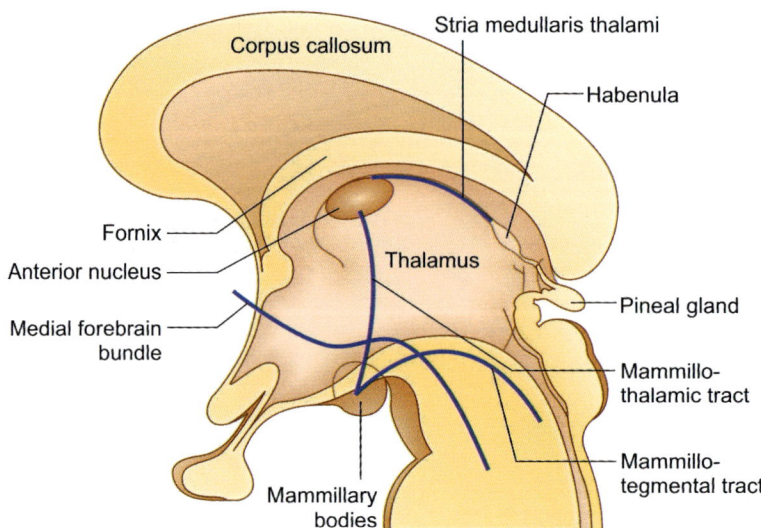

Fig. 10.8: Sagittal section of the brain shows schematic representation of fibre bundles leaving the mammillary body: the mammillothalamic bundle to the anterior group of thalamic nuclei, and mammillotegmental tract descending to the tegmental parts of the midbrain and pons. Also seen is the medial forebrain bundle

other cell types have been identified. Being quite cellular (in relation to the cortex and white matter), the pineal may be mistaken for a neoplasm. Among the cords of pinealocytes and neuroglial cell (astrocytes) ramify blood vessels and noradrenergic nerve fibres. The pinealocytes have one or more processes which end close to blood capillaries in expanded terminal buds. These buds contain vesicles containing monoamines and polypeptide hormones, which can be released directly in the blood capillaries. Fine particles of calcium, the brain sand are deposited in the pineal gland as **basophilic, extracellular concretions** in increasing amount with age (Fig. 10.9). There is, however, no evidence of pineal degeneration in the aged. These concretions due to their high calcium contents make the pineal an excellent radiological marker, particularly of the midline.

The pinealocytes consist of a cell body with 4–6 processes emerging. They produce and secrete melatonin. The pinealocytes can be stained by special silver impregnation methods. Their cytoplasm is lightly basophilic. With special stains, pinealocytes exhibit lengthy, branched cytoplasmic processes that extend to the connective septa and its blood vessels.

Functions of Pineal Body

Once considered to be a vestige of the dorsal third eye the pineal gland is now accepted as an endocrine gland, regulating practically all the other endocrine glands except the thyroid.
- The pineal gland secretes melatonin (an indoleamine) and several other similar substances. The pineal secretions are essentially inhibitory to the synthesis and release of hormones, e.g. from anterior pituitary.
- The synthetic activity in the pineal gland shows a circadian rhythm in a number of mammals. Photic stimuli seem to be involved in this rhythm the pineal being most active during darkness. Exposure to light reduces pineal activity. Neurons of the suprachiasmatic nucleus of hypothalamus, supplied directly by the axons of the retinal nerve cells, mediate these light responses.

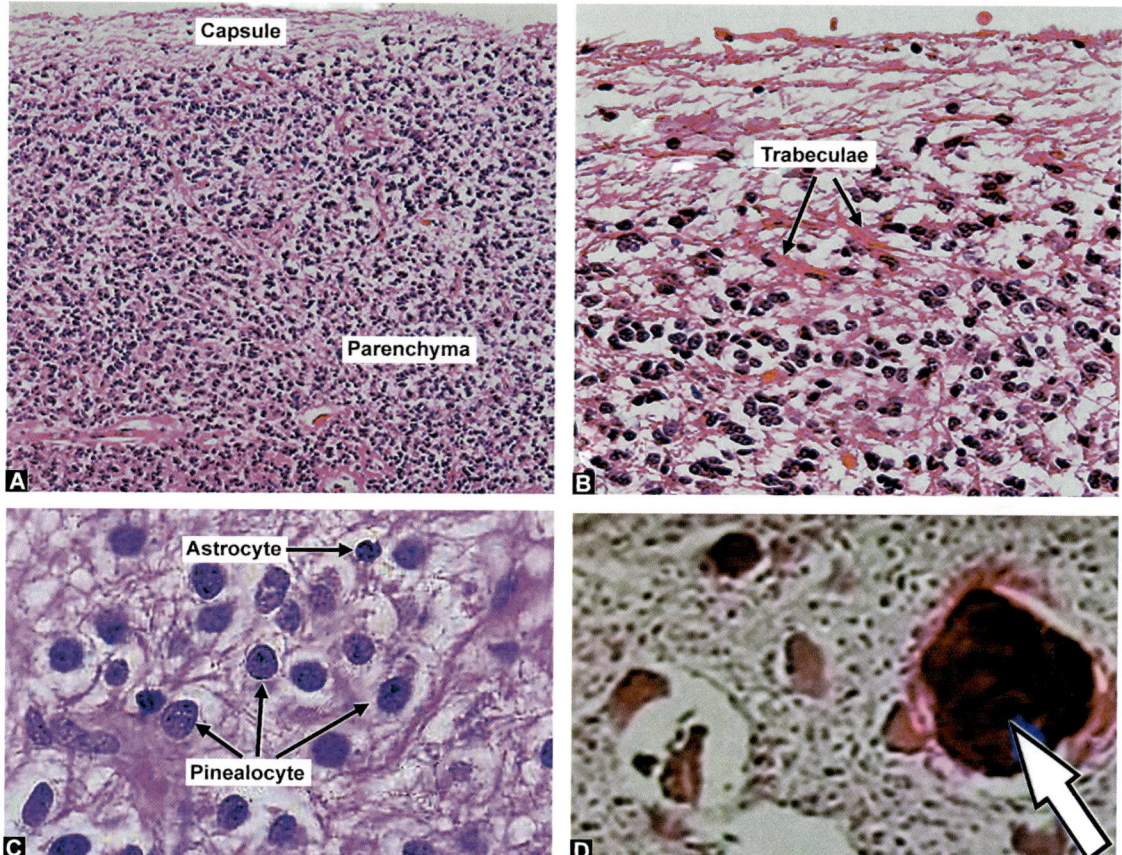

Fig. 10.9: Microscopic structure of the pineal gland: **A.** at medium magnification, **B.** as seen in very high magnification, **C.** pinealocytes are clearly visible at higher magnification, **D.** in old person although no degeneration of pineal is evident–pineal sand calcareous deposits are visible (white arrow)

Blood and Nerve Supply of Pineal Body

The pineal gland receives a profuse blood flow, second only to the kidney, supplied from the choroidal branches of the posterior cerebral artery. The gland receives a sympathetic innervation from the superior cervical ganglion—fibres reaching it through *nervus conarii*. A parasympathetic innervation from the pterygopalatine and otic ganglia is also present. Further, some nerve fibres penetrate into the pineal gland via the pineal stalk (central innervation). Also, neurons in the trigeminal ganglion innervate the gland with nerve fibres containing the neuropeptide PACAP.

Applied anatomy of pineal body

Calcium deposits make the pineal gland radio-opaque and since the gland is normally located in the median plane it serves as an important landmark on an X-ray film of the skull. An expanding lesion on one side of the brain tends to push the pineal gland to the opposite side.

Posterior Commissure

The **posterior commissure** (also known as the **epithalamic commissure**) is a rounded band of white fibres crossing the middle line on the dorsal aspect of the upper end of the **cerebral** aqueduct. The posterior commissure interconnects the pretectal nuclei, mediating the consensual pupillary light reflex, and is, therefore, important in the bilateral pupillary light reflex (Fig. 10.7).

Its fibres acquire their medullary sheaths early but their connections have not been definitively determined. Most of their connections have their origin in a nucleus, the *nucleus of the posterior commissure* (**nucleus of Darkschewitsch**), which lies in the central grey substance of the upper end of the cerebral aqueduct, in front of the oculomotor nucleus. Some are probably derived from the posterior part of the thalamus and from the superior colliculus, whereas others are believed to be continued downward into the medial longitudinal fasciculus.

Diencephalon 2
Hypothalamus and Subthalamus

- Hypothalamus
  - Nuclei of hypothalamus
  - Connections of hypothalamus
- Extrinsic Fibre Bundles
- Intrinsic Fibre Bundles
- Functions of Hypothalamus
- Clinical Manifestations of Hypothalamic Lesions
- Subthalamus or Ventral Thalamus
  - Nuclei of subthalamus
- Fibre Connections of Subthalamic Nucleus
  - Clinical aspect of subthalamus

HYPOTHALAMUS

The hypothalamus lies below and in front of the thalamus, and it is the primary regulator of homeostasis, and autonomic and endocrine functions. It occupies the floor and lateral wall of third ventricle and extends from the lamina terminalis to the posterior limit of the mammillary bodies (Fig. 11.1). The externally visible parts of hypothalamus include: the median eminence, tuber cinereum, infundibulum and the mammillary bodies.

Nuclei of Hypothalamus

A number of nuclei have been identified in the hypothalamus (Figs 11.2 and 11.3). These occupy the periventricular, medial or the lateral hypothalamic zones and have been listed according to their location in the, four, rostrocaudally disposed regions (Table 11.1).

The medial and lateral groups of hypothalamic nuclei are separated by the curving fornix which courses for its termination into the mammillary body. Each group is further divisible into nuclei, which are named from anterior to posterior as follows:

Medial group	Lateral group
Preoptic nucleus	Supraoptic nucleus
Paraventricular nucleus	Lateral nucleus
Dorsomedial nucleus	Tuberomammillary nucleus
Ventromedial nucleus	Lateral tuberal nuclei
Infundibular nucleus	
Posterior nucleus	

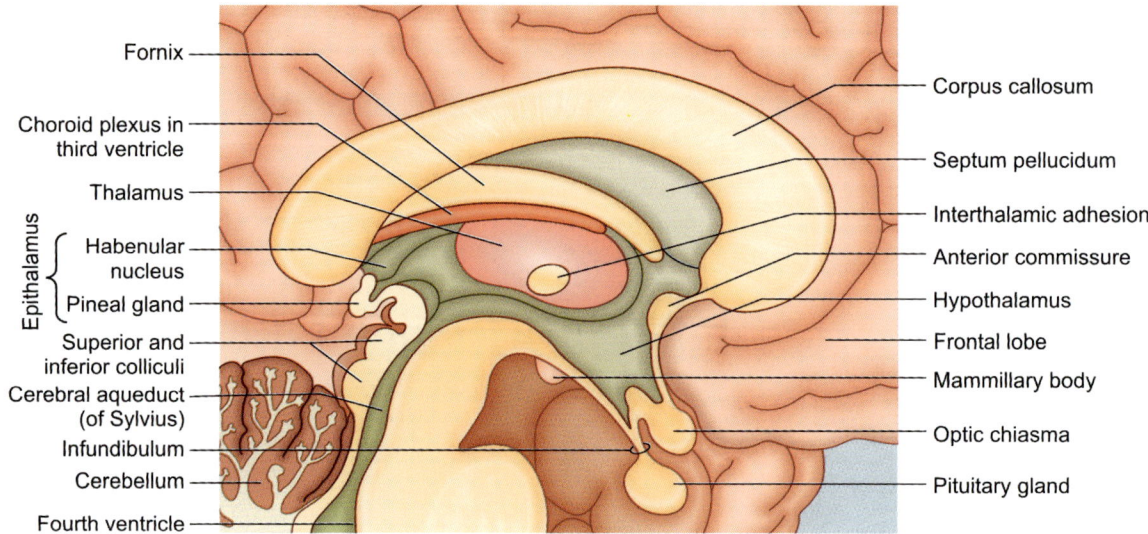

Fig. 11.1: Median sagittal section through diencephalon of the brain showing various subdivisions

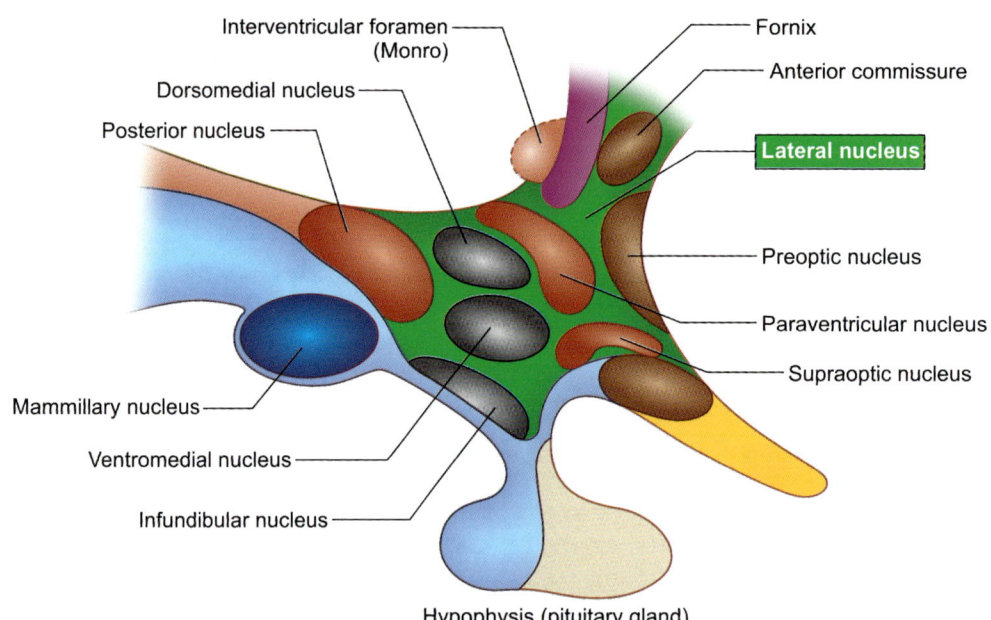

Fig. 11.2: Median sagittal section through hypothalamus showing different nuclei: lateral nucleus in green block and components of medial group of nuclei

Connections of Hypothalamus

The hypothalamus is connected mainly with the following regions of the brain:
1. Piriform (olfactory) cortex.
2. Hippocampus and amygdaloid body (limbic structures).
3. Anterior nucleus of thalamus and the subthalamic nucleus.

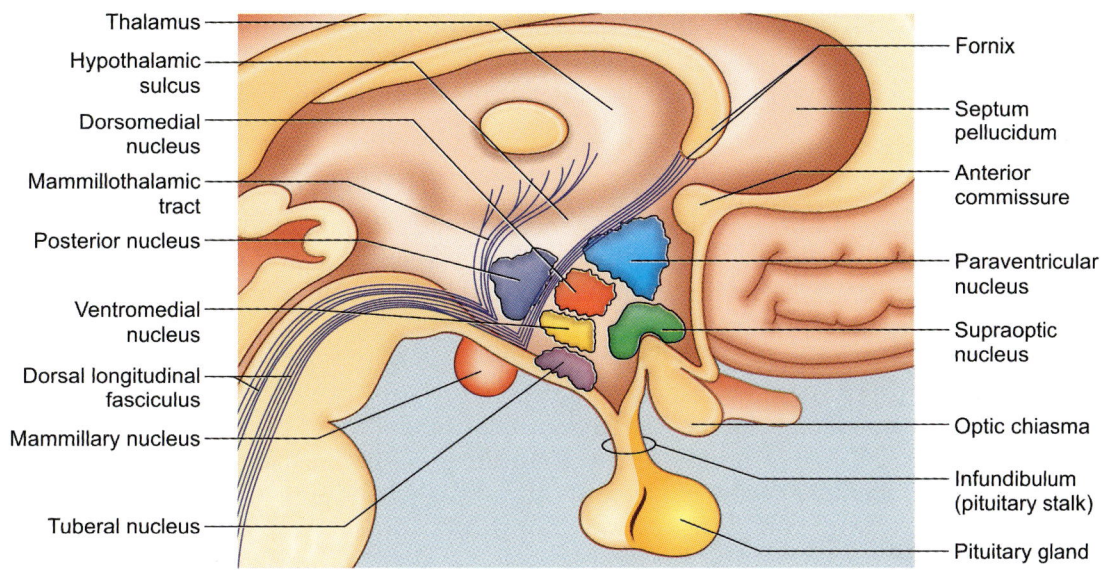

Fig. 11.3: Median sagittal section through hypothalamus showing different nuclei. The lateral nucleus is not shown

Table 11.1: Hypothalamic nuclei and their associated functions			
Regions	*Areas*	*Nuclei*	*Functions*
Preoptic	Anterior hypothalamus	• Preoptic	• Parasympathetic excitation
			• Sleep centre
			• Temperature regulation
Supraoptic		• Suprachiasmaticus	• Circadian rhythm
		• Supraoptic	• Vasopressin and oxytocin secretion
		• Paraventricular	
Tuberal	Lateral hypothalamus	• Dorsomedial	• GI stimulation and satiety centre
		• Ventromedial	• Releasing and release inhibiting
		• Infundibular (arcuate)	hormones hunger and thirst centre
		• Lateral	
		• Tuberal	
Mammillary	Posterior hypothalamus	• Mammillary (medial/lateral)	• Feeding reflexes
		• Posterior	• Sympathetic excitation
			• Wakefulness

- Brainstem reticular formation (through *periventricular fibres* and *mammillary peduncle*) and *autonomic cranial nerve nuclei.*
- *Spinal cord:* Inter-mediolateral column neurons.

EXTRINSIC FIBRE BUNDLES

Fornix

It is a curved thickly myelinated fibre bundle derived from hippocampus and applied to the inferior surface of the trunk of corpus callosum. Anteriorly it leaves the corpus callosum and curving round the anterior end of thalamus courses through the hypothalamus to terminate in the mammillary body. Efferents from the mammillary body pass to the anterior nucleus of thalamus (*mammillothalamic tract*) and the reticular nuclei of the midbrain (*mammillotegmental tract*).

Stria Terminalis

It is a curved bundle of fibres, which commences, in the amygdaloid body. It courses along the medial side of the caudate nucleus in the roof of inferior horn and the floor of the central part of lateral ventricle. Near the anterior pole of thalamus the bundle breaks up into several strands in the anterior hypothalamus.

Stria Medullaris Thalami

It forms a white ridge along the medial edge of the upper surface of thalamus. Its fibres are derived from the fornix, stria terminalis and from the preoptic nucleus of hypothalamus. The fibres end in the habenular nuclei of the same and the opposite side.

Dorsal Longitudinal Fasciculus (of Schütz)

Periventricular in position fibres connect the hypothalamus with the nuclei in the reticular formation of the brainstem and run in either direction. Its fibres originate from the paraventricular nucleus and end in relation with the autonomic cranial nerve nuclei (e.g. dorsal nucleus of vagus) and the nerve cells in the intermediolateral cell column of the spinal cord.

Medial Forebrain Bundle

This loose fibre bundle runs through the lateral hypothalamic area and includes fibres descending from the piriform cortex and the septal area. The fibres end in various hypothalamic nuclei and in the raphe nuclei of the midbrain and pons. It also contains fibres ascending to the hypothalamus from the locus coeruleus and the midbrain tegmentum. Hypothalamic efferents to autonomic nuclei in the brainstem and the spinal cord descend in it. It is a pathway for the visceral control.

Mammillary Peduncle

It is a visceral afferent fibre bundle connecting midbrain reticular formation with the mammillary body.

INTRINSIC FIBRE BUNDLES

These include:
  i. Supraoptico-hypophyseal tract from the supraoptic and paraventricular nuclei.
 ii. Paraventricular nuclei (anterior and posterior) to the posterior pituitary.
iii. Tubero-infundibular tract extending from the infundibular nucleus to end on the capillary loops of the median eminence.

FUNCTIONS OF HYPOTHALAMUS

Autonomic Control

Generally speaking, the anterior hypothalamus (preoptic region) controls the parasympathetic system while the posterior hypothalamus exercises a sympathetic control.

Regulation of Body Temperature

Regulation of body temperature is another important function of the preoptic region of the hypothalamus where heat sensitive neurons are located. The rising temperature of the arterial blood, passing through this highly vascular region stimulates these neurons, which bring about heat loss through vasodilatation and sweating. A fall in body temperature, on the other hand, decreases the activity in these neurons. Heat preserving mechanisms (peripheral vasoconstriction, piloerection) and heat generating mechanisms (shivering and increased metabolism) are initiated. Existence of an *antidrop region,* in the caudal hypothalamus is denied.

Endocrine Functions

The hypothalamus is actively involved in the secretion and release of hormones from the pituitary body. The supraoptic region is associated with the posterior pituitary while the more posteriorly located tuberal regions control the release of hormones from the anterior pituitary.

Hypothalamus and the Posterior Pituitary

The hormones ADH or vasopressin and oxytocin are secreted by the supraoptic nucleus and the large celled part of the paraventricular nucleus. The hormones are carried through axonal transport to be released on the capillaries of the posterior lobe of pituitary. The ADH regulates body water through the renal tubular reabsorption. Oxytocin causes uterine contractility during childbirth and subsequently, through reflexes initiated by sucking, brings about ejection of milk from the breast.

Hypothalamus and the Anterior Pituitary

The infundibular (arcuate) nucleus and the medial part of paraventricular nucleus produce releasing factors, which control the secretion of hormones from the adenohypophysis. These factors are carried by the tuberoinfundibular tract, and are discharged on the capillary loops in the median eminence. These are then transported through the hypophyseal portal system to a second capillary net in the anterior pituitary. Here they influence the release of anterior pituitary hormones.

Regulation of Food and Water-intake

Lateral and medial hypothalamic zones have opposite actions with regard to eating behaviours. The stimulation of lateral hypothalamic zones *(hunger or feeding centre)* will stimulate eating, while stimulation of the medially placed *satiety* centre (ventromedial nucleus) will cause the animal to eat less. The lateral hypothalamic zones also appear to have a thirst or drinking centre which when stimulated will induce copious drinking. This would restore water balance in conditions of dehydration.

Reproduction and Sexual Behaviour

The hypothalamus controls reproductive functions through the release of oxytocin from the posterior pituitary and the gonadotropic hormones of the anterior pituitary. For the various emotional aspects of the sexual behaviour, a close integration with the limbic system is necessary. Sexual drive can be stimulated from several areas of the hypothalamus especially the most anterior and the most posterior regions.

Biological Clock and Circadian Rhythms

Many functions of the body show a variation in their functional activity over the 24 hours of the day with almost clock-like regularity. Examples of such circadian rhythms include fluctuations of body temperature, sleep and wakefulness, adrenocorticosterone secretion, etc. Many of these activities are influenced by environmental light and are mediated through the suprachiasmatic nucleus (SCN). *Retinosuprachiasmatic* connections have been amply demonstrated and these are involved in the photic regulation of the circadian rhythm. Pineal gland secretion is influenced through the descending central autonomic fibres to T_1 spinal segments. The sympathetic outflow from T_1 innervates structures in the head region including the pineal gland. Loss of neurons in SCN nucleus in ageing and Alzheimer's dementia is often associated with sleep disturbance.

Emotional Behaviour

Emotional reactions in response to the changes in the internal and external environment depend upon an integrated activity of the prefrontal cortex, limbic system and the hypothalamus. Stimulation of lateral hypothalamus makes the animal irritable and produces *rage reactions* even with mild peripheral stimulation. Stimulation of the ventromedial nucleus on the contrary produces tranquillity positive and negative reward centres (*pleasure* and *displeasure centres*) have also been discovered in the hypothalamus. Stimulation of the former, located in the lateral hypothalamus, produces a sense of well-being with an occasional strong erotic content. Conversely, stimulation of the *negative reward centre* (posterior hypothalamus) causes fear and displeasure.

Sleep, Wakefulness, Alertness and Excitement

Stimulation of the regions dorsal to the mammillary body (posterior hypothalamus) excites the reticular activating system and result in wakefulness. Stimulation of the anterior hypothalamus on the other hand induces sleep.

Clinical manifestations of hypothalamic lesions

Common symptoms of hypothalamic dysfunction
- Fatigue
- Temperature dysregulation
- Weight gain
- Changes in sleep
- Pain (mainly in trigger points)
- Mood disorders
- Low libido

Signs of hypothalamic obesity disorder
- Mood disorders
- Continued weight gain (unresponsive to diet and exercise)
- Increased appetite

Hypothalamic lesions may cause either aggressive behavior (patients with lesions involving the ventromedial nuclei) or apathy, somnolence, and hypoactivity (destruction of the mammillary bodies or lesions in the medial posterior hypothalamus).

The *hypothalamus* plays a key role in regulation of endocrine (pituitary function), metabolic (food intake, energy balance, and water metabolism), and nonendocrine (body temperature, sleep/wake cycle) functions. Diseases involving the hypothalamus give rise to variable associations of endocrine, metabolic, neurologic, and other systemic.

The lesions may be categorized into two main groups:
- Common symptoms of hypothalamic dysfunction
- Signs of hypothalamic obesity disorders

Causes of *hypothalamic dysfunction* include genetic diseases neoplastic lesions (e.g., craniopharyngioma) or hematologic system disorders such as *sarcoidosis* and *Langerhans' cell histiocytosis*, traumatic, and post-irradiation brain disorders. Due to the pivotal role of the hypothalamus in regulation of food intake, obesity is a common finding in patients with *hypothalamic disorders* or in those undergoing hypothalamic-pituitary surgery.

SUBTHALAMUS OR VENTRAL THALAMUS

The **subthalamus** is the most ventral part of the diencephalon. It lies below the thalamus and dorsolateral to hypothalamus. The subthalamus continues caudally with the midbrain.

Nuclei of Subthalamus

The **subthalamus** consists of *three* nuclei:
  i. **Subthalamic nucleus** involved with integration of somatic motor function, and is the largest division.
 ii. Upward continuation of the red nucleus.
iii. Upward continuation of the substantia nigra in its posterior part.

These three structures gradually diminish, and disappear behind the mammillary bodies. The last two parts together are included in the subthalamic tegmental region of the brain.

FIBRE CONNECTIONS OF SUBTHALAMIC NUCLEUS

The subthalamic nucleus is a small brownish-coloured, biconvex lens-like grey matter mass and is seen in the coronal sections of the region, dorsolateral to the upper end of the substantia nigra and extends backwards up to the lateral aspect of the red nucleus (Fig. 11.4). A narrow area called the **zona incerta** separates the subthalamic nucleus from the lateral aspect of the thalamus.

Afferent—ansa lenticularis (fibres arising from the globus pallidus part of the lentiform nucleus that enter the dorsal aspect of the subthalamic nucleus).

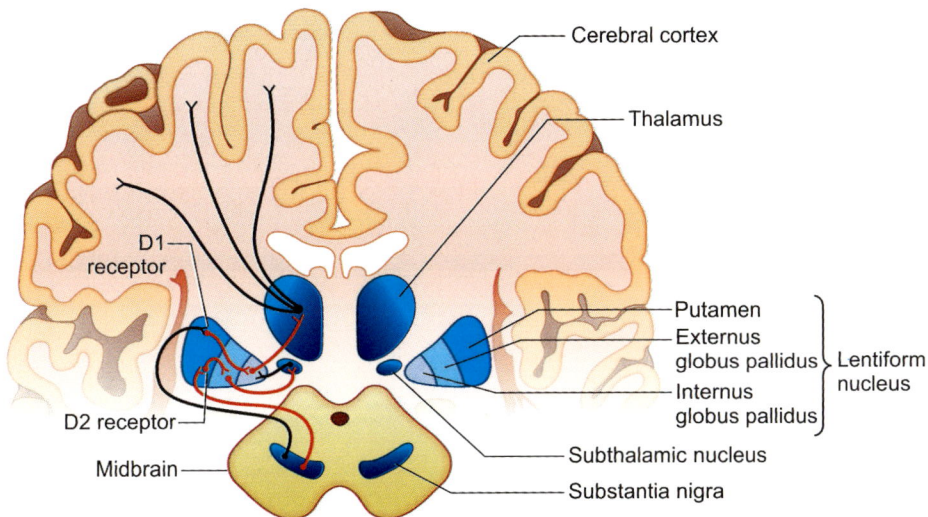

Fig. 11.4: Diagrammatic sketch shows the location of the subthalamic nucleus and its main connections

Efferents—to:
 i. Globus pallidus.
 ii. Red nucleus.
iii. Ventral nucleus of the thalamus.
iv. Reticular formation of the brainstem.

Clinical aspect of subthalamus

The subthalamic nucleus is an important constituent of the extrapyramidal system. Destruction of the subthalamic nucleus is associated with:

- Uncontrolled torsional movements, which are **choreic** in type, and exceedingly violent in character. The chorea (Gr. *choros* = dance) is a disorder of the basal nuclei of the cerebral hemispheres, and is defined *as a random, brisk, uncontrolled purposeless contraction of different muscle groups occurring continuously*. The disorder is characterized by irregular, spasmodic involuntary movements of the limbs or facial muscles, with no normal progression of movement. As an example, the person may perform a normal sequence of movements for a few seconds and the suddenly begins another sequence of movements; then another sequence after a few seconds.
- Electrical stimulation of the subthalamic nucleus causes contraction of the erector spinae and the deep muscles of the back on the opposite side.
- The subthalamic nucleus can be affected by vascular lesions involving posteromedial branches of the posterior cerebral or posterior communicating arteries, which results in a characteristic clinical condition known as **hemiballismus**. Patients with this involuntary movement disorder exhibit rapid and forceful flailing movements, which usually involve the contralateral upper extremity. These movements can be very debilitating because the patient has no control over their initiation or duration.

Diencephalon 3
Third Ventricle and Circumventricular Organs

- Boundaries of Third Ventricle
  - Anterior wall
  - Posterior wall
  - Lateral wall
  - Superior wall or roof
  - Inferior wall or floor
- Communications of Third Ventricle
  - With lateral ventricles
  - With fourth ventricle
- Recesses of Third Ventricle
- Choroid Plexus and Tela Choroidea
- Circumventricular Organs (CVOs)

The third ventricle is the cavity of diencephalon and is lined by ciliated columnar epithelium ependyma. It is a midline slit-like cavity situated between two thalami and part of hypothalamus. It extends from the lamina terminalis anteriorly to the superior end of the cerebral aqueduct of the midbrain posteriorly. The cavity of the third ventricle is traversed horizontally by a mass of grey matter termed—the interthalamic adhesion, joining the two thalami. The outline of the cavity is atypical because of the presence of several diverticula or recesses.

BOUNDARIES OF THIRD VENTRICLE

Anterior Wall

The anterior boundary (Fig. 12.1) is formed by the following:

1. The *lamina terminalis,* which is a grey, sheet extending from the upper surface of optic chiasma to the rostrum of corpus callosum. The *organ vasculosum* of lamina terminalis, the *preoptic nucleus* and the *subfornical organ* are associated with it.

2. The *anterior commissure,* which occupies the upper margin of the lamina terminalis, immediately posterior to its junction with the rostrum *of corpus callosum.*

3. The *anterior columns of fornix,* which descend just behind the anterior commissure curving downwards and backwards and sinking in the lateral walls of third ventricle on their way to the mammillary bodies.

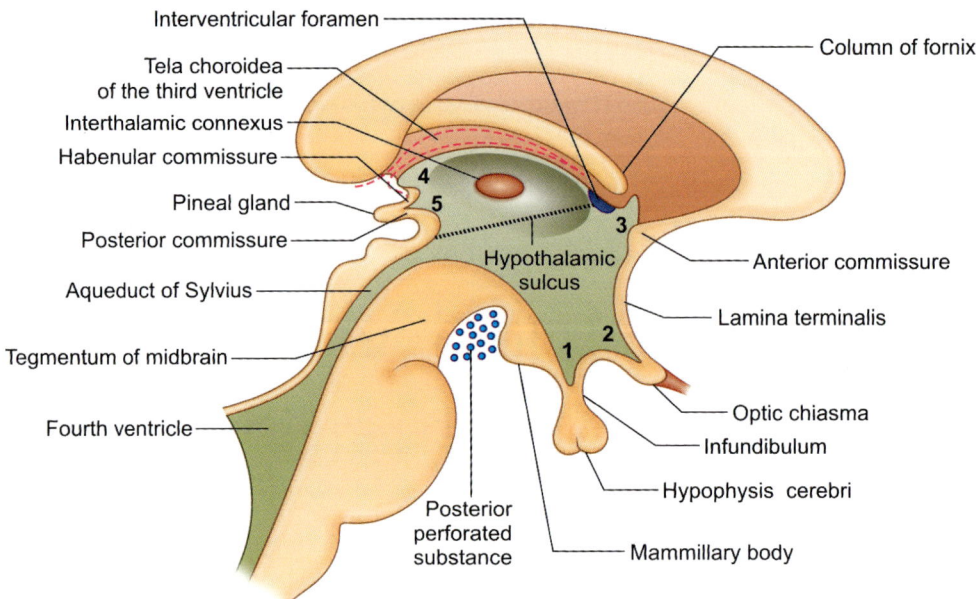

Fig. 12.1: Boundaries and recesses of the third ventricle. **1.** infundibular recess, **2.** optic recess, **3.** anterior recess or vulva, **4.** suprapineal recess, and **5.** pineal recess

Posterior Wall

The posterior boundary is formed from above downward by the following:
1. The *pineal body,* which is attached to the posterior wall of third ventricle by the pineal stalk. The cavity of the ventricle extends into the pineal stalk as the *pineal recess.*
2. The *habenular commissure,* which is formed by the fibres of the striae medullares thalami crossing over and decussating in the upper lamina of the pineal stalk.
3. The *posterior commissure* which is a rounded bundle of transverse fibres crossing within the lower lamina of the pineal stalk, immediately above the upper opening of the cerebral aqueduct. Fibres from a variety of sources including the *interstitial nucleus of Cajal* cross into it.

Lateral Wall

On either side, the lateral wall is formed by the following:
1. Marked by a curved sulcus, the **hypothalamic sulcus** extending from the interventricular foramen (of Monro) to the upper end of the cerebral aqueduct. The sulcus divides the lateral wall into a bigger upper part (thalamic) and a smaller lower part (hypothalamic). The bigger upper part of the lateral wall is composed by the medial surface of the anterior two-thirds of the thalamus. The smaller lower part of the lateral wall is composed by the hypothalamus and it is constant with the ventricular floor.
2. Both lateral walls of the third ventricle are normally closely approximated, for this reason in coronal section of the brain the cavity of the third ventricle appears as a median vertical slit.

Superior Wall or Roof

The roof *(velum interpositum)* is thin and is formed by the ependyma applied to the fold of pia mater forming the *tela choroidea of third ventricle.* The ependyma stretches between the taenia thalami of the two sides. A pair of vascular fringes, the *choroid plexuses* of the third ventricle project down from the roof into the cavity.

Inferior Wall or Floor

The floor of third ventricle is formed by the following structures, from before backwards.
1. Optic chiasma
2. Tuber cinerium
3. Infundibulum of the hypophysis cerebri
4. Mammillary bodies (corpora mammillaria)
5. Posterior perforated substance
6. Tegmentum of midbrain

All structures of the floor belong to interpeduncular fossa with the exception of the optic chiasma and tegmentum of the midbrain.

COMMUNICATIONS OF THIRD VENTRICLE

Anteriorly on every side, the third ventricle interacts with the whole lateral ventricle via interventricular foramen (of Monro) and posteriorly with the fourth ventricle via cerebral aqueduct (of Sylvius).

With Lateral Ventricles

The third ventricle communicates with the lateral ventricles through the *interventricular foramina* present in the anterosuperior part of the cavity, on either side. The foramina are crescentic and are bounded by the columns of the fornix in front and the anterior tubercles of thalami behind. These foramina allow the CSF to pass from the lateral ventricles into the third ventricle. The choroid plexus also passes through the foramina.

A hypertrophy of the choroid plexus can easily block a foramen and obstruct the flow of CSF resulting in an increase in the pressure of CSF and a dilatation of the corresponding lateral ventricle (hydrocephalus).

With Fourth Ventricle

Posteroinferiorly, the third ventricle communicates with the fourth ventricle through the cerebral aqueduct (of Sylvius).

RECESSES OF THIRD VENTRICLE (Fig. 12.1)

- **Infundibular recess:** It is a deep tunnel-shaped recess extending downward via the tuber cinereum into the infundibulum, i.e. the stalk of the pituitary gland. It is an extension of the cavity of third ventricle into the hypophyseal stalk.
- **Optic (or chiasmatic) recess:** It is an angular recess situated in the junction of the anterior wall and the floor of the ventricle just above the optic chiasma.
- **Anterior recess (vulva of the ventricle):** It is a triangular recess which extends anteriorly in front of interventricular foramen and behind anterior commissure between the diverging anterior columns of the fornix.
- *Suprachiasmatic recess.* It is a somewhat large blind diverticulum, which goes posteriorly above the stalk of the pineal gland and below the tela choroidea of the third ventricle.

- **Pineal recess:** It extends into the pineal stalk. It is a small diverticulum which widens posteriorly between the superior and inferior laminae of the stalk of the pineal gland.
- **Suprapineal recess:** It is a reasonably capacious blind diverticulum, which goes posteriorly above the stalk of the pineal gland and below the tela choroidea. It lies above the pineal stalk and is a diverticulum of the epithelial roof of the third ventricle.

CHOROID PLEXUS AND TELA CHOROIDEA

The **tela choroidea** in the roof of the third ventricle is triangular in shape. The **choroid plexus** of the third ventricle is a vascular fringed process which hangs downward from the tela choroidea as two longitudinal anteroposterior vascular peripheries. The third ventricle being a narrow slit-like space is easily obstructed by localized brain tumours or congenital defects. The obstacle results in excessive accumulation of CSF inside the brain, leading to an increased intracranial pressure in adults and in hydrocephalus in youngsters.

CIRCUMVENTRICULAR ORGANS (CVOs)

The circumventricular organs (commonly called CVOs) are structures lining the cavity of the third and fourth ventricle and possess a vascular architecture in which their capillaries have a wall devoid of blood–brain barrier. The CVOs are regions of the brain in which the capillary endothelial cells do not have tight junctions and there is a free flow of macromolecules from the blood into the brain. Most of these areas are situated close to the third ventricle. The ependymal cells in these patches are flattened and non-ciliated. These modified ependymal cells may be involved in transporting materials from the neighbouring nerve terminals and blood capillaries into the CSF. Alternatively, substances may pass from the CSF to blood vessels or deeply placed nerve cells through these regions.

The following CVOs (Fig. 12.2) are well-recognised in relation to the third ventricle (median CVOs).

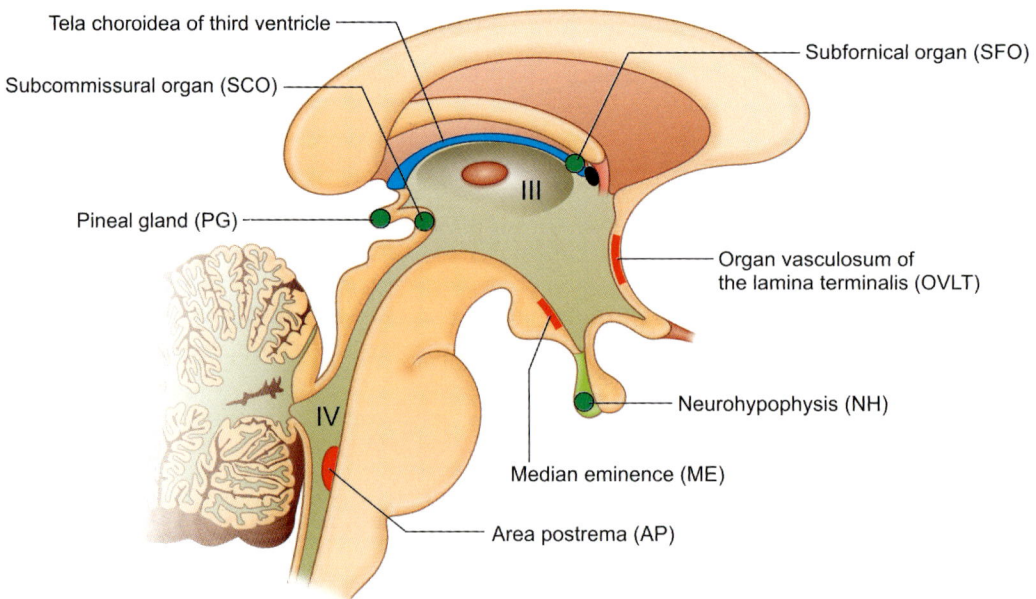

Fig. 12.2: Location of CVO described in text is shown schematically

The organum vasculosum of the lamina terminalis (OVLT), pineal (P), subcommissural organ (SCO), and subfornical organ (SFO), median eminence (ME), neurohypophysis (N) are in the midline and referred to as median CVOs. The only CVO—**area** postrema (AP) is located bilaterally in the floor of the fourth ventricle. It lacks the blood–brain barrier.

1. Organ vasculosum of the lamina terminalis (OVLT)—has been implicated in mechanisms of fever and also in the regulation of sodium metabolism.
2. Subcommissural organ (SCO).
3. Subfornical organ (SOF)—organ is a small eminence on the medial side of the column of fornix above the interventricular foramen. It responds to circulating levels of angiotensin II.
4. Median eminence (ME).
5. Infundibular recess (IR).
6. Pineal body.

The subfornical organ, vascular organ of the lamina terminalis (OVLT), area postrema, median eminence, neurohypophysis, subcommissural organ, pineal gland, and choroid plexus comprise the circumventricular organs of the human brain. All but the subcommissural organ lack a blood–brain barrier and are exposed to the general systemic extracellular fluid environment. Only the subfornical organ, OVLT, and area postrema contain neuronal cell bodies and these have both efferent and afferent neural connections with several other sites in the CNS that mediate homeostatic functions. The median eminence and neurohypophysis are sites of axonal neurosecretion of hormones into the bloodstream, while melatonin is released by the pineal and the choroid plexus is the site of cerebrospinal fluid production.

13

Telencephalon 1
Convolutions and Functional Cortical Areas

- Gross Features of Cerebral Hemispheres
  - Lobes of cerebral hemisphere
  - Surfaces and borders including convolutions
  - Types of sulci
- Cortical Areas
  - Functional cortical areas
    - Motor areas
    - Somatosensory areas
- Special Sensory Areas
  - Olfactory areas
  - Taste areas
  - Visual areas
  - Acoustic areas
- Association Areas
- Structure of Cerebral Cortex
  - General features of cerebral cortex
  - Microscopic structure of cerebral cortex

The brain consists of *three* main parts different in their size and weight in proportion to the total brain weight (98.0%; 2.0% is the weight of spinal cord). These parts are: (i) **cerebral hemispheres** (83.0%), (ii) **cerebellum** or **small brain** (10.5%), and (iii) **brainstem** (2.6%)—comprising the midbrain (0.8%), pons (1.3%), and medulla oblongata (0.5%). The **cerebral hemispheres** make us human. They include the **cerebral cortex**, the underlying **cerebral** white matter, and a complex of deep grey matter masses, the *basal ganglia* (Fig. 13.1).

GROSS FEATURES OF CEREBRAL HEMISPHERES

The *cerebral* hemispheres are two in number, but none has a hemispherical outline. Instead each so-called cerebral hemisphere is only quarter of a sphere, and is characterised by the highly convoluted external surface. The **convolutions** are termed *gyri* (singular, *gyrus*) that are separated by *fissures* and/or *grooves* called *sulci* (singular, *sulcus*). In anatomy, a **fissure** (plural *fissurae*) is a groove, natural division, deep furrow, elongated cleft, or tear in various parts of the body also generally called a sulcus, or in the brain a sulcus. A grey matter layer termed the cerebral cortex is covering the cerebral hemispheres.

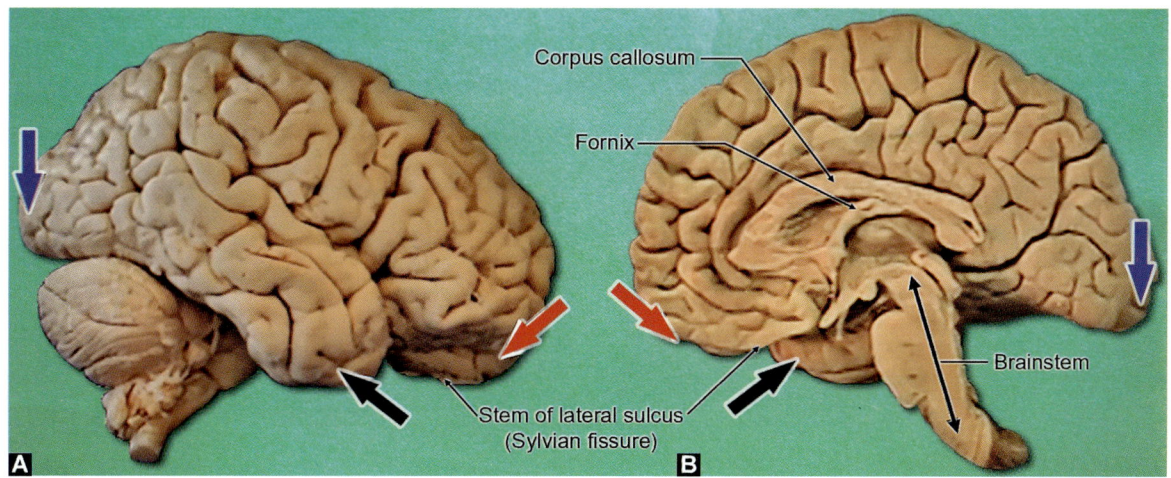

Fig. 13.1: Photographs of external appearance of whole human brain: **A.** superolateral view, **B.** medial view after bisecting the brain through superior longitudinal fissure (not seen here). In both pictures, three main poles are represented by arrows: frontal (red) directed in front, temporal (black) directed inferiorly, and occipital (blue) lying most posterior

Lobes of Cerebral Hemisphere

The cerebral hemispheres consist of six **lobes** on each side: frontal, parietal, temporal, occipital, insular, and limbic). In conventional anatomical description, four lobes (*frontal, parietal, temporal and occipital*) corresponding to the overlying skull bones (though not precisely) are described in each hemisphere. The *frontal lobe* lies in front and the *parietal lobe* behind the central sulcus (Fig. 13.2). The *temporal lobe* lies below the Sylvian fissure and the *occipital lobe* lies posterior to an imaginary line joining the parieto-occipital sulcus to the pre-occipital notch. The *insula* is

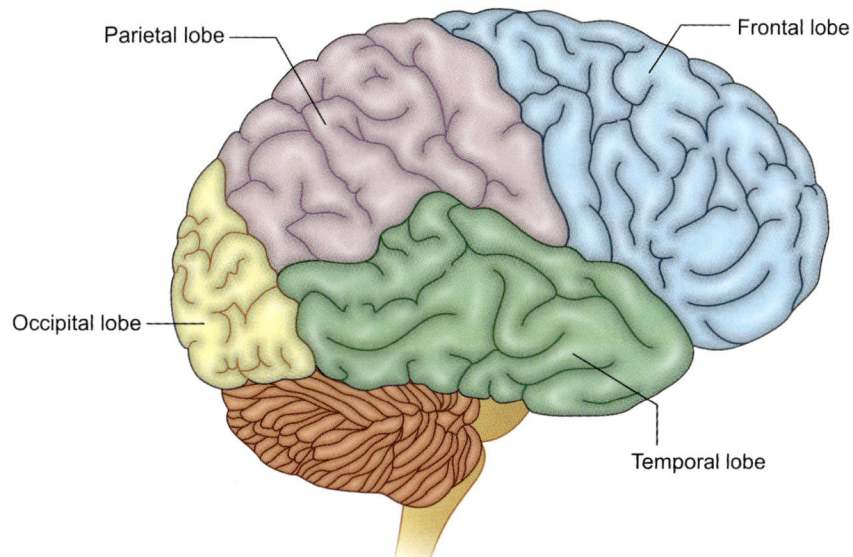

Fig. 13.2: Four commonly described lobes of cerebral hemisphere

the part buried in the lateral sulcus and is considered as the fifth lobe. The limbic lobe lies on the medial aspect of cerebral hemisphere. The insular lobe is present in the depth of lateral sulcus and may be seen only when lips of the sulcus are artificially separated.

Surfaces and Borders including Convolutions

Each cerebral hemisphere presents *three* **surfaces** (convex superolateral, uneven inferior or basal, and a flat medial), separated by *three* **borders** (inferolateral, inferomedial, and superomedial), and *three* **poles** (an anterior frontal, an inferior temporal, and a posterior occipital).

Superolateral or Convex Surface

The superolateral surface of the cerebral hemisphere is convex and extends from the *superomedial border* above, to the *inferolateral border* below. In front it extends up to the rounded *frontal* and *temporal poles,* while posteriorly it ends at the more pointed *occipital pole.* Note the *central sulcus* running downwards and forwards, from the superomedial border a little behind its mid-point to end within a short distance from the posterior limb of *lateral sulcus (Sylvian fissure).* The *Sylvian fissure* (starting on the inferior surface) courses backwards and upwards on the superolateral surface. The parieto-occipital sulcus (lying mainly on the medial surface) cuts the superomedial border about 5 cm in front of the occipital pole. The *pre-occipital notch* indents the inferolateral border about the same distance from the occipital pole.

Convolutions on Superolateral Surface

The superolateral surface presents a number of grooves or *sulci* (demarcating the *lobes* and *lobules)* and separating irregular convolutions or *gyri* (Fig. 13.3). Though largely variable, some of the sulci are fairly constant in position.
- *The lateral sulcus (Sylvian fissure)* is a deep sulcus coursing backwards and upwards on the superolateral surface. Below it, lies the *temporal lobe,* while the *frontal* and parietal *lobes lie* above it. Buried in its depth lies the *insula.*

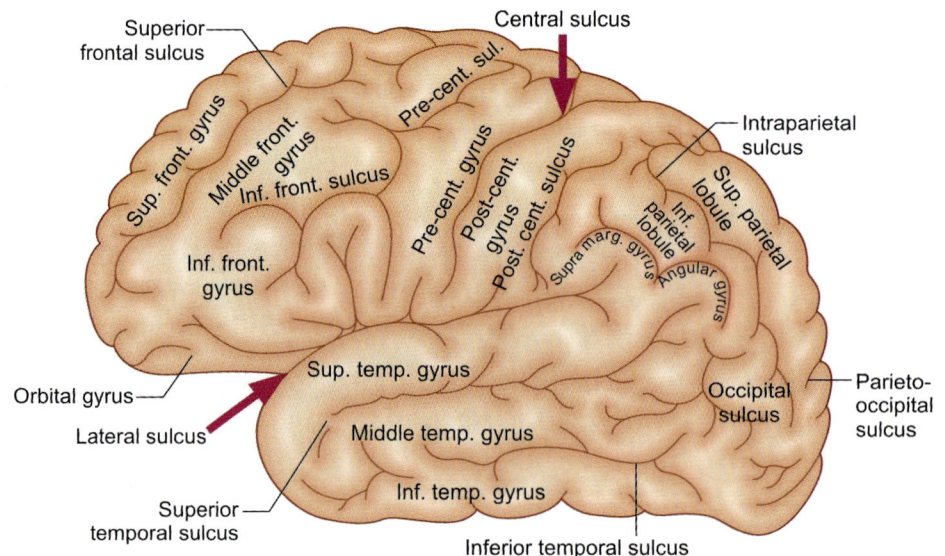

Fig. 13.3: Main sulci and gyri seen on the superolateral surface of left cerebral hemisphere

- The *central sulcus (of Rolando)*—indents the superomedial border a little behind its midpoint, and courses downwards and forwards to end just short of the lateral sulcus. The *frontal lobe* lies in front and the *parietal lobe* behind it.
- The *parieto-occipital sulcus* and the *preoccipital notch* indent, respectively, the superomedial and inferolateral borders about 5 cm in front of the occipital pole. The *occipital lobe* lies behind an imaginary line joining them. The *occipital lobe* presents a horizontally directed *lateral occipital sulcus* separating the *superior* and the *inferior occipital gyri*. The short and curved *lunate sulcus* lies close to the occipital pole.

The *frontal lobe presents* the *precentral sulcus,* in front of and parallel to the central sulcus and horizontally disposed *superior* and *inferior frontal sulci*. The *gyri* in this lobe are the *precentral* and the *superior,* the *middle* and the *inferior frontal*. Two rami *(anterior horizontal* and *anterior ascending),* from the lateral sulcus, extend into the inferior frontal gyrus, dividing it into the *pars orbitalis, pars triangularis* and *pars opercularis,* in that order from before backwards.

The *parietal lobe* has the *postcentral sulcus* behind and parallel to the central sulcus, and the *intraparietal sulcus* extending posteriorly from the postcentral sulcus. The convolutions in the parietal lobe are the *postcentral gyrus* behind the central sulcus and, the superior and inferior parietal lobules. Round the posterior upturned portions of the Sylvian fissure and the superior temporal sulcus, both of which cut into the inferior parietal lobule, are the curved *supramarginal* and *angular* gyri.

The *temporal lobe* presents *the superior* and *inferior temporal sulci* dividing this lobe into the *superior, middle* and the *inferior temporal gyri*. The *anterior* and *posterior transverse temporal gyri (of Heschl)* lie on the upper surface of the superior temporal gyrus within the lateral fissure.

The *insula,* lying at the bottom of the lateral fissure, is a raised pyramidal area surrounded by the *circular sulcus* (Fig. 13.4). Its apex directed anteroinferiorly is called the *limen insulae* (*gyrus ambiens).* The *sulcus centralis insulae* runs through the insula and divides it into an anterior

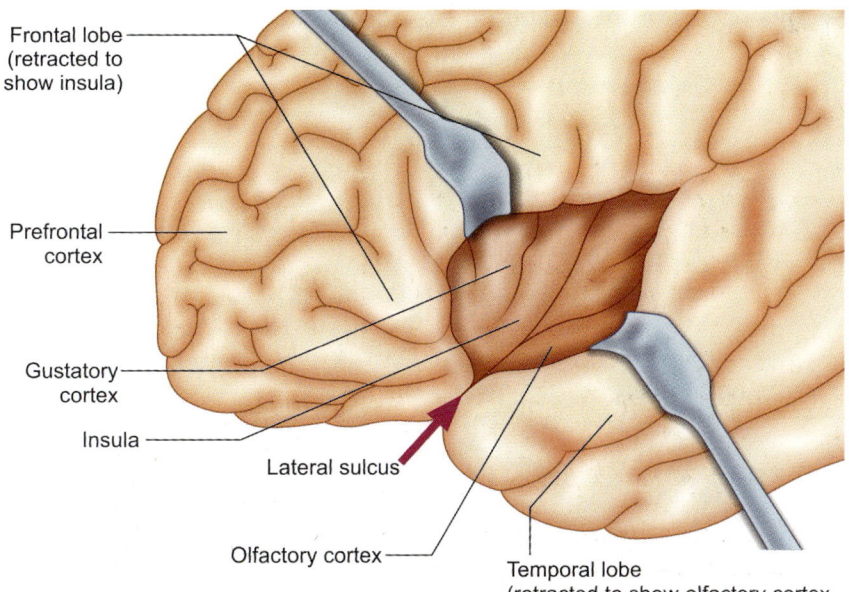

Fig. 13.4: Superolateral surface of left cerebral hemisphere. The lips of the lateral sulcus (arrow) retracted by spatulae to show insula and olfactory cortex. The gyrus longa and brevia are also seen

portion containing 3 or 4 short gyri (*gyri brevia*) and a posterior portion containing a long gyrus (*gyrus longa*).

Medial Surface

Medial view of the bisected brain (Fig. 13.5) shows the flattened *medial surface* of the cerebral hemisphere and the cut surfaces of the bisected *corpus callosum, diencephalon, brainstem* and the *cerebellum*. The *cingulate, parieto-occipital* and *calcarine* are the important *sulci* on this surface. The important convolutions are the *medial frontal gyrus*, the *paracentral lobule*, the *cingulate gyrus, precuneus, cuneus* and the *lingual gyrus*.

The *corpus callosum* joins the two cerebral hemispheres. Its cut surface is seen as a thick and curved band. Its main part is called the *trunk*. The *genu* is its anterior end where the corpus callosum bends to continue as its rostrum. The *rostrum* narrows as it passes backwards and downwards to reach the upper end of the *lamina terminalis*, in front of the anterior commissure. The thickened posterior end of the corpus callosum is called the *splenium*.

The *fornix* is also a curved white band. It is attached to the inferior surface of the corpus callosum a short distance in front of the splenium. More anteriorly it recedes from the corpus callosum to reach the anterior commissure. The *septum pellucidum* stretches between the corpus callosum and the fornix and forms the medial wall of the cavity of *lateral ventricle*. The lower free edge of the fornix binds the *choroids fissure* below which lies the *choroids plexus* of the third ventricle.

Convolutions on Medial Surface (Fig. 13.5)

The *cingulate, parieto-occipital* and *calcarine,* are the most important sulci on the medial surface of the cerebral hemisphere.

The *cingulate sulcus* parallels the curve of corpus callosum from which it is separated by the *gyrus cinguli*. The sulcus begins below the rostrum of corpus callosum in front of the *subcallosal area* and terminates opposite the splenium by turning upwards to reach the superomedial

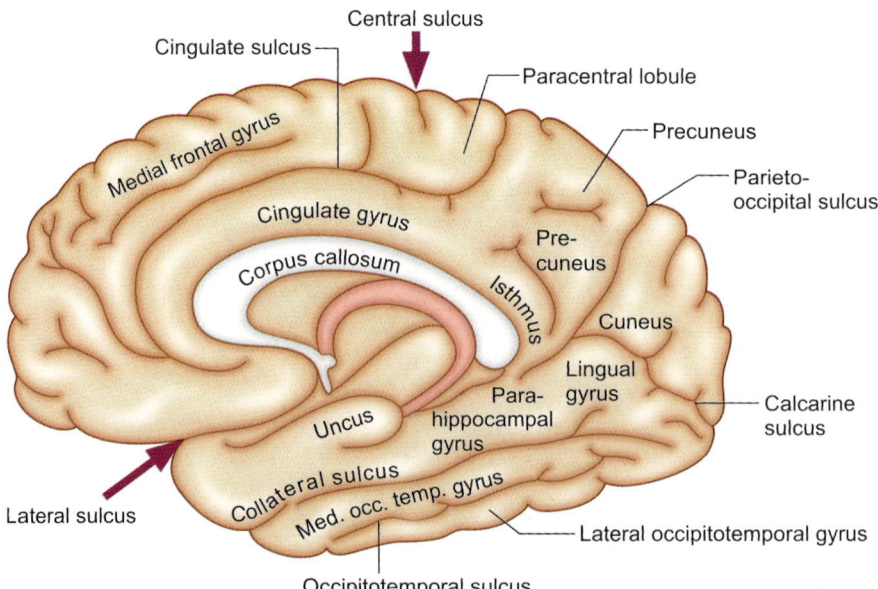

Fig. 13.5: Main sulci and gyri seen on the medial surface of right cerebral hemisphere

border, behind the central sulcus. A vertical ramus originates from the cingulate sulcus opposite the middle of corpus callosum. Between this ramus and the upturned posterior end of the cingulate sulcus lies the *paracentral lobule.* More anteriorly the *medial frontal gyrus* lies between the cingulate sulcus and the superomedial border. The gyrus cinguli passes posteriorly below the *suprasplenial sulcus* and becomes continuous with the *parahippocampal* gyrus through the narrow *isthmus.* Anteriorly, the *subcallosal area* presents the *paraterminal gyrus* in front of the lamina terminalis.

The *calcarine sulcus* starting below the splenium of the corpus callosum pursues a backwards course to the occipital pole. The *parieto-occipital sulcus* begins in the calcarine sulcus and passes upwards to the superomedial border. The *cuneus* is the wedge-shaped lobule between the calcarine and the parieto-occipital sulci. The *precuneus* lies anterior to the cuneus.

Below the calcarine sulcus lies the *lingual gyrus,* which is continuous anteriorly with the *parahippocampal gyrus.* At its anterior end the parahippocampal gyrus is recurved to form the *uncus,* limited laterally by the *rhinal sulcus.* The *dentate gyrus* is a crenated and thin strip of cortex lying above the medial part of the parahippocampal gyrus. The *collateral sulcus* lies lateral to the parahippocampal gyrus. More laterally, the *occipitotemporal sulcus* runs anteroposteriorly separating the *lateral* and the *medial occipitotemporal gyri.*

Inferior or Basal Surface

The *inferior surface* of each cerebral hemisphere is divided by a curved horizontal fissure (the stem of lateral sulcus) into an *orbital surface* in front and a *tentorial surface* behind (Fig. 13.6). The orbital surface is bounded medially by the *medial orbital border* and anterolaterally by the

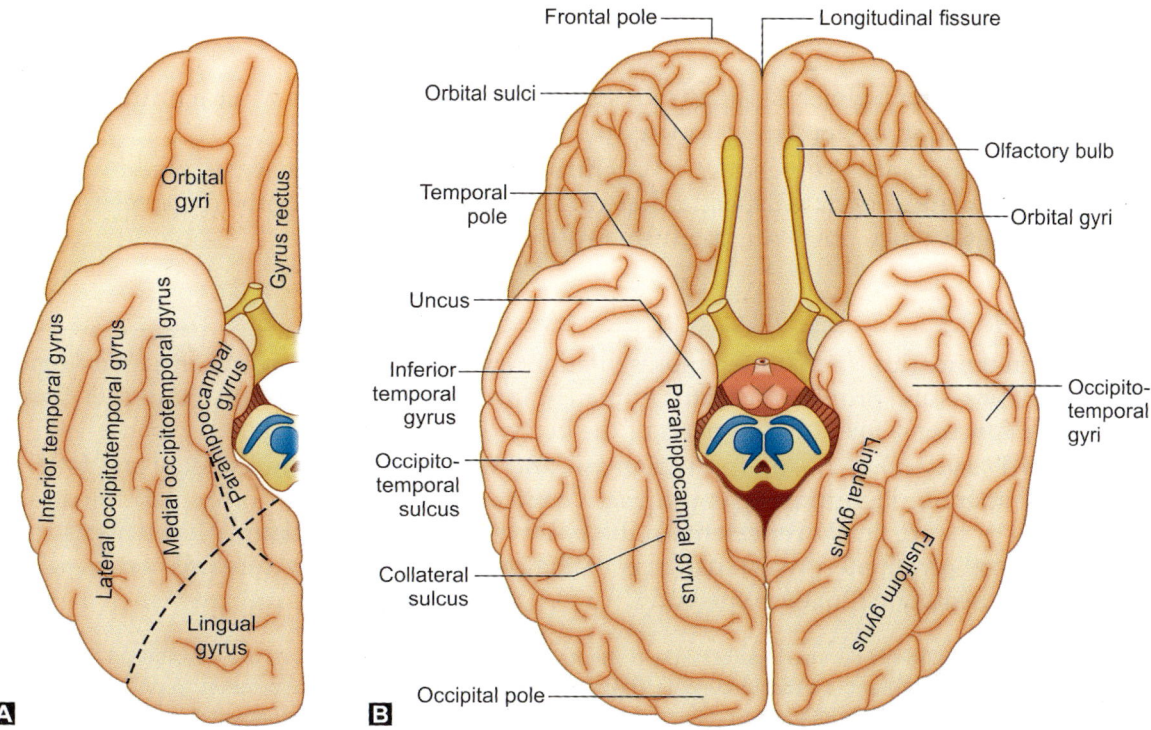

Fig. 13.6A and B: Main sulci and gyri seen on the basal (inferior) surface of cerebral hemispheres

superciliary border. It rests on the roof of orbit and presents: *orbital gyri* and *sulci* and more medially the *olfactory bulb* and *tract*. About 20 filaments of *olfactory nerve* (I cranial nerve) join the olfactory bulb. The *tentorial surface* is bounded medially by the *medial occipital* and laterally by the *inferolateral border*. It occupies the middle cranial fossa anteriorly and rests on the *tentorium cerebelli* (a fold of dura mater) posteriorly.

The stem of lateral sulcus is occupied by lesser wing of sphenoid. It begins at a depression called the *cerebral vallecula,* which lies lateral to the optic chiasma. The roof of the vallecula (*anterior perforated substance*) shows vascular foramina.

The *optic chiasma* is a transverse band of nerve fibres. The *optic nerves* (II cranial nerves) join the anterolateral angles of the chiasma. From the posterolateral angles of the chiasma begin the *optic tracts.* Each optic tract can be followed backwards, across the cerebral peduncle to the *lateral geniculate body* (a part of diencephalon).

Convolutions on Orbital Surface

The orbital surface presents the *orbital gyri* separated by a roughly H-shaped arrangement of the *orbital sulci.* Medial to it lies the olfactory bulb and tract in the *olfactory sulcus.* Further medially lies the *gyrus rectus.*

Types of Sulci

The sulci are classified as:
1. The *limiting sulci* which separate structurally different areas of the cerebral cortex, e.g. central sulcus.
2. The *axial sulci* which develop in the long-axis of a structurally homogenous area, e.g. calcarine sulcus.
3. The *operculated sulci* which separate two structurally different areas while a third structural type lies buried in its depth, e.g. lunate sulcus.
4. Some of the sulci are deep enough to produce elevations in the cavity of lateral ventricle. These are called *complete sulci,* e.g. collateral sulcus which produces the *collateral eminence.* Majority of the sulci, however, produce no such elevations inside.

CORTICAL AREAS

A **cortical homunculus** is a distorted representation of the human body, based on a neurological 'map' of the areas and proportions of the human brain dedicated to processing **motor** functions, or **sensory** functions, for different parts of the body.

The word *homunculus* is Latin for 'little man', and was a term used in alchemy and folklore long before scientific literature began using it. A cortical homunculus, or 'cortex man', illustrates the concept of heuristically representing the body lying within the brain. Nerve fibres from the spinal cord terminate in various areas of the parietal lobe in the cerebral cortex, which forms a representational map of the body.

Dr Wilder Penfield and his co-investigators Edwin Boldrey and Theodore Rasmussen are considered to be the originators of the sensory and motor homunculi. They were not the first scientists to attempt to objectify human brain function by means of a homunculus. However, they were the first to differentiate between sensory and motor function and to map the two across the brain separately, resulting in two different homunculi.

Types of Homunculi

There are two types of homunculi: motor and sensory.

A **motor homunculus** (Fig. 13.7) represents a map of brain areas dedicated to *motor* processing for different anatomical divisions of the body. The primary motor cortex is located in the precentral gyrus, and handles signals coming from the premotor area of the frontal lobes.

A **sensory homunculus** (Fig. 13.8) represents a map of brain areas dedicated to *sensory* processing for different anatomical divisions of the body. The primary sensory cortex is located in the postcentral gyrus, and handles signals coming from the thalamus.

Functional Cortical Areas

The major functional areas of the cerebral cortex have been customarily described as motor, somatosensory and special sensory namely: Visual, auditory, olfactory, taste, etc. Other cortical regions constitute the association areas (Fig. 13.9).

Motor Areas

The motor areas include, the *primary motor* (area 4), *premotor* (area 6), *frontal eye-field* (area 8), *motor speech* (areas 44 and 45), and the *supplementary motor area* (M II). Pyramidal cells of all sizes are found here but there is an almost complete absence of the granular layers in these regions. The largest pyramidal cells (of Betz) measuring more than 60 mm, are found in the cortical layer V of the area 4, being most numerous in the upper part of the precentral gyrus. The *supplementary motor area* (M II) is located in the posterior part of the medial frontal gyrus, anterior to the paracentral lobule.

1. ***The primary motor area (area 4 or MI):*** This occupies the precentral gyrus, anterior wall of the central sulcus and the paracentral lobule. Afferents are received mainly from the

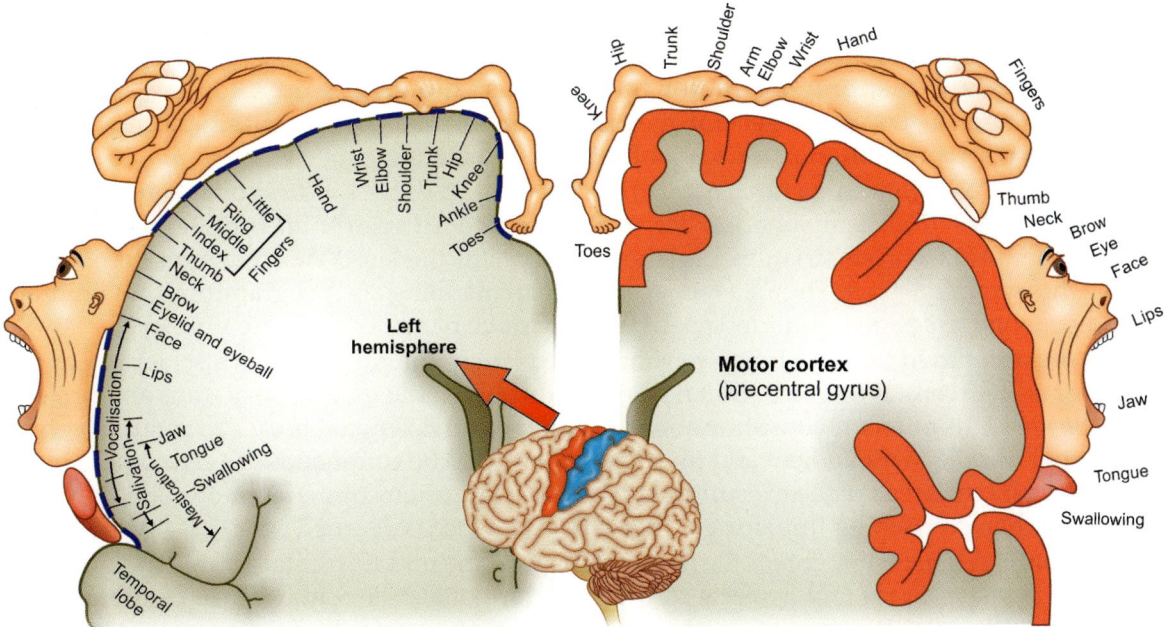

Fig. 13.7: Drawing shows a motor homunculus on superolateral surface of cerebral hemispheres

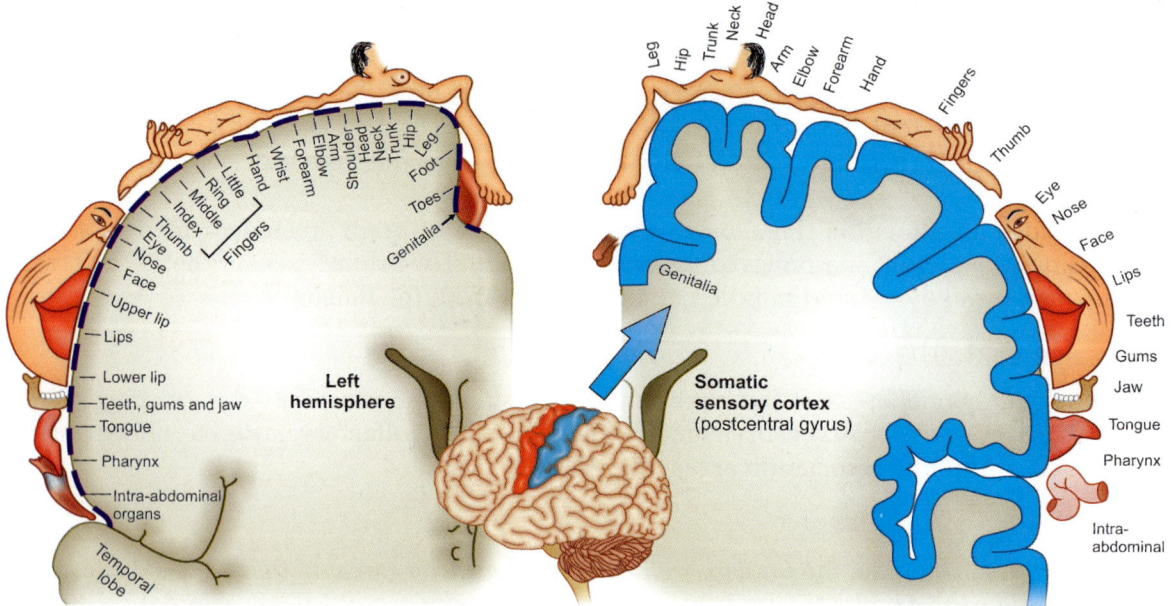

Fig. 13.8: Drawing shows a sensory homunculus on superolateral surface of cerebral hemispheres

cerebellum via the ventrolateral posterior (VLP) nucleus of thalamus. Ipsilateral connections with the somatosensory, premotor and supplementary motor areas exist. Their efferents constitute about 30% of the corticospinal and corticobulbar tracts. The area initiates and controls voluntary movements of the opposite side of the body. The body is represented upside down in this area so that the paracentral lobule is associated with the lower limb and the perineum, and the precentral gyrus with the trunk, upper limb, and head regions, in that order from above downwards. The extent of representation of a region does not depend on the bulk of the muscles but the skill with which a part is ordinarily used. This has lead to the mapping of 'motor homunculus' showing proportional somatotopic representation in the area. In general, the primary motor area 4 carries out simple movements. Lesions of area 4 result in paresis of voluntary movements.

2. *Supplementary motor area (area 6 or MII):* This is a part of the area 6 situated on the medial surface of cerebral hemisphere. Face is represented anteriorly and the leg posteriorly. Projections from corpus striatum reach here through the nucleus VA of thalamus. Its efferents join the pyramidal tract. The area is concerned with planning and programming of voluntary movements. Its lesions result in lack of urge to move or speak (akinetic mutism).

3. *The premotor area (area 6):* It lies in front of the primary motor area. It is also agranular but lacks the Betz cells. It receives striatal afferents through nucleus VL of thalamus and projects to the area 4. Its efferents constitute about 30% of the corticospinal fibres. The area is involved in programming a movement and its ongoing control. The commands are channelled to the primary motor area for the execution of movements. Lesions of the premotor area result in *apraxia* characterised by impairment in the performance of learned acts.

4. *The frontal eye field:* It occupies the posterior parts of the middle frontal gyrus. It is connected with the visual areas and projects to the superior colliculus pontine gaze centre and the oculomotor nuclei. Its stimulation produces conjugate movements of the eyes to the opposite side.

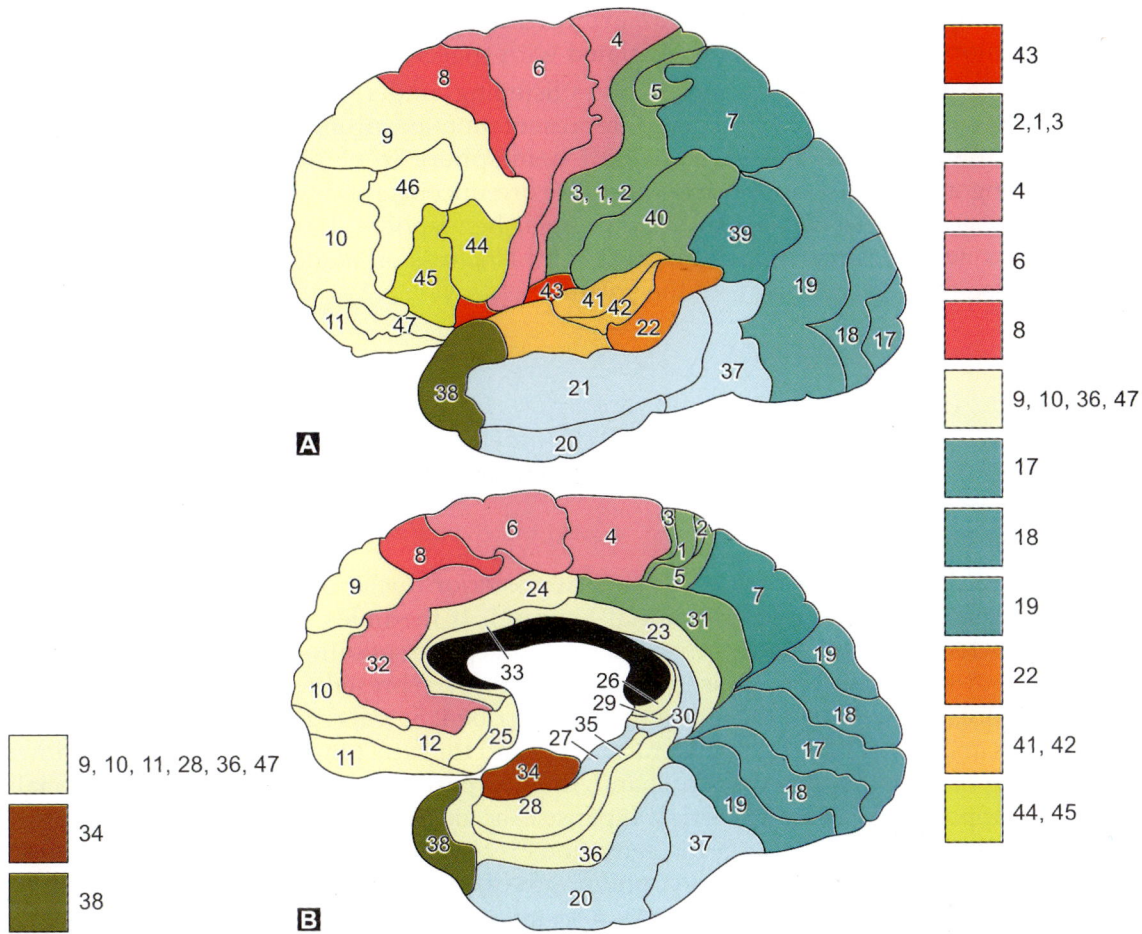

Fig. 13.9: Drawings show main cytoarchitectural areas shown in code colours on: **A.** superolateral, **B.** medial surface of cerebral hemispheres. See text for functional characteristics of individual areas

A second eye field lies in the occipital lobe, within Brodmann's areas 17 and 18. Conjugate contralateral eye-movements can also be elicited through stimulation there. The frontal and occipital and coordinate in the production of eye movements. The 18, is also involved in accommodation and are involved in slow following (smooth pursuit) and fixation movements. Efferents from the occipital eye field pass to the superior colliculus and to the motor cranial nerve nuclei innervating ocular muscles.

5. *The speech area and language functions*
   i. *Broca's motor speech area (44 and 45)* occupies the pars opercularis and pars triangularis of the inferior frontal gyrus. Its ablation produces paralysis of speech (*motor* or *expressive aphasia*) even though the muscle of the tongue and larynx are normal.
   ii. The *second speech area of Wernicke* includes: The angular gyrus (area 39), supramarginal gyrus (area 40), superior temporal gyrus (area 22) and posterior parts of the middle and inferior temporal gyri (area 37). The areas 39 and 40 are concerned with speech reception and a damage results in an inability to comprehend written or spoken words (*receptive or*

Wernicke's aphasia). Areas 22 and 37 are considered to be, respectively, auditory and visuoauditory and these are also associated with speech and language.

Speech is an intricate function and involves listening, understanding and articulation. No wonder, it has such a widespread cortical representation as outlined above. All speech areas develop in the dominant hemisphere (left hemisphere in right handed persons). The corresponding areas in the opposite hemisphere are unconcerned with speech, except when there is damage to these regions in the dominant hemisphere. Lesions of area 22 produce *'word deafness'* while lesions of area 37 cause *word blindness* or *'alexia'* (inability to read). The latter may also result from lesions of the splenium.

Somatosensory Areas

These include, (i) the primary *somatosensory area (S I)* which occupies the postcentral gyrus and the paracentral lobule (areas 3,1 and 2), (ii) the *second somatosensory area (S II)* located along the superior lip of the lateral sulcus, and (iii) the *somesthetic association cortex.*

First Somatosensory Area (S I)

This area receives projections from the ventral posterior nuclei of thalamus, which in turn receive the medial, spinal and trigeminal lemnisci. It mediates a wide range of sensory modalities including both exteroceptive and proprioceptive sensations from the opposite side of the body. A somatotopic organisation with the body represented upside down (sensory homunculus), as in the case of the motor area is described. Sacral regions lie in the paracentral lobule, trunk and upper limb on the lateral surface and the face, tongue and lips further down. Some regions of the body, like the foot, hand, fingers (particularly the index), face (especially the lips) are apportioned a greater cortical expanse in accordance with their greater involvement in the sensory perception. Though the sensations received are predominantly contralateral, bilateral (from larynx) and ipsilateral (from mouth cavity) projections also exist.

Primary somatosensory area presents a segregation of sensory modalities so that while the area 3 is activated by the cutaneous stimuli, area 2 receives proprioception. The area S I is connected with the area S II, the superior parietal lobule (area 5) and the primary and supplementary motor areas. Its efferent fibres pass in the corticospinal, corticopontine and corticostriate tracts.

Second Somatosensory Area (S II)

It occupies the posterior part of the superior lip of the Sylvian fissure. The head and face are represented most anteriorly whereas the leg is indicated posteriorly. Neurons of S II respond particularly to vibration. The more caudal regions in the area are important for the perception of pain. S II is reciprocally connected with S I.

Somesthetic Association Cortex

The areas 5 and 7 in the superior parietal lobule and the precuneus are the regions into which all the somatic sensory information from S I and S II ultimately flow. Area 5 also receives direct thalamic projections from the lateral posterior nucleus and the pulvinar. The area allows for a comprehensive assessment of the features of an object and its identification without the visual aid. Injury to these regions can lead to astereognosis and sensory neglect of the opposite side of body *(dressing apraxia).*

SPECIAL SENSORY AREAS

Olfactory Areas

The limen insulae, uncus (area 34), the underlying amygdaloid body and the entorhinal area 28 are associated with smell (primary olfactory areas, pyriform cortex). Olfactory fibres reach here through the olfactory bulb, olfactory tract and the olfactory striae. The lateral orbital gyrus receives projections from olfactory areas and is involved in behavioural reactions to recognised odours.

Note. The insula is involved in both the taste and smell sensations. It is also concerned with visceral functions.

Taste Areas

The taste areas include the lower end of the postcentral gyrus (area 43) and the adjacent insula. The taste impulses are relayed through the rostral parts of the nucleus of solitary tract and the most medial part of the nucleus VPM of thalamus into the aforesaid cortical regions.

Visual Areas

The visual areas include:

Primary Visual Area or Striate Area 17 (V 1)

The *primary visual area* (V 1) or *striate cortex (area 17)* occupies the depth of the calcarine sulcus and also extends into the cuneus above and the lingual gyrus below. Posteriorly it extends up to the occipital pole. The cortex is thin and of the granular type (koniocortex). It presents the following histological features:

- Densely packed small-sized *stellate cells* present in layers II and IV.
- *Large stellate cells*, rather than pyramidal cells present in the layer III.
- Well-developed outer band of Baillarger *(visual stria, stria of Gennari)* in the cortical layer IV.

Major input to area 17 comes from the lateral geniculate body. Other afferents are derived from the pulvinar and the intralaminar nucleus. Association fibres pass from area 17 to areas 18 and 19 and to the parietal and temporal cortices. Subcortical efferents pass to the superior colliculus and pretectum.

The striate area in each hemisphere receives impulses from the temporal half of ipsilateral and nasal half of the contralateral retina representing the contralateral half of the visual field. Within the area, the peripheral parts of retina activate the anterior regions while the macula, which is responsible for central vision of maximum discrimination, is represented over a more extensive region in the posterior part. The superior and the inferior retinal quadrants are represented in the superior and inferior halves, respectively. A destructive lesion in the striate cortex causes an area of blindness in the opposite visual field.

Parastriate Area 18 (V 2 and V 3) and Peristriate Area 19 (V 4)

The parastriate area (area 18) and the peristriate area (area 19) do not show visual stria and the stellate cells are less prominent. Stimulations in conscious persons elicit simple visual impressions such as flashes of light from the area 17, but areas 18 and 19 elicit more complex imaging.

These areas occupy the whole of the occipital lobe of the cerebral hemisphere. The lateral geniculate body projects directly to all these areas. Efferents from these areas pass to the thalamus (lateral geniculate body and the pulvinar) and to the motor nuclei of brainstem.

Areas 18 and 19 along with the posterior part of the parietal lobe, posterior part of the lateral surface and much of the inferior surface of the temporal lobe are grouped under 'visual association areas'. These regions serve to relate the present to past visual experiences, for its recognition. The association areas are also involved in the perception of depth (area 18) colour and movement (area 19). Lesions involving visual association areas result in *visual agnosia.*

Visual agnosias: Bilateral lesions of superior parts of area 19 cause visual disorientation. Moving objects may not be perceived. Extensions of lesions into the parietal lobe cause 'ocular apraxia', i.e. inability to fix the eye on a desired object. There is also 'optic ataxia', i.e. a loss of the ability to carry out visually guided movements of the hand. A combination of visual disorientation, ocular apraxia and optic ataxia, is known as the *Balint syndrome.*

Corticotectal fibres: These connect the visual areas with the superior colliculus, and with the 3rd, 4th and 6th cranial nerve nuclei. This is the pathway for fixation of gaze and for tracking a moving object in the field of vision. It also functions in accommodation convergence.

Acoustic Areas

The *primary acoustic area (A I)* corresponds to the Brodmann's areas 41 and 42. These areas occupy the anterior and posterior transverse temporal gyri of Heschl within the Sylvian fissure and also extend into the upper part of the superior temporal gyrus. Stimulation of these regions produces sounds of a simple nature such as humming, ringing or buzzing.

The *second acoustic area (A II), auditory association cortex.* It corresponds to the Brodmann's area 22 and occupies the superior temporal gyrus. Electrical stimulation of A II produces complex acoustic phenomena. The area is important for interpretation of sound.

Lesions in the acoustic areas (as also the medial geniculate body), unless bilateral do not cause deafness, since the lateral lemniscus carries fibres from the cochlea of both sides. Even extensive temporal lobe tumours have nominal effect on hearing though they may interfere with the acoustic aspects of interpretation of language, especially if involving the dominant hemisphere.

Vestibular Area

Ascending fibres from the vestibular nuclei cross and travel along the medial lemniscus to reach the VPM nucleus of thalamus. Recordings of equilibratory responses in man, implicate parts of the superior temporal gyrus anterior to the acoustic area, in the vestibular functions.

ASSOCIATION AREAS

The cortical regions not associated with sensory or motor functions are regarded as associational. The following are some of them.

The prefrontal area: This region extending up to the frontal pole includes Brodmann's areas, 8, 9 and 10. These areas have extensive connections with cortices of parietal, temporal and occipital lobes, in which all sensations flow. They also have reciprocal connections with the medial dorsal (MD) nucleus of thalamus and are associated with *higher mental functions.* The region is involved in judgment and foresight. It also monitors and exercises control over behaviour. Damage in these areas results in docility, marked lack of concentration and initiative, diminished self-criticism and disregard for others and general tenets of social behaviour.

The operation of prefrontal leukotomy devised by Egas Moniz for the treatment of various mental disorders and intractable pain, interrupts connections between the thalamus and the prefrontal area. The operation, however, leaves the patient with a changed personality and rash and reckless behaviour.

Parietal association areas: The portion of parietal lobe situated between the sensory and visual areas has connections with parts of the lateral group nuclei of thalamus. The strategic location and richness of its connections suggests its role as a prime-integrating centre. Interpretation seems to be its most important function. Lesions of parietal association area may cause agnosia, astereognosis and *astatagnosia* (loss of sense of position of body parts).

Occipital and temporal association areas: The anterior part of the temporal lobe has been related to thought and memory. Electrical stimulation in conscious patients may recall objects seen, music heard or other experiences, both in the recent and the distant past. Temporal lobe tumour patients may have visual and auditory hallucinations. Occipital lobe lesions cause visual agnosia, e.g. prosopagnosia or face blindness and dyslexia (word blindness).

The total expanse of frontal, parietal, occipital and temporal association cortices are laid down with long-term memory traces or engrams possibly as macromolecular changes in the neurons. These form the bases of learning at intellectual levels and skills acquired through practice. The limbic lobe is involved in the consolidation of recently acquired informations in the long-term memory. Total loss of the established memory is a rare possibility because the engrams are contained in several parts of the brain.

STRUCTURE OF CEREBRAL CORTEX

General Features of Cerebral Cortex

Based on the cytoarchitectural features **Brodmann (1909)** identified 52 different cortical regions. Correlation with specific functions has, however, been successful only in a limited number of these areas. Also, structurally similar areas may differ in functions.

A number of variant structural types are found in different cortical regions. Five main types are described. The *frontal, parietal* and *polar types* have all the layers and are *homotypical*. The following two types lack some of the layers and are *heterotypical*.

Agranular Type

This type lacks granular layers 2 and 4. The pyramidal cells are the predominant cell type and the largest of them (Betz cells) are found in this type of cortex. This is the motor type cortex and is found, typically, in the *precentral gyrus* (area 4).

Granular Type (koniocortex)

In this type, the granular layers 2 and particularly, the 4 are best developed while layers 3 and 5 are unidentifiable. This is the sensory type cortex and is typically found in the *postcentral gyrus* (somesthetic areas 3, 1 and 2), *transverse temporal gyrus* (auditory areas 41 and 42) and the *striate cortex* (visual area 17). The parietal and polar types closely resemble the granular types.

Microscopic Structure of Cerebral Cortex

The cerebral cortex is a mosaic of *functional units* of cell columns, 0.2 to 0.3 mm in diameter and made up of 50,000 to 150,000 cells, arranged in *six layers* (module concept). From superficial to deep these *layers* are (Fig. 13.10):

Molecular (or plexiform) Layer

It is a layer of tangentially disposed fibres derived from the *horizontal cells* of this layer and the apical dendrites of the *pyramidal cells* in the deeper layers. The cells are sparsely placed and exhibit primarily axons and dendrites.

External Granular Layer

The cortex of this layer contains non-pyramidal cells (e.g. stellate cells) having 5 to 15 µm size. However, few small pyramidal cells may be found in this layer.

External Pyramidal Layer

This layer contains mostly small and medium-sized *pyramidal cells.* The cell size ranges between 10 to 80 µm. The apical dendrites from these cells pass into the molecular layer, while the basal dendrites run tangentially in the same layers. Axons arising from the bases of these cells project on deeper cortical layers. Other axons pass into the white matter to re-enter the grey matter, at some distance, as *long* or *short association fibres.*

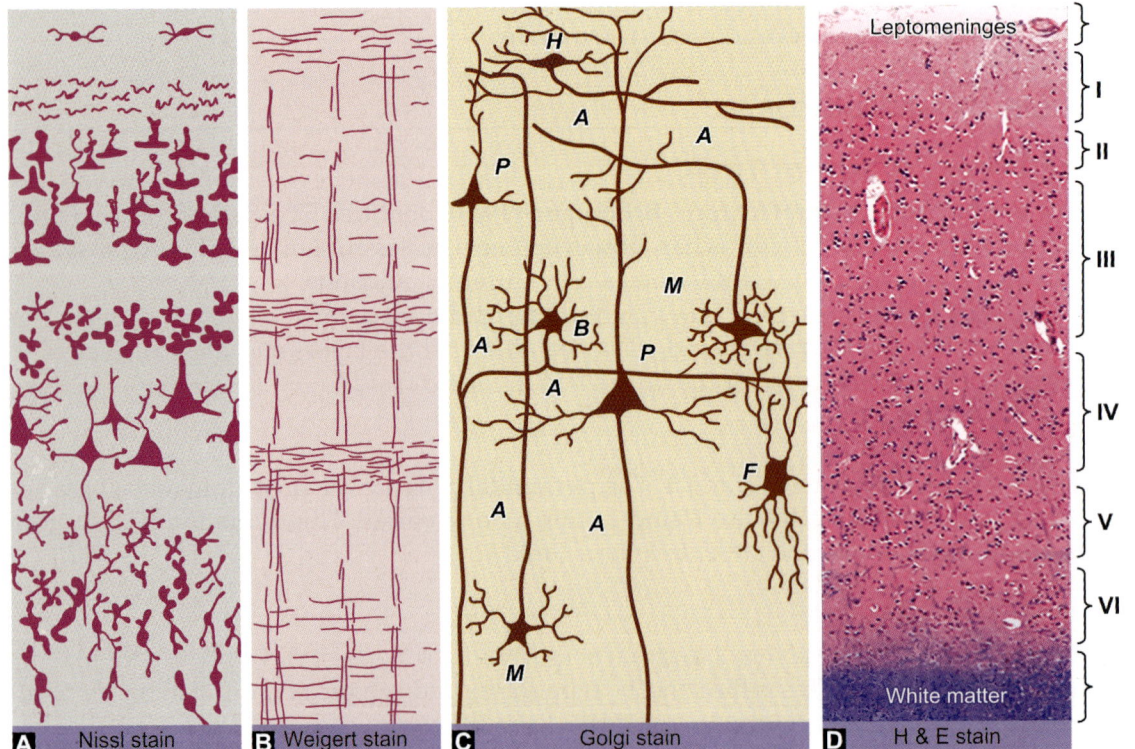

Fig. 13.10A to D: Cerebral cortical layers of neocortex are shown by using different stains. See text for details

Internal Granular Layer

This layer contains densely packed small, nonpyramidal *stellate cells* and few *pyramidal cells*. Tangentially disposed myelinated fibres in this layer form the *outer (external)* band *of Baillarger*. The layers 2, 3 and 4 are concerned with the *input signals*. The sensory signals excite first the neurons in the layer 4. Then the signals spread towards the surface and also into the deeper layers.

Internal Pyramidal (Ganglionic) Layer

This layer contains medium sized and large *pyramidal cells*. In the precentral gyrus this layer contains the *giant pyramidal cells (of Betz)*. Axons of the cells in this layer form the projection fibres to the brainstem *(corticonuclear tract)*, spinal cord *(corticospinal tract)* and the corpus striatum. Tangential fibres in this layer form the *inner band of Baillarger*.

Multiform Layer

This layer contains small and medium sized *stellate* and *pyramidal cells*. As the name suggests, this layer has a multitude of cell types. Small multipolar Martinotti cells are often prominent in this layer.

The above 6 layered arrangement is found in most parts of the cerebral cortex which constitutes the *isocortex*. Phylogenetically older cortex of the hippocampus and dentate gyrus, however, present only 3 layers and constitute the *allocortex*.

Telencephalon 2
White Matter or Fibre Tracts

- Association Fibres Tracts
  - Superior longitudinal fasciculus
  - Fronto-occipital fasciculus
  - Cingulum
  - Inferior longitudinal fasciculus
  - Uncinate fasciculus
  - Perpendicular fasciculus

- Commissural Fibres
  - Corpus callosum
  - Anterior commissure
  - Hippocampal commissure (commissure of fornix)
- Projection Fibres
  - Internal capsule

The white matter of cerebrum comprises of *three* main types of nerve fibre bundles (Fig. 14.1):

1. *Association (arcuate) fibres* connecting different regions of the cerebral cortex in the same hemisphere.
2. *Commissural fibres* which cross the median plane and connect (mostly) identical parts of the cortex in the two hemispheres.
3. *Projection fibres*, connecting the cerebral cortex with the subcortical neurons (nuclei) within the brain or the spinal cord.

ASSOCIATION FIBRES TRACTS

The association fibres (Fig. 14.2) connect one gyrus to another in the same hemisphere. These can be classified into: (i) unnamed *Short association fibres* connecting adjacent gyri, and (ii) named *Long association fibres* connecting widely placed gyri. Some of the important **long association fibres** are given below:

Superior Longitudinal Fasciculus

This fibre bundle extends from the frontal to the occipital lobe above the insula. Many of its fibres turn downwards into the temporal lobe. The fasciculus connects the gyri on the superolateral surface of the cerebral hemisphere and lies lateral to the projection fibres of the corona radiata.

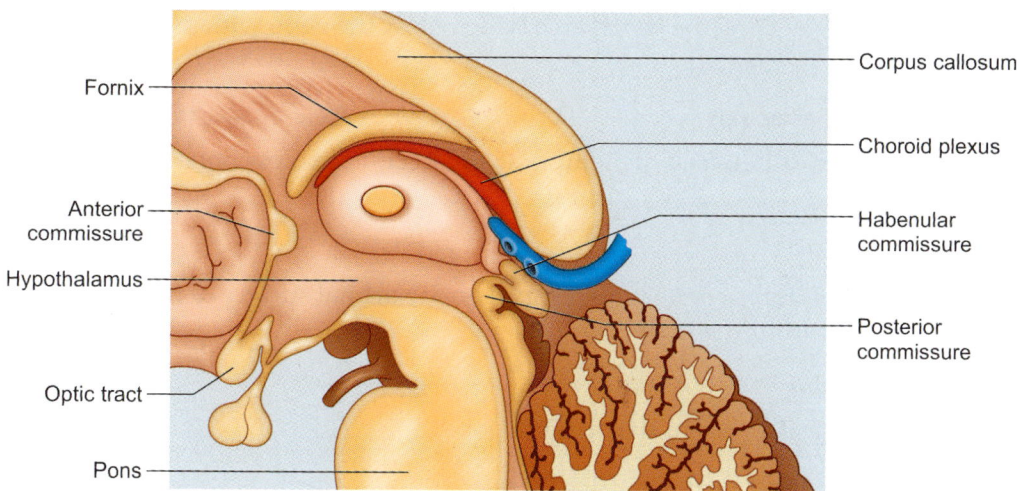

Fig. 14.1: Three white matter commissures of the cerebral hemispheres: (i) Anterior commissure—connect both temporal lobes; (ii) posterior commissure—contain fibres from pretectal nuclei connected with light reflex; and (iii) habenular commissure—connect habenular which are connected to the amygdala and hippocampus

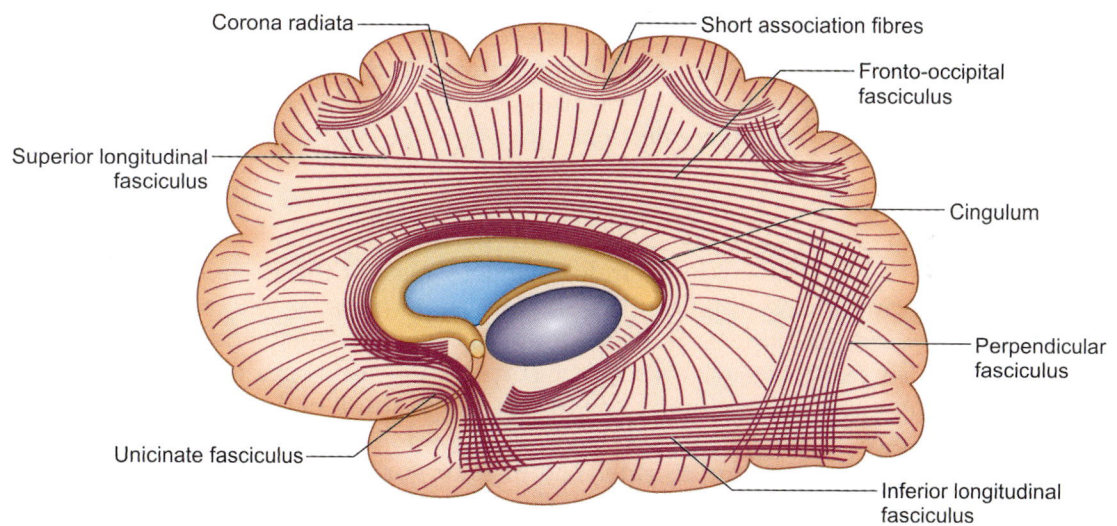

Fig. 14.2: The association fibres of cerebrum

Fronto-Occipital Fasciculus

This bundle also extends from the frontal to the occipital lobe, but it lies medial to the corona radiata and connects the gyri on the medial surface of the cerebral hemisphere.

Cingulum

This is an extensive fibre bundle which lies mainly within the gyrus cinguli. It begins in the subcallosal area, curves round the genu and posteriorly round the splenium to run within the parahippocampal gyrus in which it extends up to the uncus. It is an association fasciculus of the limbic lobe interconnecting the septal area lying below the genu with the parahippocampal gyrus.

Inferior Longitudinal Fasciculus

This fibre bundle extends between the temporal and occipital poles connecting the gyri in the corresponding lobes.

Uncinate Fasciculus

It is a curved bundle of fibres connecting the gyri on the orbital surface of the frontal lobe with those in the anterior part of the temporal lobe.

Perpendicular Fasciculus

This bundle runs vertically within the occipital lobe.

COMMISSURAL FIBRES

The commissures of the cerebral hemisphere connect corresponding gyri of two hemispheres. They include the following tracts:

Corpus Callosum

The corpus callosum is the largest commissure of the brain. It is a neocortical commissure and reaches its highest development in man. It connects corresponding cortical areas of the two hemispheres except much of the temporal lobe cortices which are connected by the *anterior commissure*. The hand areas of the primary sensory cortices and large parts of primary visual areas have no direct commissural connections.

Parts and Relations

The corpus callosum is seen as a thick, curved white band on the medial surface of a sagittally bisected brain (Fig. 14.1). It is about 10 cm long and consists of the *rostrum, genu, trunk* and *splenium*. Commencing at the upper end of the lamina terminalis, where it is narrow, the *rostrum* passes forwards and upwards, thickening rapidly as it extends to the genu. The *genu* is the most anteriorly projecting part where the corpus callosum is acutely bent. It lies about 4 cm from the frontal pole and continues backwards as the trunk of the corpus callosum. The *trunk* is the main part of the corpus callosum, its superior surface is convex from before backwards and concave from side to side. The inferior surface is reciprocally curved. The *splenium* is the thickened posterior end of the corpus callosum. It lies at an average distance of about 6 cm from the occipital pole. The splenium overhangs the pineal body in the midline and the superior colliculus and the pulvinar, on either side. Below the splenium lies the *transverse cerebral fissure* through which a fold of pia mater passes forwards to form the tela chodoidea of the third ventricle.

The outer (dorsal) surface of the corpus callosum seen in the depth of the longitudinal cerebral fissure is clothed by a thin sheet of grey matter called the *indusium griseum*. Embedded in this grey layer are *lateral* and *medial longitudinal striae* (two fine bundles of myelinated nerve fibres, on either side of the midline (Fig. 14.3). Along this surface of the corpus callosum is found a pair each of the anterior cerebral arteries and veins coursing around.

The inner surface of the corpus callosum on either side forms the roof of central part and the anterior wall and floor of the anterior horn of lateral ventricle. In the midline, posteriorly,

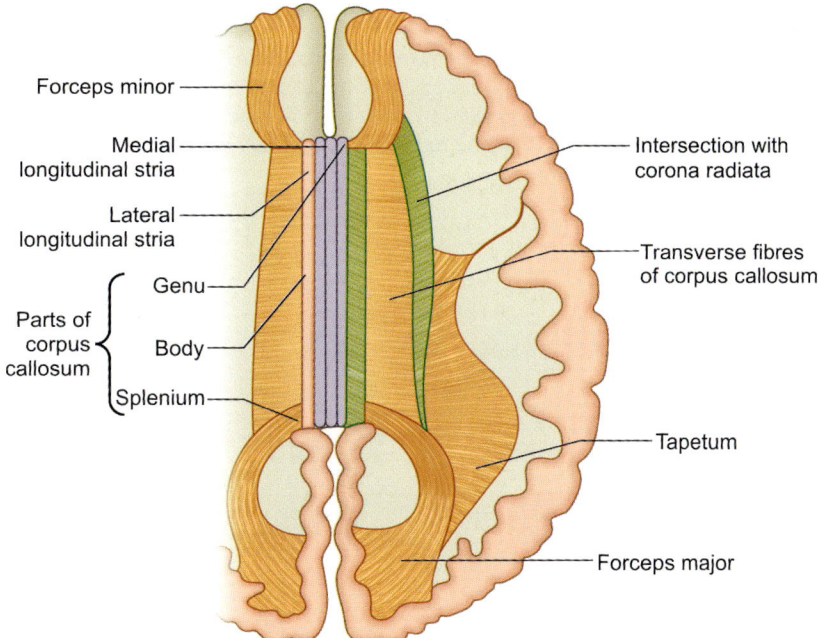

Forceps minor

Medial longitudinal stria

Lateral longitudinal stria

Genu

Parts of corpus callosum { Body

Splenium

Intersection with corona radiata

Transverse fibres of corpus callosum

Tapetum

Forceps major

Fig. 14.3: Corpus callosum dissected and viewed from the superior aspect

the body of fornix is attached to this surface. More anteriorly the fornix gradually recedes from this surface and the septum pellucidum attaches it to the corpus callosum.

Fibres of Corpus Callosum

i. The *rostrum* transmits fibres connecting the gyri on orbital surfaces of opposite frontal lobes.

ii. The *genu* transmits fibres connecting the superolateral and medial surfaces of the frontal lobes of the two sides. These fibres spread forwards and laterally from the genu in each hemisphere and constitute the *forceps minor* (Fig. 14.3).

iii. The *trunk* of the corpus callosum transmits fibres connecting widespread areas on the superolateral and medial surfaces of the two hemispheres. Most of these fibres are intersected by the projection fibres of the corona radiata. Fibres traversing the posterior part of the body and the anterior part of splenium are, however, not intersected by the corona radiata and constitute the *tapetum*. The tapetal fibres pass into the lateral regions of the temporal and occipital lobes, forming the lateral wall of the inferior horn and the roof and lateral wall of the posterior horn of the lateral ventricle.

iv. The *splenium* transmits fibres which extend backwards to the occipital pole. These fibres form the *forceps major* and produce an elevation called the *bulb* in the medial wall of the posterior horn of lateral ventricle.

Anterior Commissure

The **anterior commissure** (also known as the precommissure) is a white matter tract (a bundle of axons) connecting the two temporal lobes of the **cerebral** hemispheres across the midline, and placed in front of the columns of the fornix (Figs 14.1 and 14.4).

Functional Significance of Corpus Callosum

The corpus callosum helps in the inter-hemispheric transfer of informations. The split-brain experiments of Sperry (Noble Prize – 1981) have revealed that after the transection of the corpus callosum (and the anterior commissure), memory stored in one hemisphere cannot be recalled by the other hemisphere. Thus objects palpated by the left hand (with eyes closed) could not be named since the right sensory cortex could not 'ask' the language area located in the left hemisphere for the object's 'name'.

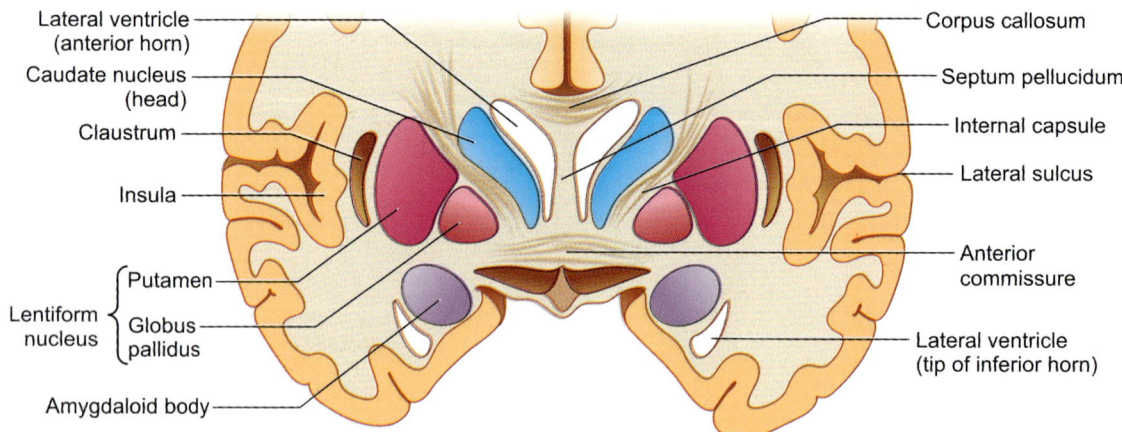

Fig. 14.4: Coronal section of the cerebral hemispheres to show corpus callosum and anterior commissure—the two commissures described in the text. Other important structures visible in the immediate vicinity of these two commissures are: the head of the caudate nucleus (in blue) separated by internal capsule from the components of the lentiform nucleus (in magenta). Also notice the septum pellucidum between the anterior horns (clear space) of lateral ventricles

Its fibres twined like strands of a rope, when traced laterally separate into two bundles. The anterior bundle curves forwards into the olfactory tract. These fibres interconnect the opposite olfactory bulbs. The posterior bundle curves backwards and laterally grooves the anteroinferior aspect of the lentiform nucleus, to finally spread-out within the temporal lobe. The anterior commissure connects the olfactory and basal limbic structures of the two hemispheres.

Hippocampal Commissure (Commissure of Fornix)

The fibres joining the crura of fornix form the hippocampal commissure, below the posterior part of corpus callosum. A horizontal cleft (*ventricle of the fornix*) separates the commissure from the corpus callosum. The commissure connects the hippocampus of the two sides.

PROJECTION FIBRES

The projection fibres connect more or less vertically the cerebral cortex with the corpus striatum, diencephalon, brainstem and the spinal cord. The fibres are both ascending and descending and appear to diverge (radiate) from the periphery of the corpus striatum to form the *corona radiata*. These fibres intersect the commissural fibres of corpus callosum. Lower down, the fibres collect into a thick white band called the *internal capsule* which cuts through the corpus striatum dividing it into the lentiform and the caudate nuclei. Apart from the corona radiata (Fig. 14.5) and the internal capsule (Fig. 14.6), the **fornix** (connecting the hippocampus with the mammillary bodies) and the **stria terminalis** (connecting the amygdala with the habenular nuclei) are other projection fibre bundles of the cerebrum.

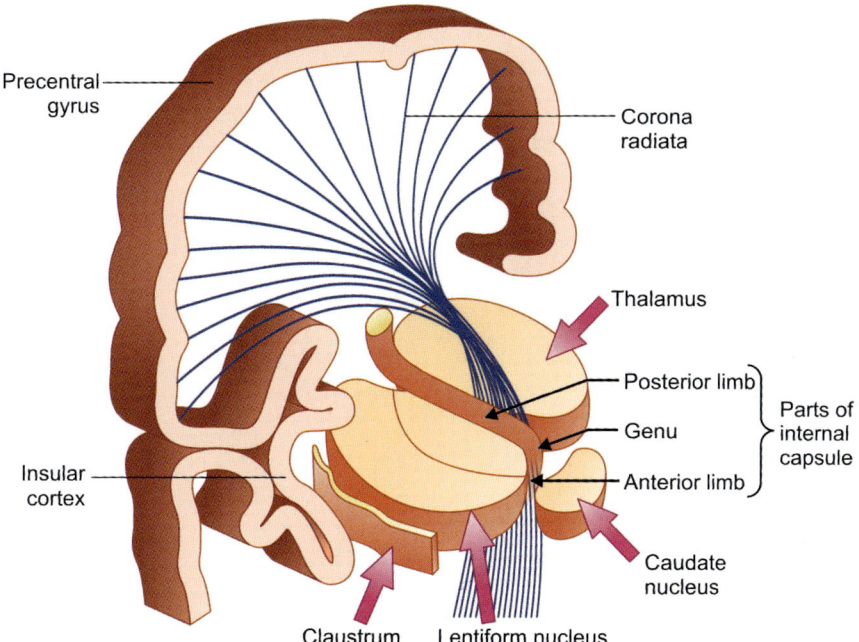

Precentral gyrus

Corona radiata

Thalamus

Posterior limb

Genu

Anterior limb

} Parts of internal capsule

Insular cortex

Claustrum   Lentiform nucleus

Caudate nucleus

Fig. 14.5: Coronal section of the left cerebral hemispheres to show the fibres constituting the corona radiata being arranged as the internal capsule descending further in relation to the thalamus and the two basal nuclei (caudate and lentiform nuclei). Out of the five parts of the internal capsule three parts are shown here

Projection fibres from the primary sensory and motor cortex form the largest input to the basal nuclei (Chapter 15). The thalamus receives projection fibres from all parts of the cerebral cortex (corticothalamic fibres). Other major projection systems are:

i. *Corticopontine*—to the ipsilateral nuclei pontis.
ii. *Corticonuclear*—to contralateral motor and somatic sensory cranial nerve nuclei in pons and medulla oblongata.
iii. *Corticospinal*—to ventral horn motor neurons.

Internal Capsule

The internal capsule (Figs 14.6 and 14.7) is a thick and curved lamina of myelinated nerve fibres covering the medial and inferior aspects of the lentiform nucleus. It separates the lentiform nucleus from the caudate nucleus and the thalamus medially, and the inferior horn of the lateral ventricle inferiorly. Its fibres are continuous superiorly with the corona radiata and inferiorly with the cerebral peduncle.

Parts and Fibres in Internal Capsule

In a horizontal section of the cerebral hemisphere the internal capsule presents the form of a V-shaped (white) band accommodating the lentiform nucleus between its widely separated parts.

Various constituents (ascending and descending) traversing through the different parts of the internal capsule are summarized in Table 14.1.

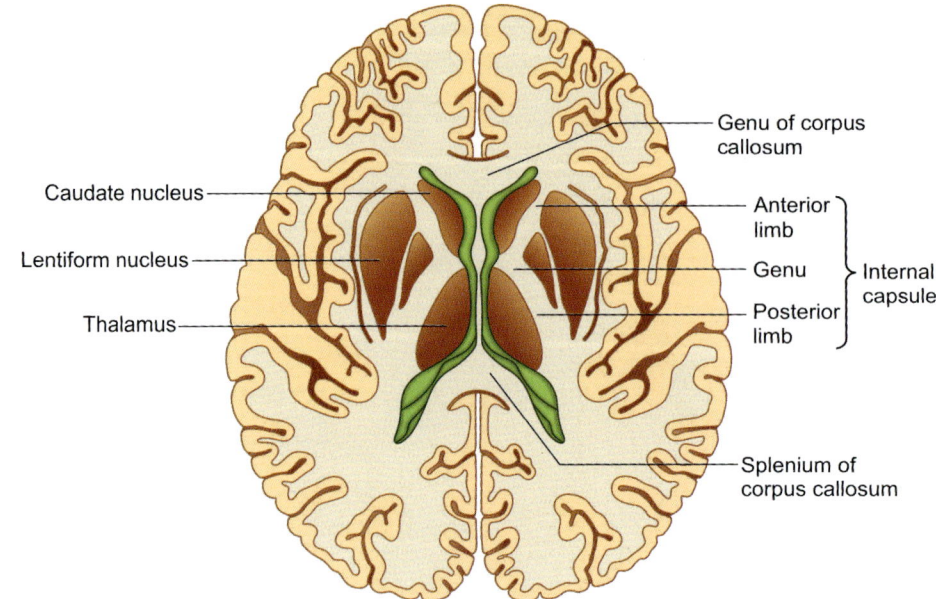

Fig. 14.6: Horizontal section of cerebral hemispheres at the level across the corpus callosum

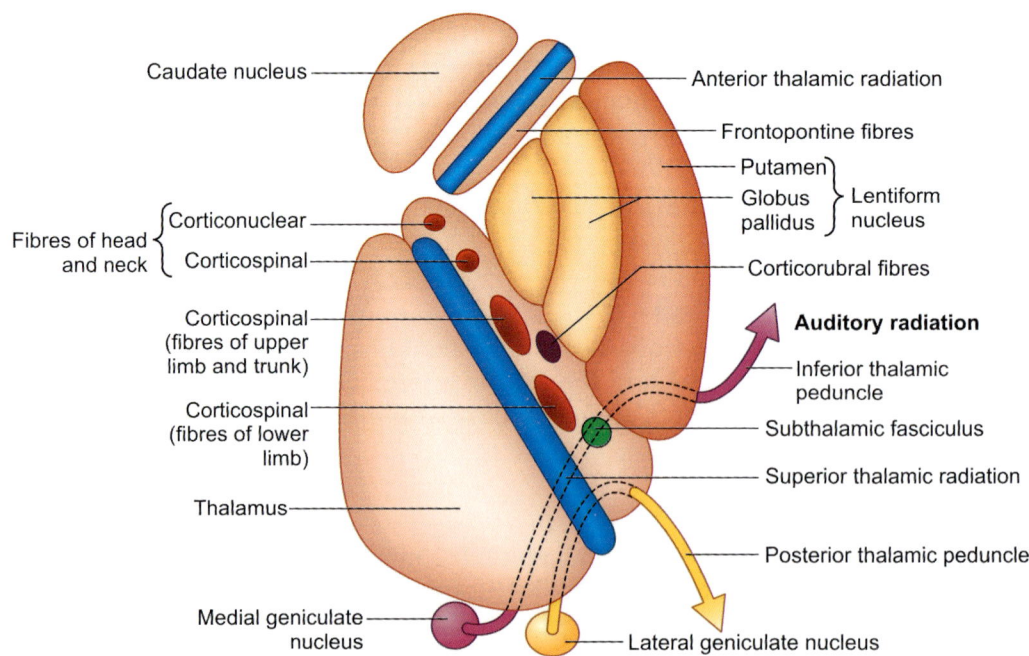

Fig. 14.7: The parts of the internal capsule and their components in a horizontal section

Table 14.1: Fibres of different parts of internal capsule

Parts	Ascending fibres	Descending fibres
Anterior limb	Anterior thalamic radiations from anterior and medial nuclei of thalamus (reciprocal) to the frontal lobe	Frontopontine fibres Corticostriate fibres
Genu	Thalamocortical fibres (from VA-VL thalamic nuclei to cortical areas 6 & 8)	Frontopontine fibres Corticonuclear fibres
Posterior limb	• Superior thalamic radiations (thalamocortical fibres from VPL and VPM nuclei of thalamus to areas 3, 1, and 2 in the postcentral gyrus) • Nonspecific thalamoparietal projections	Corticospinal fibres (in scattered bundles). Anterior limb fibres in front, trunk and posterior limb fibres behind Frontopontine fibres from areas 4 and 6 Corticorubral fibres (extrapyramidal) Subthalamic fasciculus (lenticulothalamic fibres)
Posterior thalamic radiations	• Optic radiations • Thalamo-occipital fibres	Parietopontine fibres Occipitopontine fibres Occipitotectal fibres

Arterial Supply of Internal Capsule

The following arteries supply the internal capsule. The **blood supply** of the **internal capsule** is variable but is commonly from:

   i. Small perforating branches of the middle cerebral artery.
  ii. Anterior cerebral artery.
 iii. Lateral lenticulostriate arteries.
  iv. Recurrent artery of Heubner respectively.

Telencephalon 3
Basal Nuclei of Cerebral Hemispheres

INTRODUCTION TO BASAL NUCLEI

The **basal nuclei** (*erroneously* termed basal ganglia) are a fundamental group of structures found deep within the cerebral hemispheres and the brainstem. In contrast to the cortical layer that lines the surface of the forebrain, the basal ganglia are a collection of distinct masses of grey matter lying deep in the brain not far from the junction of the thalamus (Fig. 15.1). They lie to the side of and surround the thalamus. The basal ganglia consist of left and right sides that are virtual mirror images of each other.

These structures are connected by strands of grey matter, traversing the anterior limb of the internal capsule and impart a striped appearance to this region, hence originated the term '**corpus striatum**'. Basal nuclei are strongly interconnected with the cerebral cortex, thalamus, and brainstem, as well as several other brain areas.

MAIN COMPONENTS OF BASAL NUCLEI

In terms of anatomy, the basal ganglia are divided into *four* distinct structures, depending on how superior or rostral they are (in other words depending on how close to the top of the head they are): Two of them, the **striatum** and the **pallidum**, are relatively large; the other two, the **substantia nigra** and the **subthalamic nucleus**, are smaller (Fig. 15.2). The subthalamic

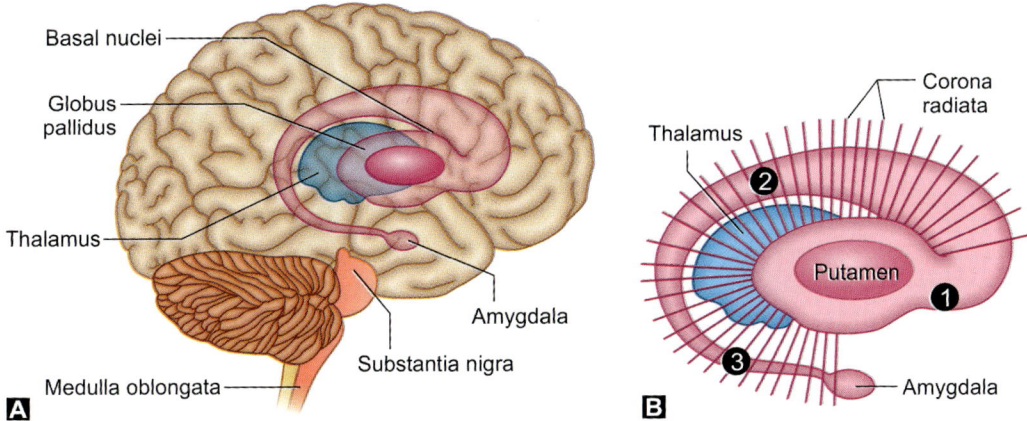

Fig. 15.1: A. Basal nuclei (ganglia) and related structures of the brain–lateral view. **B.** The numbers 1 to 3 indicate the head, body, and tail of the caudate nucleus, respectively. Notice that the corona radiata fibres descend between the putamen laterally and thalamus and head of caudate nucleus medially

nucleus and substantia nigra lie farther back (posteriorly) in the brain than the striatum and pallidum. The striatum (full name corpus striatum comprises the caudate nucleus and the outer putamen part of the lentiform nucleus. The pallidum (strictly speaking the globus pallidus, of the lentiform nucleus, which itself consists of an inner part (*globus pallidus internus*) and outer part (*globus pallidus externus*).

Each of these components has a complex internal anatomical and neurochemical organisation. The largest component, the striatum (dorsal and ventral), receives input from many brain areas beyond the basal ganglia, but only sends output to other components of the basal ganglia. The pallidum receives input from the striatum, and sends inhibitory output to a number of motor-related areas. The substantia nigra is the source of the striatal input of the neurotransmitter dopamine, which plays an important role in basal ganglia function. The subthalamic nucleus receives input mainly from the striatum and cerebral cortex, and projects to the globus pallidus.

The differences between striatum (caudate nucleus plus putamen of lentiform nucleus) and pallidum (globus pallidus) are summarized in Table 15.1.

Caudate Nucleus

The caudate nucleus is a comma-shaped mass of grey matter that is related to the floor of the anterior horn and body of the lateral ventricle, and also in the roof of the inferior horn of the lateral

Table 15.1: Differences between striatum and pallidum components of basal nuclei

Striatum (caudate nucleus plus putamen)	Pallidum (globus pallidus)
Pinkish colour	Pale colour
Permeated by delicate (fine) bundles of finely medullated or non-myelinated fibres	Encapsulated and traversed by numerous coarse heavily myelinated fibres
Neurons are of *two* kinds: small, multipolar, receptive; and large, multipolar efferent **20 : 1**	Majority of neurons are larger in size and multipolar
Dendritic spines ++++	Dendritic spines are rare
Synapses are axosomatic	Synapses are dendritic

ventricle (Chapter 16). It has *three* parts: (i) **Head** massive, rounded, projecting into the anterior horn of the lateral ventricle. (ii) **Body** is the portion arching upwards, backwards, and laterally. Its medial surface is related to thalamus, thalamostriate vein, and stria terminalis. The lateral surface is related to the fronto-occipital fasciculus above and corona radiata below. (iii) **Tail** of the caudate nucleus runs forwards in the roof of the inferior horn of the lateral ventricle.

Lentiform Nucleus

The lentiform (lens-shaped) nucleus is rather wedge-shaped. It lies deep to the insula with the *external capsule* separating it from the claustrum. The internal capsule covers it medially, separating it from the caudate nucleus anteriorly and the thalamus posteriorly. Its dark coloured lateral part, called the putamen is separated by the *external medullary lamina* from the medially placed paler portion called the *globus pallidus*. An *internal medullary lamina* divides the globus pallidus into external and internal segments. Along the anterior, superior and posterior margins, the lentiform nucleus is related to the fibres of the corona radiata which converge to the periphery of the corpus striatum. The fibres of the anterior commissure passing backwards into the temporal lobe groove its anteroinferior aspect. The lentiform nucleus lies above the inferior horn of the lateral ventricle from which it is separated by the sublentiform fibres of the internal capsule, tail of the caudate nucleus and the stria terminalis.

Corpus Striatum

The caudate nucleus and the putamen are similar in structure and contain, mainly, small multipolar inhibitory (GABAergic) cells. They also contain large cholinergic neurons. Both these parts are highly cellular, richly vascular and contain only finely myelinated nerve fibres.

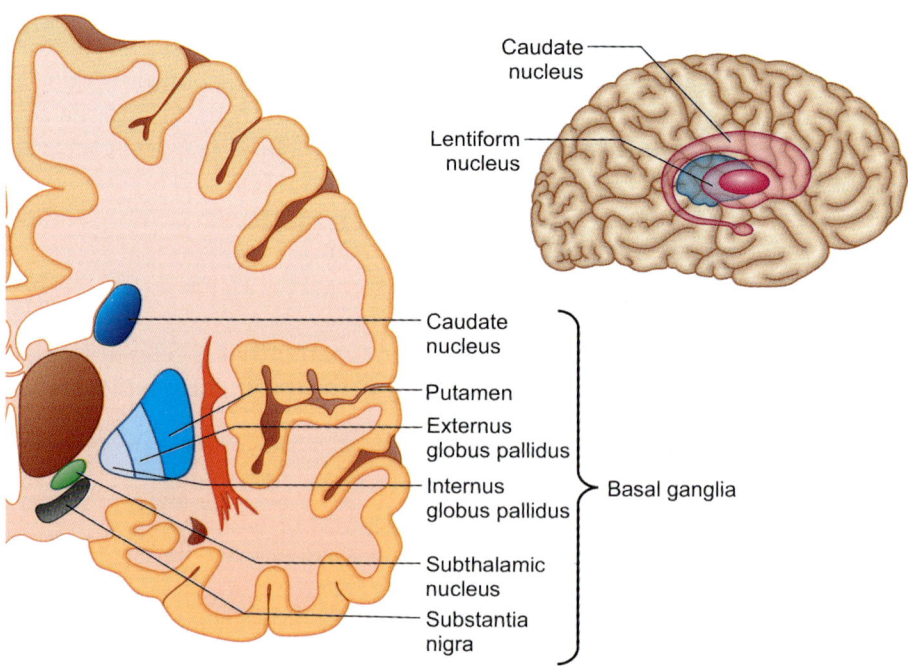

Fig. 15.2: Basal nuclei (ganglia) and related structures of the brain in a corona section through a cerebral hemispheres. All constituents of basal nuclei are identifiable

They appear pinkish grey in contrast to the pale colour of the globus pallidus which is traversed by numerous coarse and heavily myelinated nerve fibres, and contains a rather scattered population of large multipolar cells.

Connections of Corpus Striatum

The caudate and putamen (striatum), the main receiving stations, get afferents from the cerebral cortex, amygdala, thalamus and the substantia nigra. These parts project to the globus pallidus (pallidum) which gives origin to the main outflow pathways. These ultimately target the cerebral cortex (supplementary motor area, prefrontal area and cingulate cortex) and the superior colliculus.

Striatal Afferents

1. *Corticostriate fibres*: All parts of the cerebral cortex send fibres, mostly ipsilateral, to the striatum. The most profuse contributions arise from the frontal and parietal lobes, while the occipitotemporal areas contribute the least. Sensorimotor cortices project mainly to putamen. Fibres reach the striatum through both the external and the internal capsules and are predominantly excitatory.
2. *Amygdalostriate fibres:* These pass to the caudate nucleus through the stria terminalis.
3. *Thalamostriate fibres:* Thalamostriate fibres are derived from the intralaminar nuclei of thalamus. These conduct sensory and cognitive informations which are processed here and passed onto the supplementary motors cortex.
4. *Nigrostriate fibres:* The nigrostriatal fibres, which utilise dopamine as the neurotransmitter, pass from the pars compacta of the substantia nigra to the striatum. In Parkinson's disease, due to degeneration of these nigral neurons the striatum is deprived of its dopaminergic input.

Striatal Efferents

The majority of striatofugal fibres pass to both segments of the pallidum. Other fibres pass to the substantia nigra pars reticulata, which in turn projects to the superior colliculus and brainstem reticular formation.

Pallidum

The *pallidum* consists of a large structure called the globus pallidus (pale globe) together with a smaller ventral extension called the ventral pallidum. The globus pallidus appears as a single neural mass, but can be divided into two functionally distinct parts, called the internal (or medial) and external (lateral) segments, abbreviated GPi and GPe. Both segments contain primarily GABAergic neurons, which therefore have inhibitory effects on their targets (Fig. 15.3). The two segments participate in distinct neural circuits. The GPe receives input mainly from the striatum, and projects to the subthalamic nucleus. The GPi receives signals from the striatum via the 'direct' and 'indirect' pathways. Pallidal neurons operate using a disinhibition principle. These neurons fire at steady high rates in the absence of input, and signals from the striatum cause them to pause or reduce their rate of firing. Because pallidal neurons themselves have inhibitory effects on their targets, the net effect of striatal input to the pallidum is a reduction of the tonic inhibition exerted by pallidal cells on their targets (disinhibition) with an increased rate of firing in the targets.

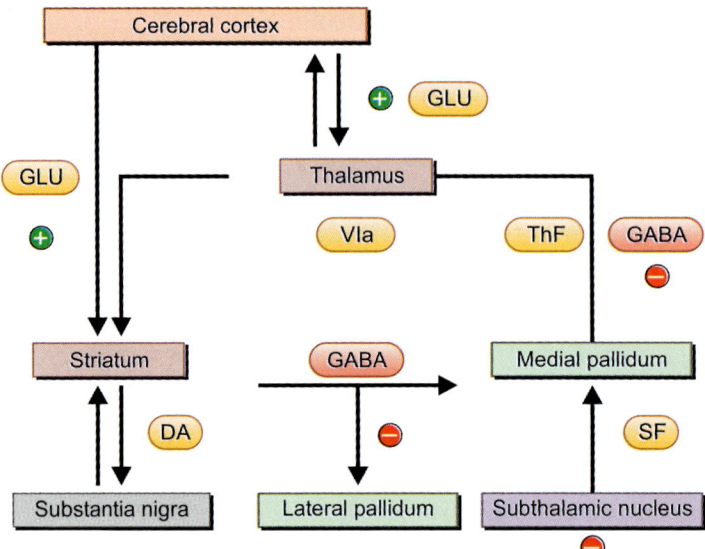

Fig. 15.3: Summary of principal connections of the basal nuclei and associated neurotransmitters. GLU = glutamate, DA = dopamine, GABA = gamma aminobutyric acid, SF = subthalamic fasciculus, ThF = thalamic fasciculus, (+) = excitatory neurons, and (–) = inhibitory neurons

Connections of Pallidum

Pallidal Afferents

The majority of these are derived from the striatum, but afferents are also received from the subthalamic nucleus (*subthalamic fasciculus*), substantia nigra and the intralaminar nuclei of thalamus.

Pallidal Efferents

1. The most important efferents are the *ansa lenticularis* and the *fasciculus lenticularis*. The ansa lenticularis loops round the ventral edge of the internal capsule before curving dorsally to reach the *prerubral field (Forel's field H)* in the rostral subthalamus. The fibres of the fasciculus lenticularis, on the other hand, course through the internal capsule to join the fibres of the ansa lenticularis and form the *thalamic fasciculus*. The thalamic fasciculus ends in the anterior division of the ventral lateral nucleus (VLa) of the thalamus and also the nucleus centromedianum. The nucleus VLa projects to the supplementary motor area involved in the mental planning of movements. The nucleus centromedianum projects to the sensoriomotor cortex. Other pallidal efferents project to the ventral anterior and dorso-medial nuclei of thalamus which in turn project to the prefrontal cortex.
2. Reciprocal connections between the subthalamic nucleus and the globus pallidus constitute the *subthalamic fasciculus* which passes through the internal capsule.

OTHER PARTS OF BASAL NUCLEI

Substantia Nigra

The substantia nigra is a midbrain grey matter portion of the basal ganglia that has two parts: the pars compacta (SNc) and the pars reticulata (SNr). *Substantia nigra* is Latin for 'black

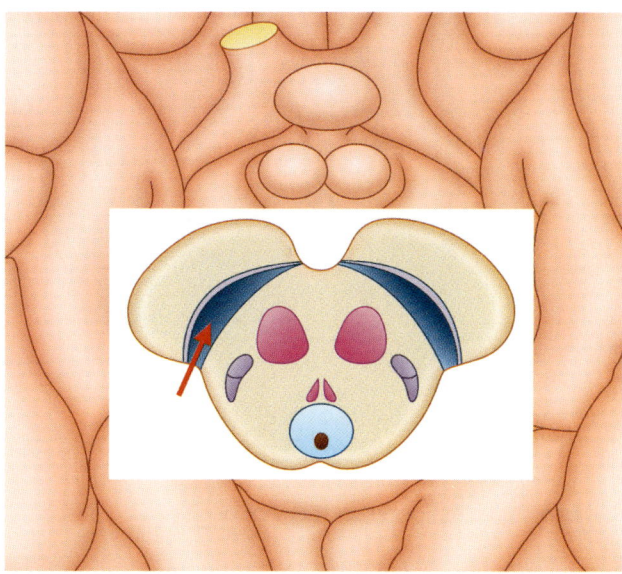

Fig. 15.4: Location of substantia nigra (red arrow) in a transverse section through midbrain superimposed at basal surface of a portion of brain

substance', reflecting the fact that parts of the substantia nigra appear darker than neighbouring areas due to high levels of neuromelanin in dopaminergic neurons. SNr often works in unison with GPi, and the SNr-GPi complex inhibits the thalamus. Substantia nigra pars compacta (SNc) however, produces the neurotransmitter dopamine, which is very significant in maintaining balance in the striatal pathway. The circuit portion below explains the role and circuit connections of each of the components of the basal ganglia.

Although the substantia nigra appears as a continuous band in brain sections (Fig. 15.4), anatomical studies have found that it actually consists of two parts with very different connections and functions: the pars compacta (SNpc) and the pars reticulata (SNpr). The pars compacta serves mainly as an output to the basal ganglia circuit, supplying the striatum with dopamine. The pars reticulata, though, serves mainly as an input, conveying signals from the basal ganglia to numerous other brain structures.

Subthalamic Nucleus

The subthalamic nucleus (Fig. 15.5) is a diencephalic grey matter portion of the basal ganglia, and the only portion of the ganglia that produces an excitatory neurotransmitter, glutamate. The role of the subthalamic nucleus is to stimulate the SNr-GPi complex and it is part of the indirect pathway. The subthalamic nucleus receives inhibitory input from external part of the globus pallidus and sends excitatory input to GPi.

ARTERIAL SUPPLY OF BASAL NUCLEI

The basal nuclei are supplied by the following arteries:
1. Striate branches of the middle cerebral artery.
2. Recurrent branch of the anterior cerebral artery.
3. Branches from the anterior choroidal artery.
4. Central branches from the posterior communicating artery.

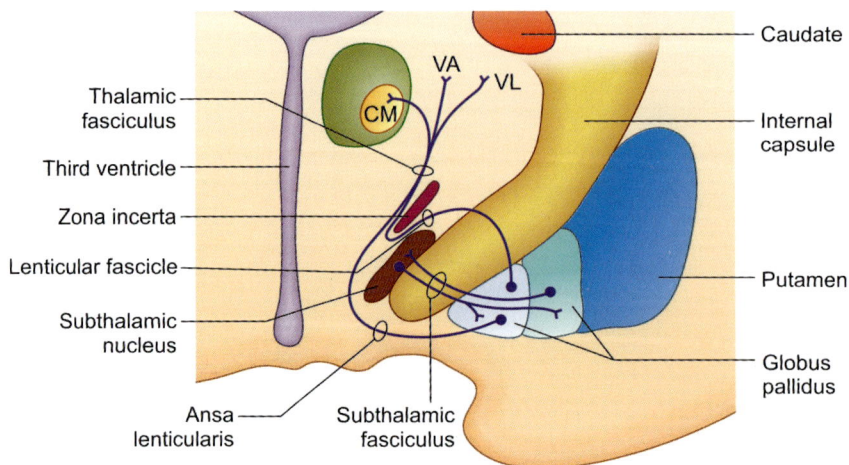

Fig. 15.5: Location of subthalamic nucleus and summary of principal connections of the basal ganglia and associated neurotransmitters.

The striate arteries (Fig. 15.6) include a medial and a lateral group of branches from the middle cerebral artery. Arteries of both the groups pierce the anterior perforated substance, supply the lentiform nucleus and pass through it and the internal capsule to end in the caudate nucleus. The recurrent branch of the anterior cerebral artery supplies the head of caudate nucleus. The branches of the anterior choroidal artery supply the posterior part of the body and the tail of caudate nucleus, the globus pallidus and the amygdaloid body. The central branches from the posterior communicating artery supply the medial most part of the globus pallidus.

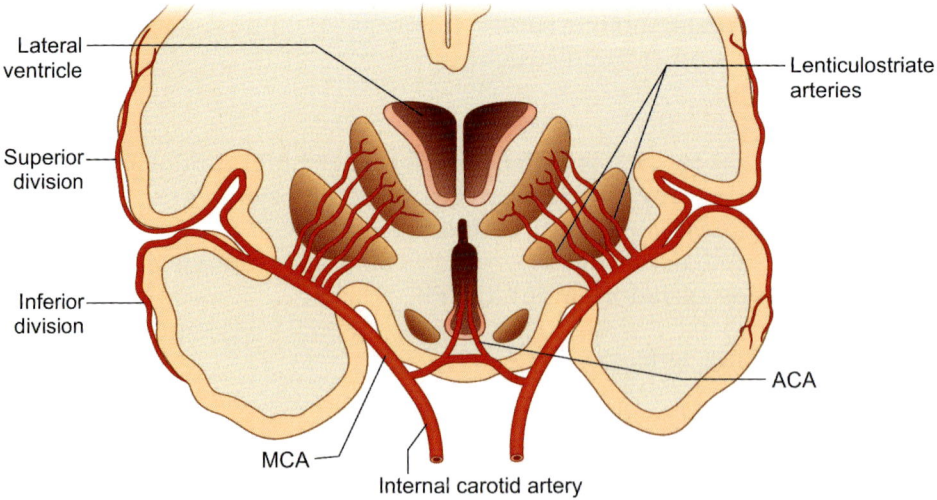

Fig. 15.6: Arterial supply of major parts of basal nuclei. ACA: anterior cerebral artery, MCA: middle cerebral artery

FUNCTIONS OF BASAL NUCLEI

The basal ganglia are associated with a variety of functions, including control of voluntary motor movements, procedural learning, habit learning, eye movements, cognition, and emotion. The basal ganglia primarily act for normal brain function and behaviour in action selection—in helping to decide which of several possible behaviours are to be executed at any given time. In more specific terms, the basal ganglia's primary function is likely to *control* and *regulate* activities of the motor and premotor cortical areas so that voluntary movements can be performed smoothly. Experimental studies show that the basal ganglia exert an inhibitory influence on a number of motor systems, and that a release of this inhibition permits a motor system to become active. The *'behaviour switching'* that takes place within the basal ganglia is influenced by the prefrontal cortex, which plays a key role in executive functions.

Motor Functions

Salient Points

1. Globus pallidus is active during rest and suppresses abnormal movements in the body.
2. The corpus striatum is active during voluntary movements.
3. The striatal activity is dependent on the dopaminergic input from the substantia nigra.

Detailed Account

Cortical excitation of the striatum results in the inhibition of the medial pallidal segment by striatal efferents. Inhibitory influences of the pallidal efferents on thalamus are removed and increased thalamocortical excitation of the motor cortex initiates voluntary movements. Additional cortical inputs to the striatum result in the inhibition of the lateral pallidal segment. Removal of the inhibition of the subthalamic nucleus and its increased activity excites the medial pallidal segment. The thalamus is inhibited. This indirect loop is considered to suppress involuntary movements. In Parkinson's disease there is loss of dopaminergic input to the striatum. Consequent loss of striatal inhibition of medial pallidum results in ultimate inhibition of thalamocortical activity and akinesia. In Huntington's disease, initial loss of striatal neurons projecting to the lateral pallidum would result in excessive inhibition of the subthalamic nucleus leading to a lack of suppression of abnormal movements, the end result being chorea. As the disease progresses, there is further loss of striatal neurons leading to disinhibition of the medial pallidal segment resulting in akinesia and rigidity.

Cognitive Functions

Through its projections to the prefrontal cortex (which are mediated through the dorsomedial nucleus of thalamus the corpus) striatum is involved in cognitive functions.

Motor Components

1. *Initiation of voluntary movements:* The basal ganglia play an important role in motor functions. The major output from the basal ganglia (through the ventral lateral anterior nucleus of thalamus) is directed to the supplementary motor cortex. Through these projections the motor cortex receives the drive for the initiation of movements. Disorders of the basal ganglia are characterised by difficulties in the initiation of voluntary movements (bradykinesia).
2. *Control of muscle tone:* Efferents from the basal nuclei through the substantia nigra and brainstem reticular formation exercise control over the spinal cord gamma efferent neurons which innervate the intrafusal fibres in the muscle spindles. Efferents from the spindles

influence the alpha motor neurons and thus, the extrafusal muscle tone is controlled. Disorders of basal ganglia manifest as increased muscle tone and rigidity.

3. *Suppression of involuntary movements:* A normally functioning corpus striatum ensures an evenly balanced resting muscle tone between the synergists and the antagonists. The normal functioning is guaranteed by a balance between the inhibitory (dopaminergic) and excitatory (cholinergic) neurons of the straitum. Reduced activity of the dopaminergic pathways leads to oscillatory bursts of activity in the ventrolateral anterior (VLA) thalamic neurons. The latter generate rhythmical activity in the cortical motor centres. This is responsible for tremors and other abnormal involuntary movements (dyskinesias) which characterise diseases of the corpus striatum, e.g. Parkinson's disease and Huntington's chorea. The dyskinesias include: (i) *choreiform movement*, which are brisk, jerky and non-repetitive movements of axial or proximal limb musculature, (ii) *athetoid movements*, which are slow and writhing movements involving the distal limb musculature, and (iii) *ballism* which are violent flinging type of limb movements involving shoulder or hip muscles.

CLINICAL DISORDERS AFFECTING BASAL NUCLEI

The dysfunction involving constituents of basal nuclei results in a wide range of neurological conditions including disorders of behaviour control and movement. Those of behaviour include obsessive–compulsive disorder, and addiction. Huntington's disease, primarily involves damage to the striatum, for normal brain function and behaviour dystonia, and more rarely hemiballismus. The basal nuclei have a limbic sector whose components are assigned distinct names. There is considerable evidence that this limbic part plays a central role in reward learning that uses the neurotransmitter dopamine. A number of highly addictive drugs, including cocaine, amphetamine, and nicotine, are thought to work by increasing the efficacy of this dopamine signal.

1. **Parkinson's disease (paralysis agitans):** It is a degenerative motor disorder characterised by rigidity, tremors, bradykinesia (slowness of movements) and loss of automatic associated movements, such as arm swinging. Neuronal degeneration in the substantia nigra leading to a dysfunction of the nigrostriatal dopaminergic system is responsible for the disease (Fig. 15.7). Repetitive head injuries sustained by boxers may result in progressive

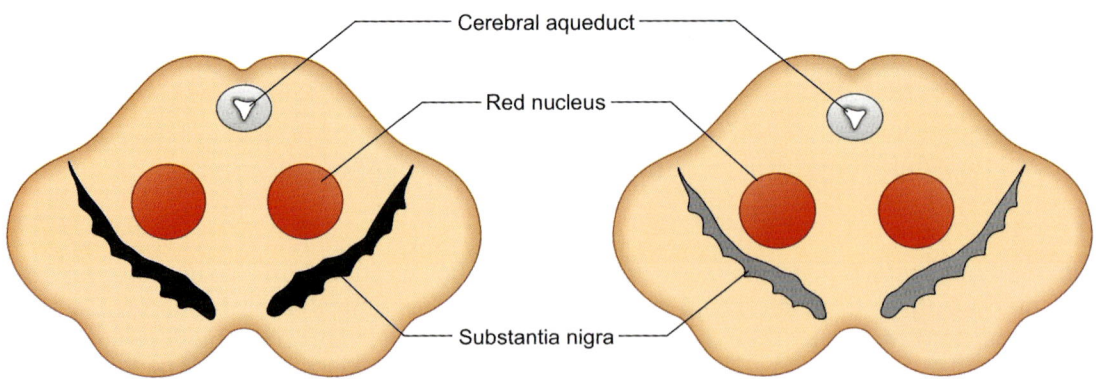

A Non-Parkinson's (normal brain)   **B** Parkinson's (brain with lesion)

Fig. 15.7A and B: The substantia nigra in a normal (non-Parkinson's) and a patient suffering with Parkinson's disease. Notice reduction in the colour of the substantia which is less or almost colourless in the diseased condition

parkinsonism. L-dopa, a dopamine precursor is a useful drug but it helps only as long as there are enough nigral neurons left to convert it into dopamine.

2. **Sydenham's chorea (St. Vitus'dance):** It is a rare childhood disease occurring mostly in girls. There are brisk, jerky and purposeless movements of the proximal limb muscles. Minute haemorrhages are seen in the corpus striatum.

3. **Huntington's chorea:** This is a rare hereditary disorder characterised by degeneration of GABA and acetylcholine utilising neurons in the striatum. The person suffers from widespread, arrhythmic, involuntary movements of the choreiform type.

4. **Hemiballismus:** This is most commonly caused by vascular lesions of the subthalamic nucleus. There are violent flinging types of movements of the extremities on the opposite side of the body.

5. **Extrapyramidal symptoms of antipsychotic drugs:** Antipsychotic drugs such as the phenothiazines, cause dopamine receptor blockade. This causes drug-induced parkinsonism.

6. **Wilson's disease:** It is a familial disorder with a defect of copper metabolism. High content of copper causes toxic degeneration of the basal ganglia, producing rigidity, tremors and involuntary movements. Manganese and prolonged treatment with reserpine also produce Parkinson like symptoms.

Therapeutic ablation of the ventrolateral thalamus has helped in alleviating contralateral rigidity and tremors in disease conditions.

16

Telencephalon 4
Lateral Ventricles and Choroid Plexuses

- Lateral Ventricles
  - Central part or body
  - Anterior or frontal horn
  - Posterior or occipital horn
  - Inferior or temporal horn
- Choroid Plexuses of Lateral Ventricles

- Choroid Fissure
  - Boundaries of the choroid fissure
- Radiological Procedures Related to Lateral Ventricles
  - Pneumoencephalography
  - Ventriculography
  - CT scan and magnetic resonance imaging (MRI)
  - Age changes

The forebrain consists of three cavities: Two lateral ventricles, one in each cerebral hemisphere; and one midline cavity in the diencephalon—the third ventricle. Each lateral ventricle communicates with the cavity of the third ventricle through the interventricular foramen (of **Monro**); the third ventricle communicates through the aqueduct of Sylvius (in the midbrain) to the cranial end of the fourth ventricle—a rhomboidal tented cavity of the hindbrain (Fig. 16.1).

LATERAL VENTRICLES

The two lateral ventricles are cavities of the telencephalon and lie within the lower and medial parts of the cerebral hemispheres. They are lined with ependyma and are completely closed cavities except for the *interventricular foramina (of Monro)* through which they communicate with the third ventricle. Each lateral ventricle consists of a *body* (central part) and three *horns: anterior, posterior,* and *inferior.* The anterior horn, central part and the inferior horn of lateral ventricle present a continuous C-shaped curve while the posterior horn, developing later, projects backwards from the junction of the central part with the inferior horn (Figs 16.1 and 16.2).

Central Part or Body

It lies mainly within the parietal lobe of the cerebral hemisphere and extends from the interventricular foramen to the level of splenium of corpus callosum. It is triangular in cross-section and has a roof, a floor and a medial wall (Fig. 16.3).

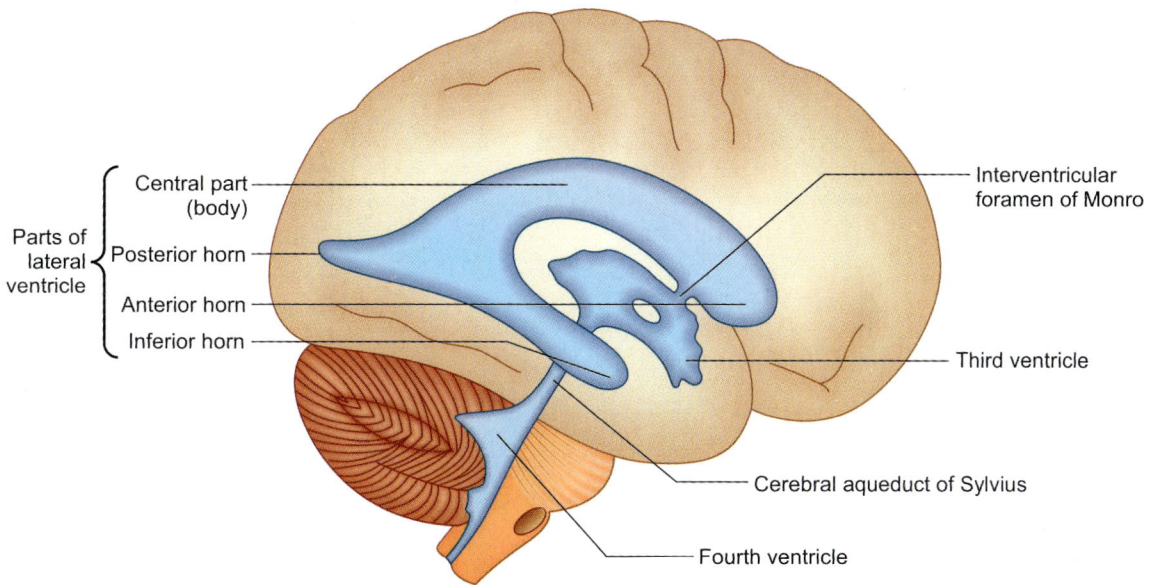

Fig. 16.1: Surface projection of the ventricles on the brain—left lateral view (*Courtesy:* Nafis Ahmad Faruqi)

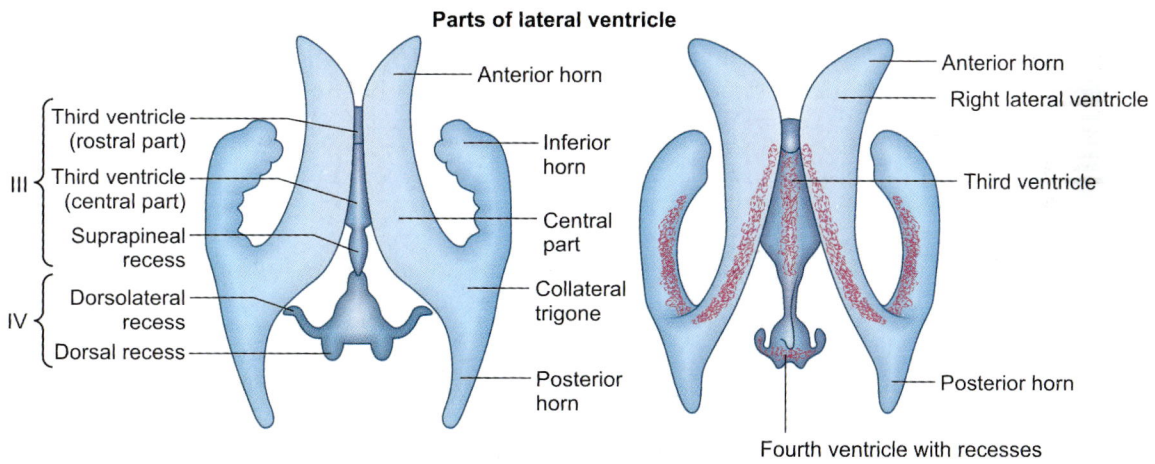

Fig. 16.2: Ventricles of the brain viewed from above. The right diagram shows choroid plexuses also

Roof: Formed by the inferior surface of the trunk of corpus callosum.

Floor: Formed by the following from the medial to lateral:
1. Thalamus (lateral part of upper surface).
2. Thalamostriate vein.
3. Stria terminalis.
4. Body of caudate nucleus.

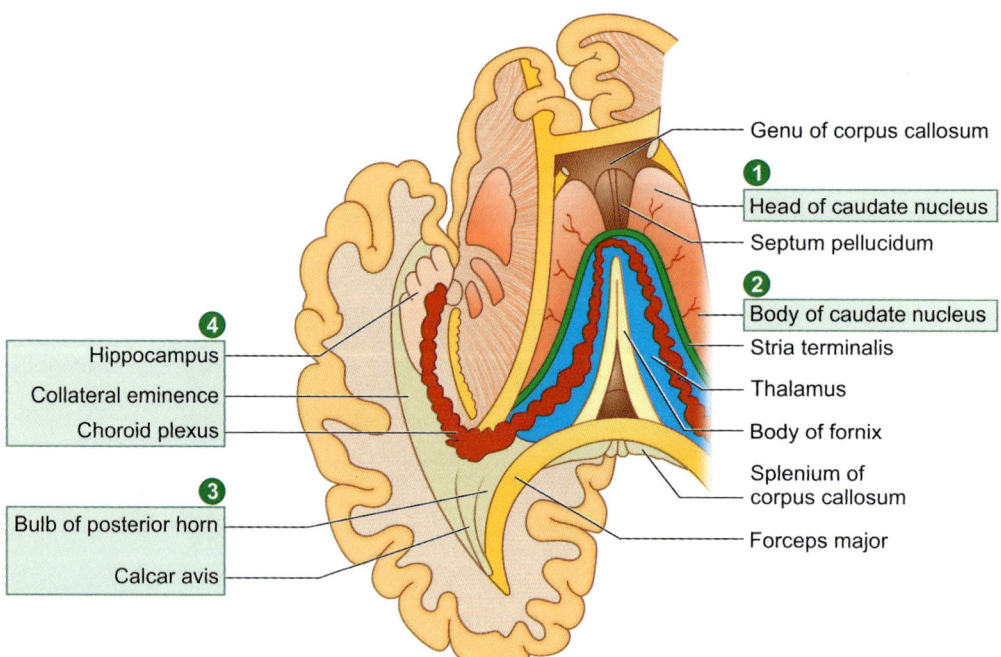

Fig. 16.3: A dissection of cerebrum to expose the central part or body of lateral ventricles from above. The numbers 1 to 4 indicate: anterior horn, body, posterior horn, and temporal horn of the lateral ventricle

Medial wall: Formed by the septum pellucidum with the fornix attached to its lower margin. Posteriorly, where the septum ends, the fornix is directly applied to the corpus callosum and the medial wall is considerably reduced in height.

Anterior or Frontal Horn

It extends into the frontal lobe from the level of the interventricular foramen to the genu of corpus callosum. The cavity has a roof, floor and a medial wall (Fig. 16.4).

Roof: Formed by the inferior surface of the trunk of corpus callosum.

Floor: Formed by the:
1. Upper surface of the rostrum of corpus callosum medially.
2. Head of the caudate nucleus laterally.

Medial wall: Formed by the septum pellucidum.

Posterior or Occipital Horn

It extends backwards for a variable distance into the occipital lobe. It has a roof and lateral and medial walls (Fig. 16.5).

Roof and lateral wall: The fibres of the tapetum of corpus callosum form the roof as well as the lateral wall. Lateral to the tapetum lies the optic radiation and further laterally the inferior longitudinal fasciculus.

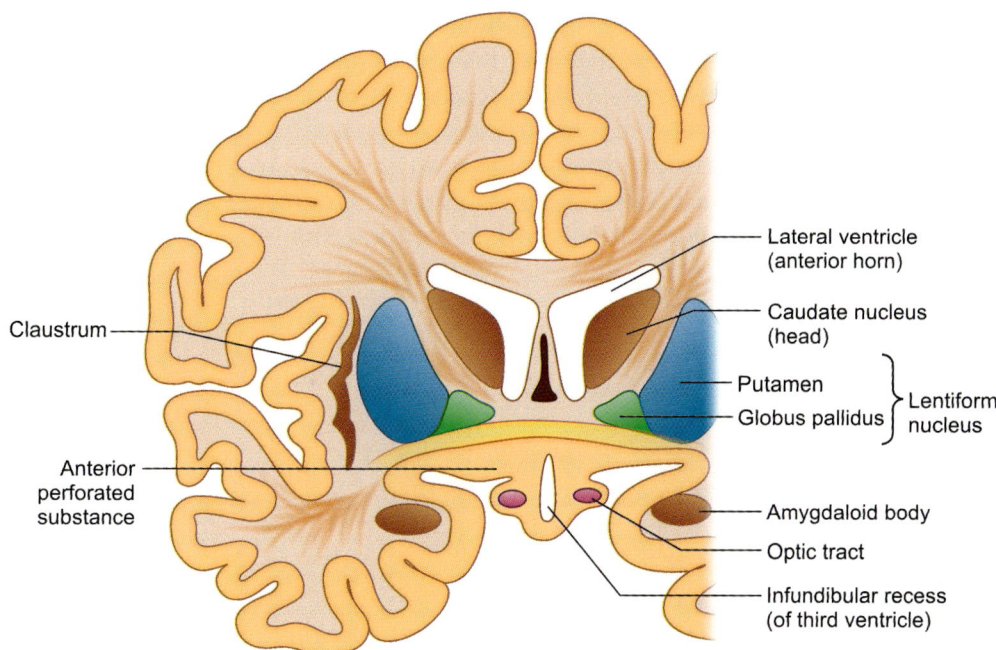

Fig. 16.4: Coronal section through the cerebral hemispheres opposite the anterior horns of the lateral ventricle (*Courtesy:* Nafis Ahmad Faruqi)

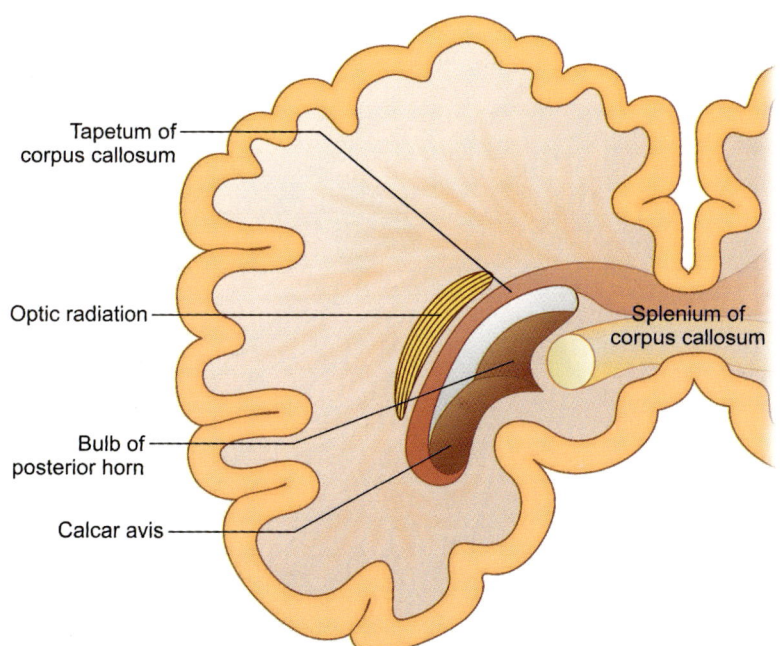

Fig. 16.5: Coronal section of cerebral hemisphere through the posterior horn of the lateral ventricle

Medial wall: The medial wall presents the following two elevations:
1. *Above: Bulb of the posterior horn* produced by the *forceps major.*
2. *Below: Calcar avis* produced by the calcarine sulcus.

Inferior or Temporal Horn

The inferior horn (Fig. 16.6) runs downwards and forwards into the temporal lobe, reaching almost up to the amygdaloid body. It is the direct continuation of the central part of lateral ventricle so that the caudate nucleus and stria terminalis, seen in the floor of the central part continue into the roof of the inferior horn. The fornix seen in the central part is the continuation of the fimbria of the inferior horn. The inferior horn has a roof, a lateral wall and a floor.

Roof: From medial to lateral side it presents:
1. *Stria* terminalis (from amygdala)
2. *Tail* of *caudate nucleus*
3. *Tapetum* of the corpus callosum.

Lateral wall: The tapetum forms the lateral wall also.

Floor: It is formed by the following:
1. The *hippocampus (Ammon's horn):* This bulging structure expands anteriorly to form the *pes hippocampi.* Its fibres form a white layer called the *alveus* on its surface and collect into the *fimbria* lying along its medial border.
2. The *collateral eminence:* It is produced by the collateral sulcus. Posteriorly it widens to form the *collateral trigone* at the junction of the inferior and posterior horns.

CHOROID PLEXUSES OF LATERAL VENTRICLES

The choroid plexus is a highly vascular and fringed structure responsible for the secretion of the cerebrospinal fluid. It is formed by a fold of pia mater containing a plexus of blood vessels

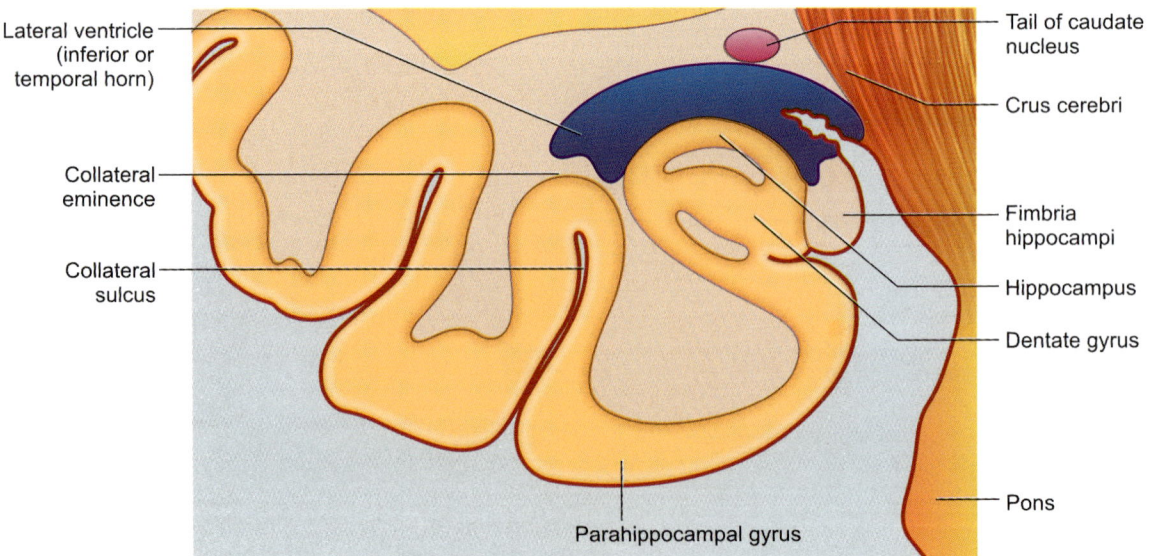

Fig. 16.6: Coronal section of cerebral hemisphere through the inferior horn of the lateral ventricle

and covered by the ventricular ependyma. Microvilli are present on the free surface of the ependymal cells. The choroid plexus is present only in the central part and the inferior horn of lateral ventricle (Fig. 16.2). The plexus in the central part lies within the lateral margin of the tela choroidea of third ventricle, which is tucked into the lateral ventricle through the choroid fissure. Anteriorly the choroid plexus passes through the interventricular foramen to become continuous with the choroid plexus of the third ventricle. Posteriorly it is continuous with the plexus present in the inferior horn. The *arteries* for the choroid plexus are derived from the, anterior choroidal branches of the internal carotid and the posterior choroidal branches of the posterior cerebral arteries. These vessels enter the choroid plexus through the choroid fissure of the inferior horn of lateral ventricle.

CHOROID FISSURE

The choroid fissure is a C-shaped developmental cleft present on the medial aspect of the cerebral hemisphere. It leads into the central part and inferior horn of the lateral ventricle. The choroid plexus projects into the lateral ventricle through the fissure. It is the first cerebral groove to appear during development and is visible during the eighth embryonic week.

No nervous tissue develops in the region of this linear groove and, therefore, the pia mater is in direct contact with the ventricular ependyma. Subsequently a fold of pia mater, containing vessels, invaginates into the ventricular cavity to form the choroid plexus.

Boundaries of the Choroid Fissure

The choroid fissure lies in tile concavity of the C-shaped curve of the fornix and the fimbria. Its boundaries are:
1. In the central part of the lateral ventricle:
   a. *Superiorly*—fornix.
   b. *Inferiorly*—thalamus.
2. In the inferior horn:
   a. *Superiorly*—stria terminalis.
   b. *Inferiorly*—fimbria hippocampi.

RADIOLOGICAL PROCEDURES RELATED TO LATERAL VENTRICLES

The lateral ventricles can be demonstrated radiologically in the living by introducing air (pneumoencephalography) or a radio-opaque substance into the ventricles (ventriculography) or else by the newer imaging techniques.

Pneumoencephalography

Pneumoencephalography was a common medical procedure in which most of the cerebrospinal fluid was drained from around the brain by means of a lumbar puncture and replaced with air, oxygen, or helium to allow the structure of the brain to show up more clearly on an X-ray image. In this procedure, air (which is radiolucent) is introduced through the lumbar puncture, in the sitting position, rises in the subarachnoid space to reach the cerebello-medullary cistern. It finds its way through the foramina of Magendie and Luschka into the fourth ventricle and thereafter the other ventricles of the brain. The dark shadows of air in the ventricles are outlined in an X-ray (Fig. 16.7). Newer techniques such as MRI and CT make pneumoencephalography obsolete.

Ventriculography

In this procedure a radio-opaque dye is injected directly into the lateral ventricle. A needle introduced through a trephine hole in the skull enters the inferior horn in the temporal lobe. An amount of CSF is withdrawn and an equivalent amount of the radio-opaque dye is injected. The ventricle presents a radio-opaque shadow.

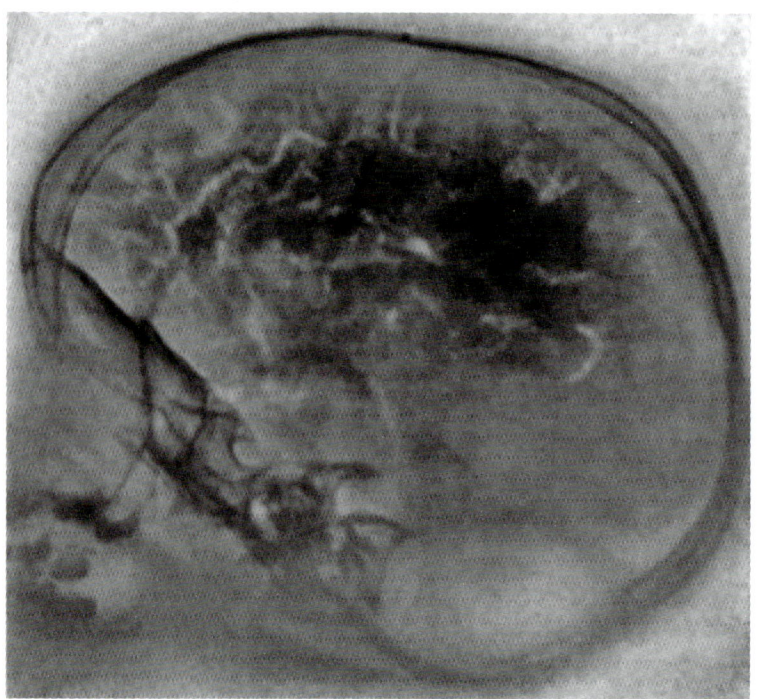

Fig. 16.7: Pneumoencephalography (MRI and CT make it obsolete)

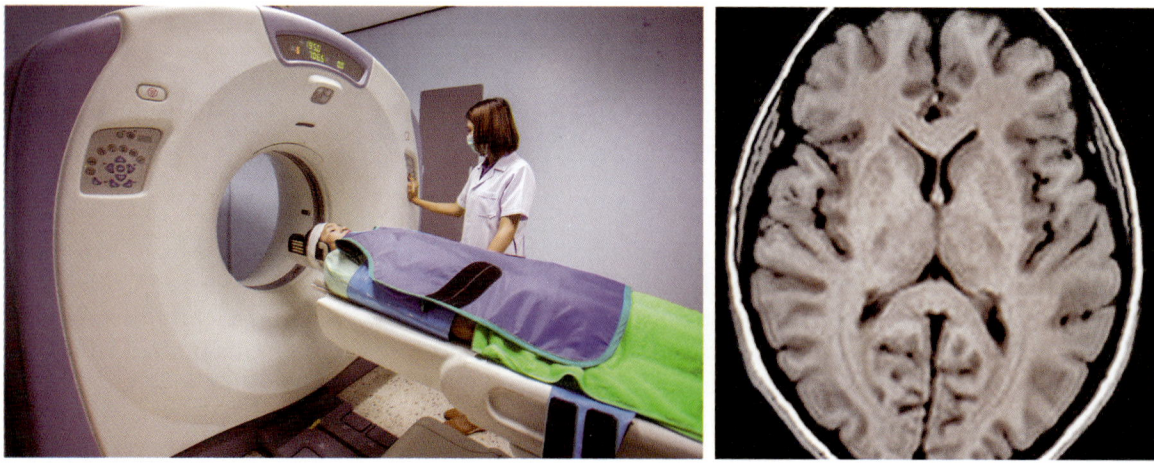

Fig. 16.8: Magnetic resonance imaging (MRI) and CT of brain are newer techniques that have made the older procedure like pneumoencephalography obsolete

CT-Scan and Magnetic Resonance Imaging (MRI)

Visualisation of the ventricles can be more conveniently and efficiently accomplished by computerised tomography (CT-scan) and MRI, which are noninvasive procedures (Fig. 16.8).

Age Changes

In the young, the walls of the lateral ventricle are almost in apposition so that the cavity is a mere cleft. With increasing age the cavity expands and attains considerable size. Neuronal destruction around the ventricular cavity (cortical atrophy) is responsible for the large-sized ventricle in the elderly people.

Meninges of Central Nervous System and Cerebrospinal Fluid

- Dura Mater
  - Cranial or cerebral dura mater
  - Dural septa (folds)
  - Dural venous sinuses
  - Spinal dura mater
- Arachnoid Mater
  - Cerebral arachnoid mater
  - Spinal arachnoid mater
- Pia Mater
  - Cerebral pia mater
  - Spinal pia mater
- Subarachnoid Space and Cisterns
  - Subarachnoid cisterns
- Cerebrospinal Fluid (CSF)
- Clinical Significance
  - Distribution of CSF
  - Collection of CSF

The brain and the spinal cord both are soft in consistency and are protected by *three* fibrous envelopes or *meninges* (singular, meninx = membrane). From without inwards these are the *dura mater, arachnoid m*ater and the *pia mater* (Fig. 17.1). The dura mater is the outer, thick, tough and opaque membrane (dura = tough; mater = mother). It is also called the *pachymeninx* (pachy = thick) and is mesodermal in origin. The arachnoid is intermediate in position. It is thin, transparent and spider-web like (arachnoid = spider-web). Both the dura and the arachnoid mater invest the brain and spinal cord loosely. The pia mater (pia = tender, or affectionate) is the inner membrane. It forms a close investment for the brain and the spinal cord and also dips into the fissures and sulci on their surfaces. Blood vessels form a plexus in the pia mater and carry pial sheaths as they enter the brain and the spinal cord. The arachnoid and pia together constitute the leptomeninges (lepto = thin). These are ectodermal in origin and are derived from the neural crest.

DURA MATER

Cranial or Cerebral Dura Mater

The cerebral dura mater is made up of an outer endosteal and inner meningeal layers. These two layers are fused except where they separate to enclose venous sinuses and also where the

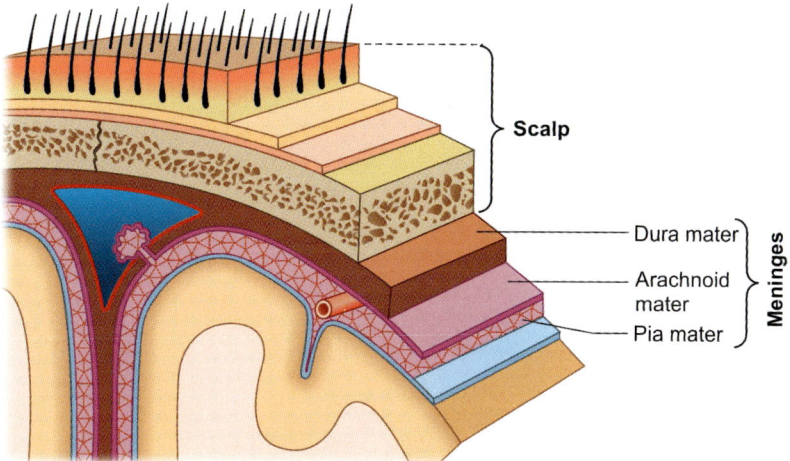

Fig. 17.1: Coronal section through the skull showing the meninges of the brain. Notice these form a 'PAD' from within out. Above the outermost and toughest dural layers are the layers of the scalp

inner layer is folded to form the dural septa. The dura mater can be stripped off from the cranial vault, e.g. when an extradural haematoma is formed between the bone and dura. It is, however, adherent to the bones at the base of the skull. The branches of the middle meningeal artery and the accompanying veins stand out in relief on the external surface of the dura mater. They groove the skull and are torn conditions of fracture. The blood escapes in the extradural space to form a haematoma.

Dural Septa (folds)

The dura mater gives septa, which divide the cranial cavity into compartments to lodge different parts of the brain. The septa restrict displacement of brain within the skull. The four dural septa are the *falx cerebri, tentorium cerebelli, falx cerebelli* and the *diaphragma sellae* (Fig. 17.2).

The *falx cerebri* is sickle-shaped and is sagittally oriented. It dips into the longitudinal cerebral fissure between the two cerebral hemispheres. Narrow in front where it is attached to the crista galli of the ethmoid bone, it broadens posteriorly to be attached to the upper surface of the tentorium cerebelli. Its outer attached border encloses the *superior sagittal sinus;* the inner (inferior) free border contains the *inferior sagittal sinus.* The *straight sinus* runs along its line of attachment to the tentorium cerebelli.

The *tentorium cerebelli* forms a sloping roof for the posterior cranial fossa. Along its outer attached border lie the *transverse* and the *superior petrosal sinuses.* Its inner free border forms the *tentorial notch,* through which passes the midbrain. The tentorium cerebelli supports the occipital lobes of the cerebral hemispheres and separates them from the cerebellar hemispheres.

The *falx cerebelli* is a small, sickle-shaped dural fold attached to the internal occipital crest. It projects into the cerebellar vallecula.

The **diaphragma sellae** is a small circular fold roofing over the pituitary fossa. It has a hole in its centre for the passage of the stalk of the pituitary body.

Nerve Supply

Branches of the trigeminal nerve supply supratentorial dura while the upper three cervical nerves supply the dura in the posterior cranial fossa. Pain arising in the former is referred to forehead. Pain from the latter goes to the occiput.

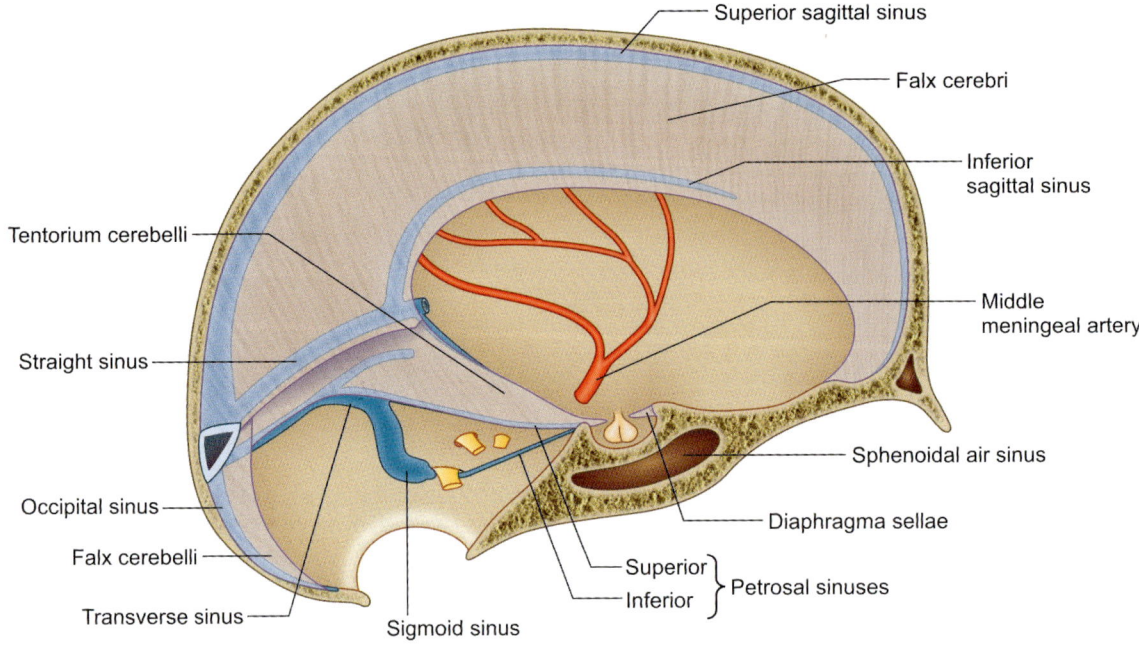

Fig. 17.2: Sagittal section through the skull showing the dural septa and associated venous sinuses

Dural Venous Sinuses

These drain blood from the brain and the cranial bones and are both paired and unpaired (Fig. 17.3). The *unpaired venous sinuses* include: (1) superior sagittal, (2) inferior sagittal, (3) straight, and (4) occipital sinus.

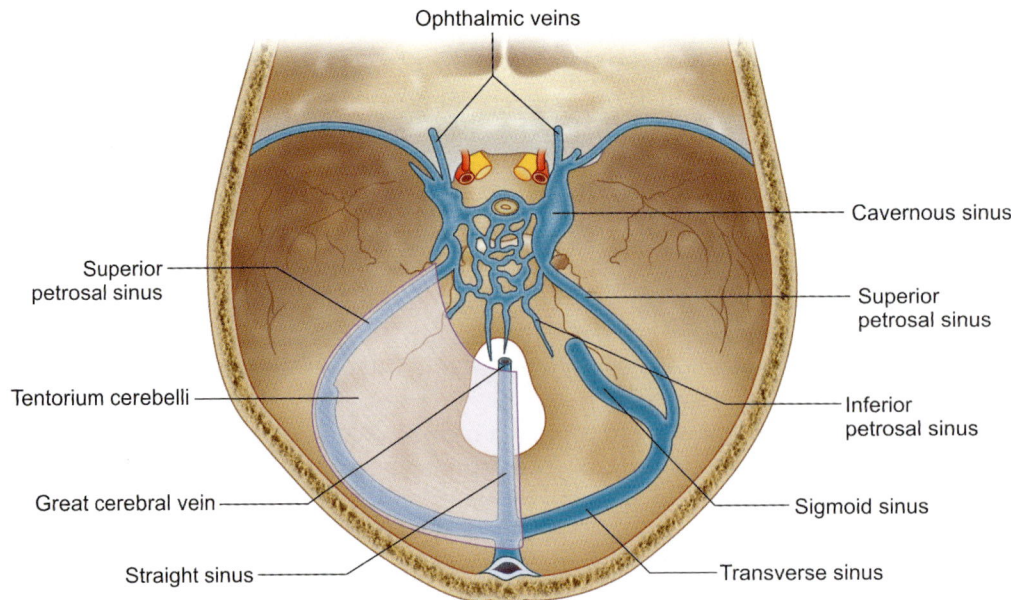

Fig. 17.3: Interior of the cranium showing some of the dural venous sinuses

The *paired sinuses* are: (1) sphenoparietal, (2) cavernous, (3) superior petrosal, (4) inferior petrosal, (5) transverse, and (6) the sigmoid sinuses.

1. The **Sphenoparietal sinus** lies along the lesser wing of sphenoid bone and drains into the cavernous sinus.
2. The **cavernous sinus** lies by the side of the body of the sphenoid and drains through the superior petrosal sinus into the sigmoid sinus and through the inferior petrosal sinus directly into the internal jugular vein. The internal carotid artery, with the abducens nerve (inferolateral to it) passes through the sinus. The oculomotor, trochlear, ophthalmic and maxillary nerves run in the lateral wall of the sinus. Infections reaching the sinus from nose or paranasal sinuses cause 'cavernous sinus thrombosis' which presents with pain in the eye and involvement of associated cranial nerves.
3. The **superior petrosal sinus** lies along the superior border of the petrous temporal bone.
4. The **inferior petrosal sinus** lies in the groove between the petrous temporal bone and the clivus.
5. The **transverse sinuses** lie along the attached margin of the tentorium cerebelli. The right transverse sinus is usually a continuation of the superior sagittal sinus while the left one is a continuation of the straight sinus. Both transverse sinuses continue into the sigmoid sinuses.
6. The **sigmoid sinus** runs a S-shaped course posterior to the base of the petrous temporal bone and continues as the internal jugular vein.

Spinal Dura Mater

It is a continuation of the meningeal layer of cerebral dura mater into the vertebral canal. It envelops the spinal cord and the cauda equina and ends inferiorly opposite the second sacral vertebra. The spinal dura mater represents only the inner, or meningeal, layer of the cerebral dura; the outer, or endosteal layer ceases at the margins of the foramen magnum. An interval, termed the *extradural space* separates the spinal dura with the periosteum lining the vertebral canal where the spinal cord lies.

Contents of extradural space are: (i) areolar tissue with some quantity of fat that extends laterally on each side for a short distance through the intervertebral foramina. This space is known to clinicians as the *epidural space*, and (ii) plexus of veins.

Between the spinal dura mater and the arachnoid mater lies another potential space called the subdural space. This space contains a film of serous fluid avoiding friction between the adjacent membranes.

ARACHNOID MATER

Cerebral Arachnoid Mater

The cerebral arachnoid mater is a thin, transparent and loose investment that does not dip into the fissures of the brain except the longitudinal cerebral fissure.

The **arachnoid granulations** are granular masses derived from the arachnoid mater. They pierce the dura mater to protrude into the superior sagittal sinus and its lateral extensions (Fig. 17.4). In early life these are microscopic projections called the *arachnoid villi*. The subarachnoid space containing the CSF extends into them. The arachnoid granulations and the villi help in the drainage of the CSF into the venous sinuses. Meningiomas are tumours arising from the arachnoid villi. They most commonly occur along the superior sagittal sinus.

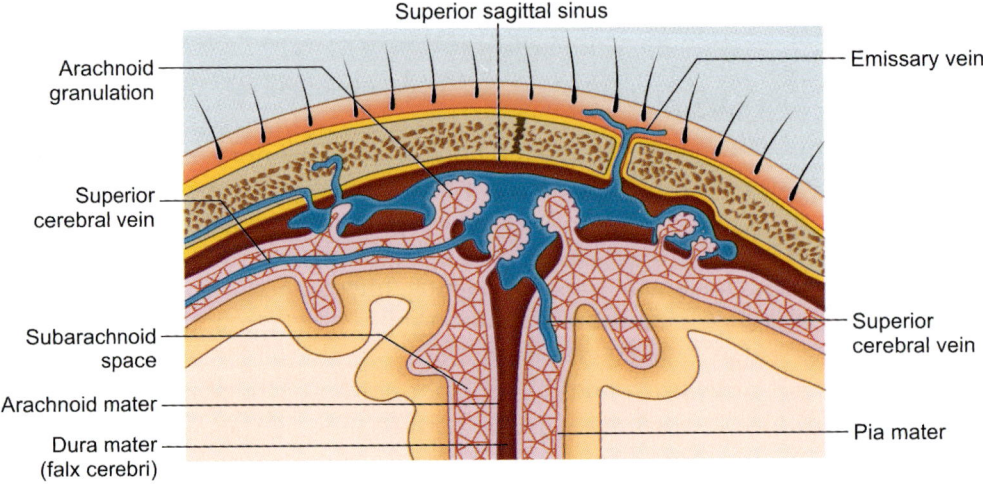

Fig. 17.4: A coronal section showing arachnoid granulations in the superior sagittal sinus

Spinal Arachnoid Mater

It is the continuation of the cerebral arachnoid mater and extends from the foramen magnum to the level of the second sacral vertebra (Figs 17.5 and 17.6).

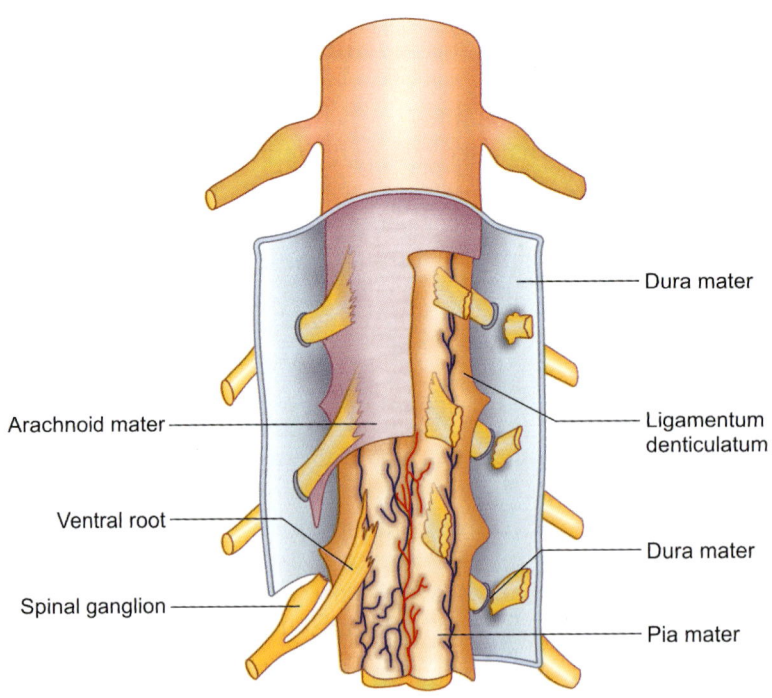

Fig. 17.5: Meninges of the spinal cord and the ligamentum denticulatum

PIA MATER

Cerebral Pia Mater

The cerebral pia mater invests the brain closely, covering its convolutions and dipping into the fissures and sulci. A fold of pia mater invaginates through the transverse cerebral fissure, below the splenium of the corpus callosum. It forms the *tela choroidea of the third ventricle.* Vascular fringes project from this fold into the third and the lateral ventricles to form their *choroid plexuses.*

Another fold of pia mater invaginates between the cerebellum and the dorsal aspect of the medulla oblongata to form the *tela choroidea of the fourth ventricle.* Choroid plexuses project from this fold into the cavity of fourth ventricle.

The choroid plexuses secrete cerebrospinal fluid that fills the ventricles of the brain and also escapes out to fill the subarachnoid spaces.

Spinal Pia Mater

The spinal pia mater invests the spinal cord closely and dips into its anterior median fissure. Inferiorly, from the lower end of the spinal cord it extends as the thread-like *filum terminale.* The filum anchors the spinal cord to the back of coccyx. A sheet-like extension of pia mater from either side of spinal cord and having tooth-like projections along its lateral margin forms the *ligamentum denticulatum* (Fig. 17.5). It has 21 pairs of teeth, which pierce the arachnoid mater to be attached to the dura mater. The ligamentum denticulatum serves to suspend the spinal cord in the subarachnoid space.

SUBARACHNOID SPACE AND CISTERNS

The subarachnoid space lying between the arachnoid and the pia mater contains cerebrospinal fluid. The space is traversed by the subarachnoid trabeculae and the large blood vessels of the brain. It is greatly reduced over the cerebral gyri but angular intervals exist opposite the sulci. At places, the space is greatly enlarged to from the *subarachnoid cisterns.* The spinal subarachnoid space is wider and devoid of the subarachnoid trabeculae. Inferiorly, from the second lumbar to the second sacral vertebra, it is most extensive and forms the *lumbar cistern.*

Subarachnoid Cisterns

Some of the important subarachnoid cisterns (Fig. 17.7) are given below:
1. *Cerebellomedullary cistern (cisterna magna):* It lies between the cerebellum and the dorsal aspect of the medulla oblongata. The fourth ventricle opens into it through its dorsal aperture *(foramen of Magendie).* A sample of CSF can be collected by a needle introduced into this cistern (*cisternal puncture*).
2. *Pontine cistern:* It lies on the ventral aspect of the pons and lodges the basilar artery. It communicates dorsally with the cerebellomedullary cistern, superiorly with the interpeduncular cistern and inferiorly with the spinal subarachnoid space.
3. *Interpeduncular cistern:* It is formed due to the arachnoid mater stretching between the temporal lobes of the two sides. It lodges the circulus arteriosus.
4. *Cistern of great cerebral vein (cisterna ambiens* or *superior cistern):* It is formed due to the arachnoid bridging the interval between the splenium of the corpus callosum and the upper surface of the cerebellum. It lies dorsal to the midbrain and lodges the pineal gland and the great cerebral vein.

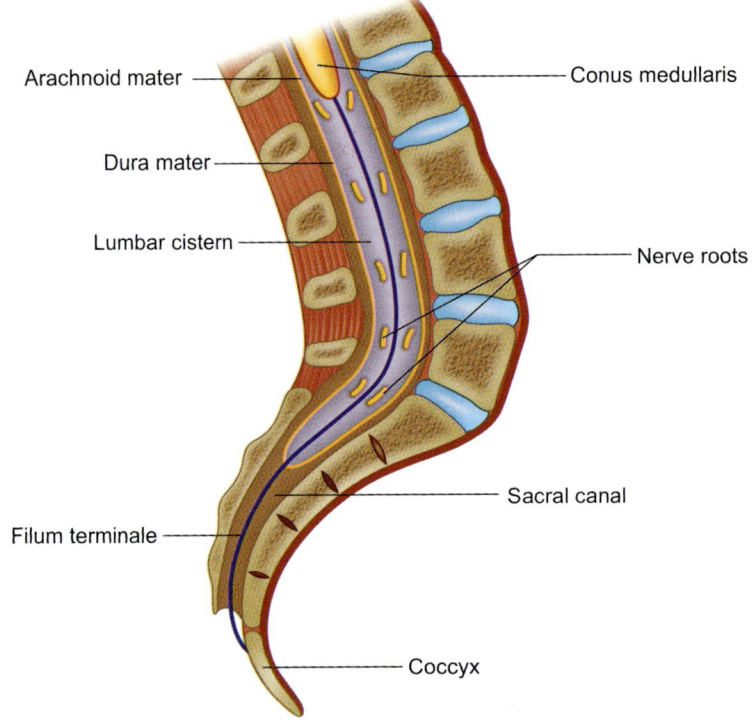

Arachnoid mater

Dura mater

Lumbar cistern

Filum terminale

Conus medullaris

Nerve roots

Sacral canal

Coccyx

Fig. 17.6: Sagittal section through the lower part of the vertebral canal

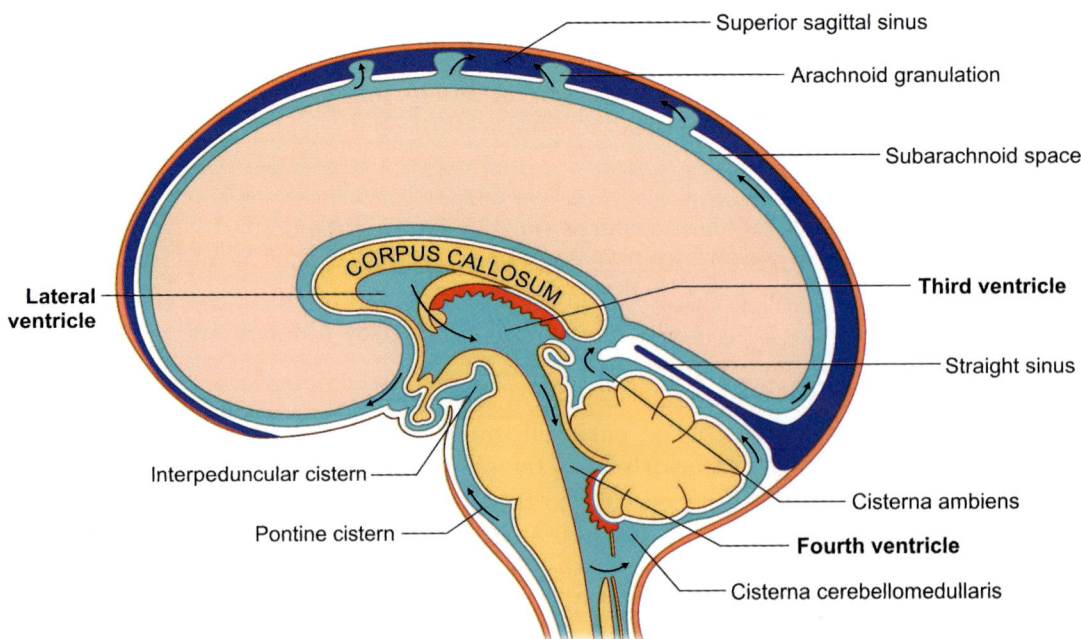

Superior sagittal sinus

Arachnoid granulation

Subarachnoid space

CORPUS CALLOSUM

Third ventricle

Lateral ventricle

Straight sinus

Interpeduncular cistern

Pontine cistern

Cisterna ambiens

Fourth ventricle

Cisterna cerebellomedullaris

Fig. 17.7: Principal subarachnoid cisterns and the circulation of CSF

5. *Cistern of lateral sulcus:* It is formed due to the arachnoid bridging over the lateral sulcus. It lodges the middle cerebral artery and the middle cerebral veins.
6. *Lumbar cistern:* It is the most dependent and the widest part of the spinal subarachnoid space. It contains the cauda equina formed by the lower spinal nerve roots. It is the most convenient and the safest site for the tapping of CSF. A needle is introduced (usually) between the spines of the third and the fourth lumbar vertebrae to enter the space, (lumbar puncture).

CEREBROSPINAL FLUID (CSF)

It is a clear, colourless, slightly alkaline fluid filling the ventricles of the brain and spinal cord and the subarachnoid space. It is secreted (mainly) in the ventricles of the brain, by the choroid plexuses produced by the specialised ependymal cells in the choroid plexuses. The CSF secreted in the lateral ventricles passes into the third ventricle through the interventricular foramen of Monro. From the third it passes into the fourth ventricle through the cerebral aqueduct (of Sylvius). Through a dorsal aperture (foramen of Magendie) and two lateral apertures (foramina of Luschka) of the fourth ventricle, the CSF escapes into the cerebellomedullary and the pontine cisterns. There is also a connection from the subarachnoid space to the bony labyrinth of the inner ear via the perilymphatic duct where the perilymph is continuous with the cerebrospinal fluid. From the cerebellomedullary and pontine cisterns CSF passes downwards into the spinal subarachnoid space and superiorly through the tentorial notch into the supratentorial compartment. It next ascends over the superolateral surface of the cerebral hemisphere to drain through the arachnoid granulations into the superior sagittal sinus. The circulation of the CSF is facilitated by the pulsations of arteries running in the subarachnoid space.

Circulation of CSF

The CSF enters the third ventricle through the interventricular foramen (of Monro). Thereafter, it descends to the fourth ventricle through the cerebral aqueduct (of Sylvius). It enters the subarachnoid space though median and lateral apertures in the roof of the fourth ventricle. Flow of CSF in the central canal of the spinal canal is negligible. Some CSF descends through foramen magnum reaching the lumbar cistern in 12 hours. Small amount of CSF is absorbed into the spinal veins but most returns to subarachnoid space in cranium (Fig. 17.8).

It ascends further through the tentorial notch and around the cerebrum. Finally, the CSF is absorbed into the venous sinuses. CSF moves in a single outward direction from the ventricles, but multi-directionally in the subarachnoid space. Fluid movement is pulsatile, matching the pressure waves generated in blood vessels by the beating of the heart. Some authors dispute this, posing that there is no unidirectional CSF circulation, but cardiac cycle-dependent bi-directional systolic-diastolic to and fro craniospinal CSF movements.

Biochemical Composition

- Specific gravity is 1.007.
- Higher in CSF than plasma: Sodium and chloride (720–750 mg/100 ml).
- Lower in CSF than plasma: Proteins (major protein in CSF is albumin; 20–40 mg/100 ml), glucose (normal CSF glucose level is 50–75 mg/100 ml about 60 to 80% of the blood glucose concentration), potassium, cholesterol, phosphorus, bicarbonate, sulphate and enzymes.
- CSF normally **does not contain** erythrocytes.
- Normal CSF consists of varying proportions of small lymphocytes and monocytes (0–5/mm^3).
- Major Ig in normal CSF is IgG, which normally originates from the serum.

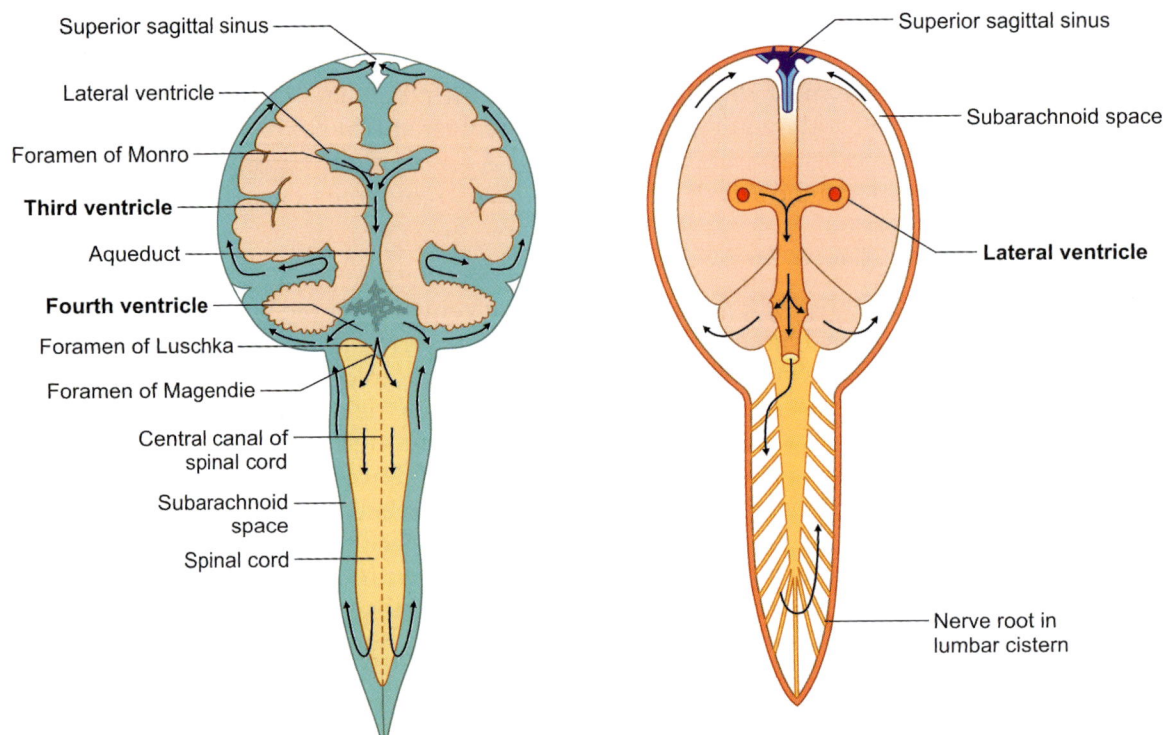

Fig. 17.8: Principal subarachnoid cisterns and the circulation of CSF

Functions of CSF

1. Protection. The CSF supports the brain and the spinal cord and maintains a uniform pressure over them. The buoyant effect of the fluid environment greatly decreases the tendency of various forces (e.g. gravity) to deform the brain. A brain weighing 1500 g in air weighs less than 50 g in the CSF, where it is easily able to maintain its shape.
2. Regulation of intracranial pressure.
3. Providing nutrients.
4. Removing waste products. Metabolic functions have also been assigned to the CSF.
5. CSF acts as a cushion or buffer for the brain, providing basic mechanical and immunological protection to the brain inside the skull.
6. CSF also serves a vital function in cerebral autoregulation of cerebral blood flow.

CLINICAL SIGNIFICANCE

Distribution of CSF

There is about 125 to 150 ml of CSF at any one time and about 500 ml is generated everyday. This CSF circulates within the ventricular system of the brain. The majority of CSF is produced from within the two lateral ventricles. From here, CSF passes through the interventricular foramina to the third ventricle, then the cerebral aqueduct to the fourth ventricle. From the fourth ventricle, the fluid passes into the subarachnoid space through four openings—the central canal of the spinal cord, the median aperture, and the two lateral apertures. CSF is present within the subarachnoid space, which covers the brain, spinal cord, and stretches below the end of the spinal cord to the sacrum. There is a connection from the subarachnoid space to the bony labyrinth of the inner ear making the cerebrospinal fluid continuous with the perilymph in 93% of people.

Collection of CSF

A sample of CSF can be taken via lumbar puncture. This can reveal the intracranial pressure, as well as indicate diseases including infections of the brain or its surrounding meninges.

Hydrocephalus

It is a condition seen in the newborns and infants where the head is enormously increased in size and the sutures gape widely. There is an abnormal increase in the amount of CSF (normal quantity 125 ml). The CSF pressure is also raised (normal pressure 125 mm H_2O). An over-production, defective absorption or an obstruction to the flow of CSF are the possible causes. Sites of obstruction include foramen of Monro, cerebral aqueduct and the foramina in the fourth ventricle. A developmental anomaly where the foramina of Magendie and Luschka are closed by membranes also gives rise to hydrocephalus (Dandy-Walker syndrome). This is an example of *internal* or *non-communicating type* of hydrocephalus, the obstruction being within the ventricular system of the brain. Arnold-Chiari malformation is a congenital condition of herniation of medulla and tonsil of cerebellum through the foramen magnum. Exit of CSF from the fourth ventricle is blocked, producing internal hydrocephalus. An obstruction outside the ventricular system, e.g. at the tentorial notch gives rise to the *external* or *communicating type* of hydrocephalus.

In the adult, after the closure of the sutures, the condition manifests itself by an increase in the CSF pressure, widening of the ventricles and thinning of the brain tissue. Increased CSF pressure also produces papilloedema or choked optic disc.

Blood Supply of Central Nervous System

- Significance of Blood Supply to Brain
- Vertebrobasilar System
  - Branches of vertebral artery
  - Branches of basilar artery
- Internal Carotid System
  - Branches of internal carotid artery
  - Circle of Willis
- Applied Anatomy of Blood Supply to Brain
  - Subarachnoid haemorrhage
  - Cerebral angiography
- Arterial Supply of Spinal Cord
  - Anterior spinal arteries
  - Posterior spinal arteries
  - Radicular arteries
- Venous Drainage of Brain
  - External (superficial) veins
  - Internal (deep) veins
- Venous Drainage of Spinal Cord

SIGNIFICANCE OF BLOOD SUPPLY TO BRAIN

The CNS is metabolically very active and requires a constant supply of well-oxygenated blood. Although the brain weighs only 2% of the body weight, it consumes 20% of the body's total oxygen requirement. The brain is critically dependent on a continuous blood supply. After just 15 seconds of complete cessation of blood supply to the brain one loses consciousness and after about 4 minutes irreversible neuronal damage occurs. Cardiac arrest due to coronary thrombosis is the commonest cause of the latter.

The average rate of cerebral blood flow is 50 ml/100 g/minute (lower values are obtained in the elderly). With increased neuronal activity the regional cerebral blood flow increases. Regional blood flow can be measured with the help of positron emission tomography (PET-scan).

There are two main arterial systems supplying the brain: 1. the vertebrobasilar system, and 2. the carotid system. Out of about 800 ml of blood flowing to the brain per minute, 200 ml flows through the vertebrobasilar and 600 ml through the carotid system.

VERTEBROBASILAR SYSTEM

The *vertebral artery*, one on either side, is the first branch of the subclavian artery. It ascends in the neck and enters the cranial cavity through the foramen magnum. Ascending along the sides and front of the medulla oblongata the arteries of the two sides come together and unite opposite the lower border of pons to form the *basilar artery* (Figs 18.1 and 18.2). The basilar

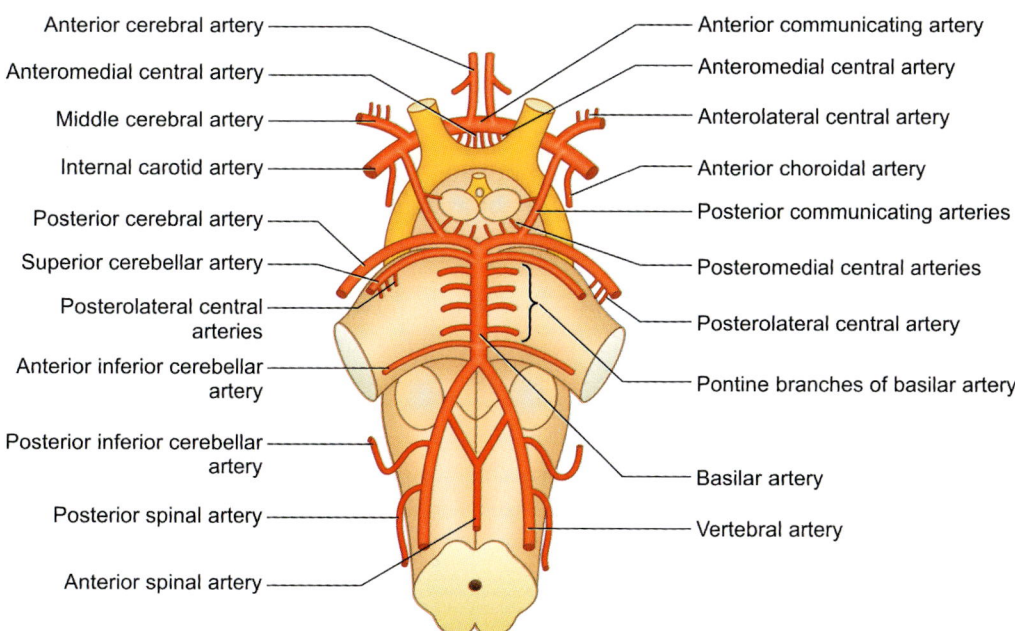

Fig. 18.1: Arteries on the ventral aspect of the brainstem and the arterial circle of Willis

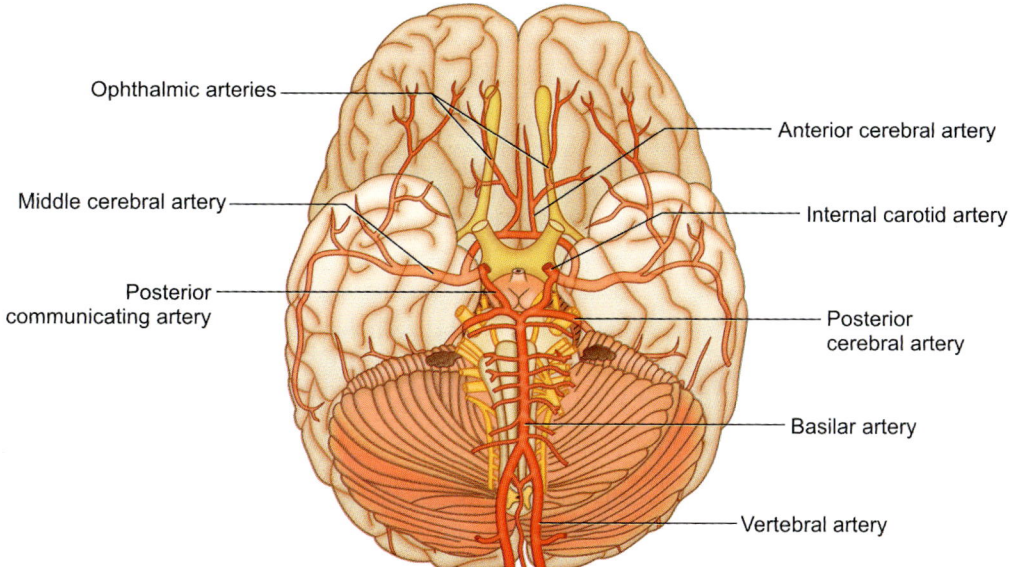

Fig. 18.2: Arteries of the brain seen in ventral view: The circle of Willis

artery runs upwards in the basilar groove on the ventral aspect of the pons to terminate at its upper border by dividing into a pair of *posterior cerebral arteries* (PCA).

Branches of Vertebral Artery

Anterior Spinal Artery

The anterior spinal arteries of the two sides unite to form a single midline artery, which descends in the anterior median fissure of the medulla oblongata and the spinal cord to its lower end. It supplies the ventral medulla and the ventral portion of the spinal cord.

Posterior Spinal Artery

It descends downwards to supply the dorsal portion of the lower medulla and then courses on the surface of the spinal cord along the line of attachments of the dorsal nerve roots.

Posterior Inferior Cerebellar Artery (PICA)

It courses backwards and ascends behind the IX and X nerve roots to reach the inferior surface of the cerebellum and supply it. It also supplies the dorsal medulla and the choroid plexus of the fourth ventricle.

Medullary Arteries

Several small direct medullary branches are distributed to the upper ventral medulla oblongata.

Branches of Basilar Artery

Anterior Inferior Cerebellar Artery (AICA)

It arises at the commencement of the basilar artery and courses laterally along the lower border of pons to reach and supply the anterior part of the inferior surface of the cerebellum. The artery also supplies the upper medulla and the lower pons.

Labyrinthine Artery

The basilar or from the anterior inferior cerebellar artery, this artery enters the internal accoustic meatus to supply the internal ear.

Pontine Branches

These are several small arteries which pierce the ventral surface of the pons to supply it.

Superior Cerebellar Artery

It arises near the termination of the basilar artery and follows the upper border of the pons to supply the superior surface of the cerebellum. Branches are also distributed to the pons, colliculi, pineal body and the tela chroidea of the third ventricle.

Posterior Cerebral Artery

This artery courses laterally above the pons and across the ventral aspect of the cerebral peduncle. It runs parallel to and the above the superior cerebellar artery from which it is separated by the oculomotor nerve medially and the trochlear nerve laterally. The artery, next winds round the lateral aspect of the cerebral peduncle to reach the tentorial surface of the

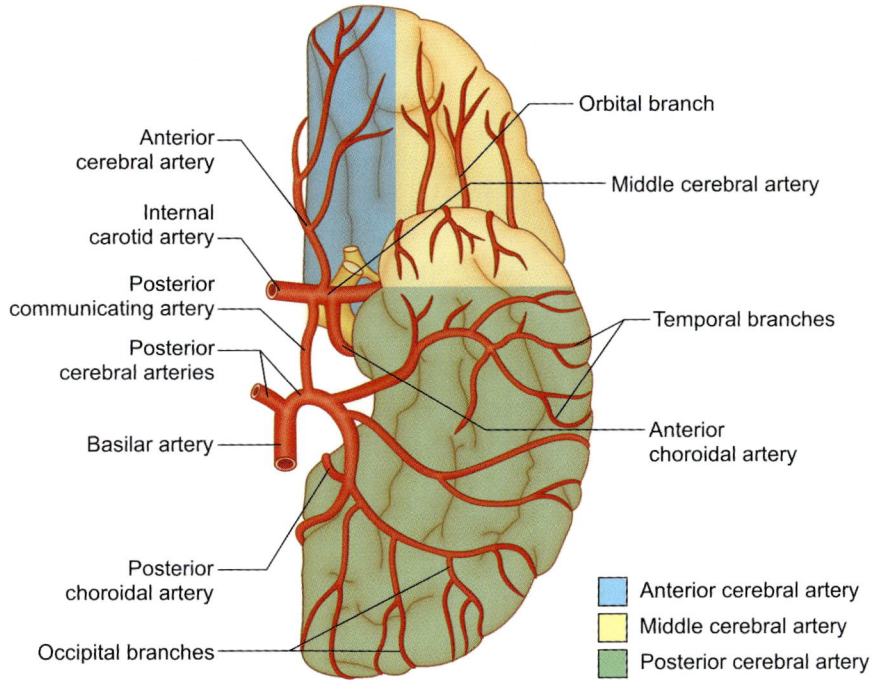

Fig. 18.3: Cerebral arteries, their branches and the areas of distribution on the inferior surface of the left cerebral hemisphere

cerebral hemisphere. The artery is joined by the posterior communicating branch of the internal carotid artery in its proximal part (Fig. 18.3). It gives the following branches:

- *Thalamoperforating (posteromedial central) arteries:* These arteries arise from the posterior cerebral and the posterior communicating arteries. They pierce the posterior perforated substance to supply the thalamus and the globus pallidus.
- *Thalamogeniculate (posterolateral central) arteries:* These arteries supply the lateral and medial geniculate bodies and the posterior part of thalamus.
- *Posterior choroidal arteries:* These are several branches some of which course over the lateral geniculate body and supply it before entering the inferior horn of lateral ventricle. Others wind round the posterior end of thalamus to supply its dorsal regions and pass through the transverse fissure into the tela choroidea of third ventricle. These arteries supply choroid plexuses of third and the lateral ventricles.
- *Cortical branches (temporal, occipital and parieto-occipital):* Supply the whole of the occipital lobe, inferior surface and the lower part of the lateral surface of the temporal lobe (except the temporal pole) and the precuneus (Figs 18.4 and 18.5). The territory of distribution includes the visual area. The macula is, however, not affected in an obstruction of the posterior cerebral artery (sparing of the macula).

INTERNAL CAROTID SYSTEM

The *internal carotid artery,* derived from the common carotid, enters the skull through the carotid canal. Within the cranial cavity it courses through the cavernous sinus lying alongside the body of sphenoid. It terminates at the cerebral vallecula lateral to the optic chiasma by dividing

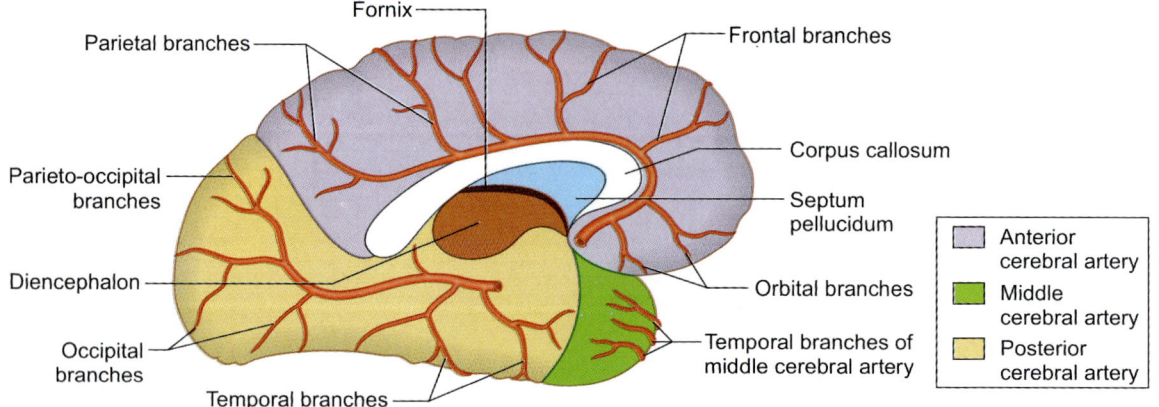

Fig. 18.4: Branches of three cerebral arteries and the areas of their distribution on the medial surface of the left cerebral hemisphere

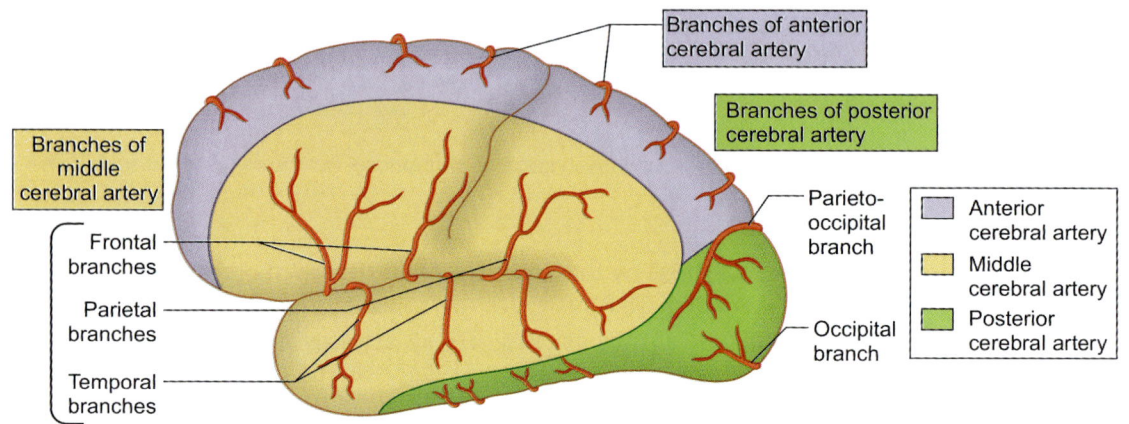

Fig. 18.5: Branches of three cerebral arteries and the areas of their distribution on the superolateral surface of the left cerebral hemisphere

into the *anterior* and *middle cerebral arteries* (Fig. 18.5). The artery presents about half a dozen bends in its course through the carotid canal and the cranial cavity. The bends are seen as the *'carotid siphon'* in a carotid angiogram.

Branches of Internal Carotid Artery

Anterior Cerebral Artery

It arises lateral to the optic chiasma and passes medially above the optic nerve to reach the longitudinal cerebral fissure. Here it comes close to its fellow of the opposite side and is connected to it by the anterior communicating artery. Beyond this communicating the anterior cerebral arteries follow the curve of the corpus callosum almost to the splenium. Following branches arise from it.

- ***The anteromedial central branches*** *arise* from the anterior cerebral and the anterior communicating arteries, pierce the lamina terminalis and the anterior perforated substance and supply the septum pellucidum, anterior part of the lentiform and the head of the caudate nucleus. The branch to the caudate head *(recurrent artery of Heubner)* also supplies rostral part of the internal capsule. Its occlusion results in hemiparesis with brachial predominance.

- *The cortical branches* are distributed to different areas of the cerebral hemisphere and are named, according to the territory supplied, as under:
  a. *Orbital branches* for the olfactory bulb, olfactory tract and the medial part of the orbital surface of cerebral hemisphere
  b. *Frontal branches*
  c. *Parietal branches* which distribute to the medial surface and upper part of the superolateral surface of the respective lobes of the cerebral hemisphere, as far back as the parieto-occipital sulcus (Fig. 18.5).

These cortical branches are also named *frontopolar, pericallosal* and *callosomarginal.* **The anterior cerebral artery is thus, the main artery supplying the medial surface of the cerebral hemisphere of its side.**

Middle Cerebral Artery

This artery, larger than the anterior cerebral, courses laterally and then backwards in the Sylvian fissure on the surface of insula. It gives the following branches.

- *The anterolateral central branches* arise from the proximal part of the artery, pierce the anterior perforated substance and supply the corpus striatum and the internal capsule. These branches *(lenticulostriate arteries)* form two sets, a *lateral* and a *medial.* One of the lateral striate arteries is larger and most susceptible to bleed in the presence of arteriosclerosis and hypertension. It is called the *'Charcot's artery of cerebral haemorrhage'.*
- *The cortical branches* include *orbital, frontal, parietal* and *temporal* (Figs 18.3 and 18.4). These branches are distributed to the lateral part of the orbital surface and the lateral surfaces of the frontal, parietal and temporal lobes, except for the strips along the inferolateral and the superomedial borders of cerebral hemisphere. The middle cerebral is thus, the main artery of the superolateral surface of the cerebral hemisphere.

Anterior Choroidal Artery

It arises from the internal carotid artery close to its termination and courses backwards across the optic tract and the cerebral peduncle to enter the inferior horn of the lateral ventricle and supply the choroid plexus. In its course it also gives branches to the cerebral peduncle, hypothalamus, optic tract, optic radiation, lateral geniculate body and posterior part of internal capsule.

Posterior Communicating Artery

It arises close to the anterior choroidal artery and passes backwards to join the posterior cerebral artery. Perforating branches from the artery supply the thalamus and the hypothalamus.

Circle of Willis (Circulus Arteriosus)

This is the name given to a hexagonal or heptagonal anastomotic arrangement of the arteries at the base of the brain lying within the cisterna interpeduncularis. It is formed by the proximal portions of the two posterior cerebral arteries joined to the two internal carotid arteries by the posterior communicating arteries. More anteriorly it is formed by the proximal portions.

Branches of Circulus Arteriosus

Six groups of *central* branches arise from the circle of Willis and vessels close to it. These include:

1. An anteromedial group
2. and 3. right and left anterolateral groups
4. A posteromedial group
5. and 6. right and left posterolateral groups (Table 18.1).

Table 18.1: Central branches of circulus arteriosus (of Willis)			
Group(s)	*Source/group*	*Perforating through*	*Distribution area*
Anteromedial	Anterior cerebral art.	Anterior perforating substance	Hypothalamus (anterior part)
Anterolaterals	Middle cerebral art.	Anterior perforating substance	• Caudate nucleus (head) • Internal capsule • Lentiform nucleus • External capsule • Claustrum
Posteromedial (thalamoperforating)	Posterior cerebral art. Posterior communicating art.	Posterior perforating substance	• Thalamus (anterior and medial) • Hypothalamus (middle and posterior parts) • Subthalamus • Crus cerebri
Posterolaterals	Posterior cerebral art.	Area lateral to crus cerebri	• Thalamus (posterior part) • Metathalamus • Tectum • Cerebral peduncle

APPLIED ANATOMY OF BLOOD SUPPLY TO BRAIN

Cerebrovascular disorders are quite commonly encountered in the general practice. In its mildest form it presents with a momentary or short duration *cerebrovascular insufficiency* leading to an attack of fainting (with a feeling of weakness and dizziness) or syncope (loss of consciousness). These attacks are caused by defective vasovagal reflexes or by strong emotions.

Cerebrovascular diseases with a temporary or permanent neurological deficit are called *cerebrovascular accidents* (CVAs) or strokes. These are caused by blockage (cerebral thrombosis or embolism) or haemorrhage from an artery of the brain. *Transient ischaemic attacks* (TIAs) are often the forerunners of a major stroke. TIAs are reversible within 24 hours and do not leave any functional or neurological deficits.

Subarachnoid Haemorrhage

Subarachnoid haemorrhage is usually non-traumatic. It results from rupture of an aneurysm in the circle of Willis or one of its major branches. The common symptoms include: a sudden severe headache, stiffness of neck and loss of consciousness result. Diagnosis is established by CT scanning. A **subarachnoid haemorrhage** is a surgical emergency and if the patient survives, angiographic investigation and surgical treatment are required.

Cerebral Angiography

The arteries of the brain can be visualised by injecting a contrast medium through a catheter pushed up through the common carotid artery. The contrast medium is injected and radiographs are taken at 1 second interval. Cerebral angiography helps to: 1. determine abnormalities of blood vessels, 2. localise brain tumours and 3. find out vascular patterns of tumours.

ARTERIAL SUPPLY OF SPINAL CORD

The spinal cord is supplied by the anterior and posterior spinal arteries derived from the vertebral arteries, and the radicular arteries derived from the spinal branches of the regional arteries (Fig. 18.6).

Anterior Spinal Artery

It is unpaired, descends opposite the anterior median fissure and supplies the ventral two-thirds of the cross-sectional area of the spinal cord.

Posterior Spinal Arteries

One on either side, these descend along the attachments of the dorsal nerve roots. These supply the posterior funiculus, posterior grey column and posterior portions of the lateral funiculus.

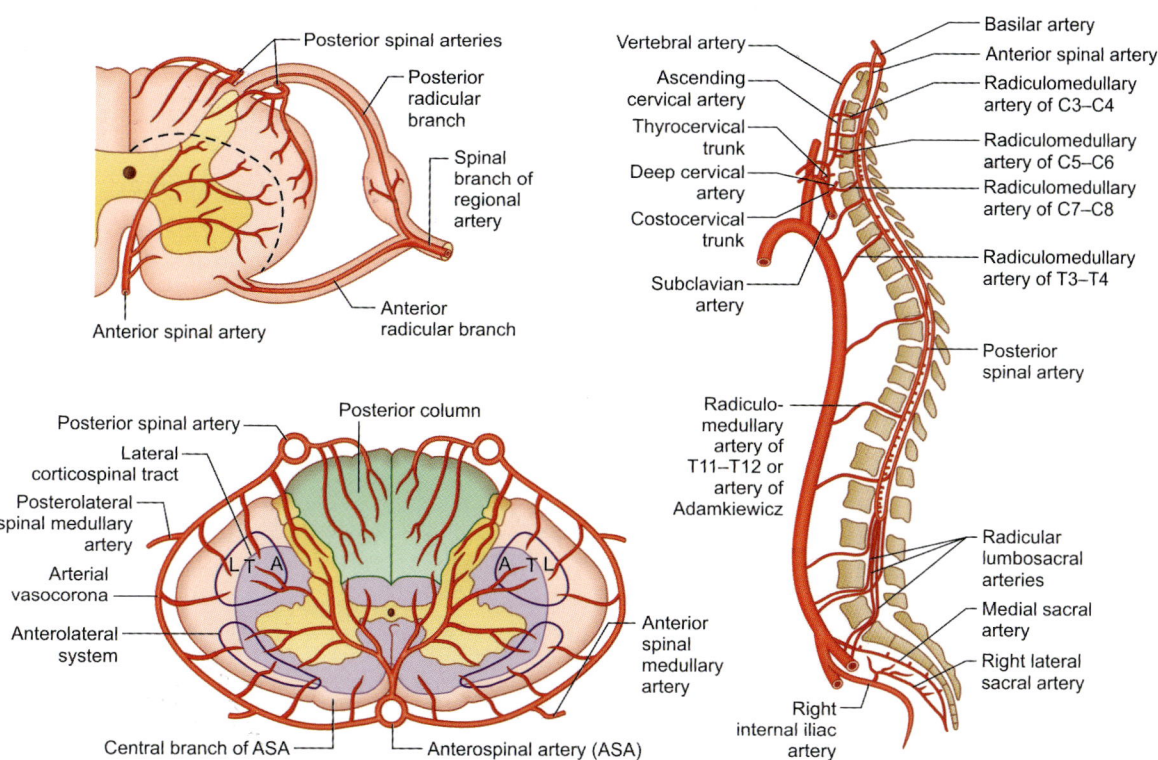

Fig. 18.6: Branches of three spinal arteries and their branches for supply of spinal cord

Radicular Arteries

These arise from the spinal branches of vertebral, lumbar and lateral sacral arteries. An *anterior* and a *posterior radicular branch* accompanies the corresponding nerve roots. One of the anterior radicular arteries, the *arteria radicularis anterior magna (of Adamkiewicz)* is larger than the others and usually enters from the left side along the tenth thoracic ventral nerve root. It supplies the lumbar enlargement of the spinal cord. Often it is the principal source of blood supply to the lower one-third of spinal cord.

VENOUS DRAINAGE OF BRAIN

The veins of the brain are thin-walled, valveless and capable of considerable distension. Most veins lie on the surface of the brain in the subarachnoid space and pierce the arachnoid and the dura to drain in the intracranial venous sinuses. The veins of the cerebrum can be divided into an *external* and an *internal group*.

External (superficial) Veins

Superior Cerebral Veins

These are about a dozen in number and drain the upper parts of the superolateral and the medial surfaces of the cerebral hemisphere. They end in the superior sagittal sinus. The anterior of these veins course almost vertically. The more posterior ones, which have an oblique direction, turn forwards to open in the sinus against the current of the blood-flow. This arrangement safeguards against the collapse of these veins in conditions of raised intracranial pressure.

Inferior Cerebral Veins

These veins drain the lower parts of the superolateral surface of the cerebral hemisphere and terminate into the superficial middle cerebral vein. The more posterior of these veins and those draining the inferior surface, drain into the transverse, superior petrosal and the cavernous sinuses (Fig. 18.7).

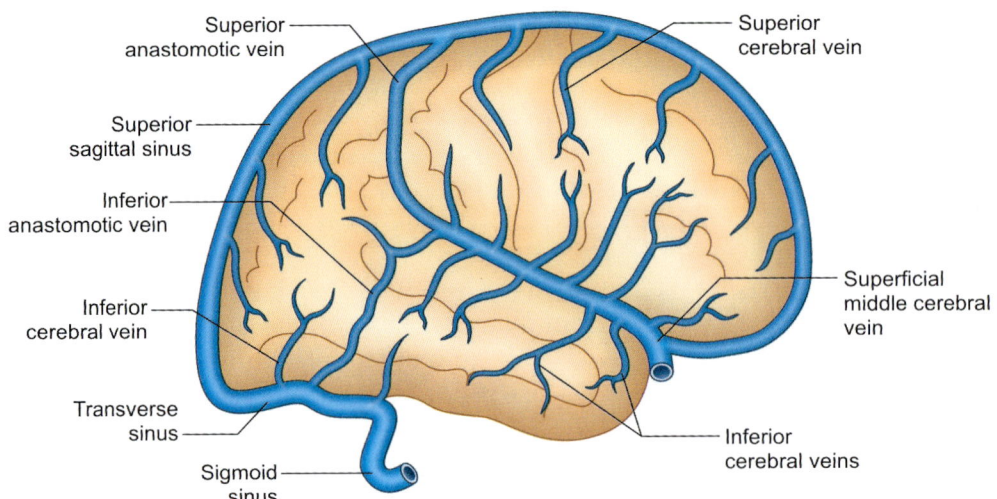

Fig. 18.7: Veins on the superolateral surface of the right cerebral hemisphere

Superficial Middle Cerebral Vein

It runs opposite the Sylvian fissure and drains the middle regions of the superolateral surface. It terminates into the cavernous sinus. Posteriorly, a *superior anastomotic vein (of Trolard)* connects it to the superior sagittal sinus and an *inferior anastomotic vein (of Labbe)* connects it to the transverse sinus.

Basal Vein (of Rosenthal)

It is formed on either side in the region of the cerebral vallecula, by the union of (i) the *deep middle cerebral vein* which drains the insula and courses in the depth of the Sylvian fissure, (ii) an *anterior cerebral vein,* which accompanies the artery of the same name, and (iii) the *striate veins* which emerge at the anterior perforated substance from within the cerebral substance. The basal veins of the two sides course backwards, wind round the cerebral peduncle and join the *great cerebral vein* on the dorsal aspect of the midbrain.

Internal (deep) Veins

On either side an *internal cerebral vein* is formed opposite the interventricular foramen, by the union of the *thalamostriate* and the *choroid veins.* The two internal cerebral veins run backwards, side by side, between the layers of the tela choroidea of the third ventricle. Posteriorly, near the splenium of corpus callosum they join to from the *great cerebral vein (of Galen).* The great cerebral vein escapes through the transverse cerebral fissure, receives a basal vein, on either side, and finally terminates into the straight sinus.

The veins of the cerebellum and the brainstem drain into the basal and great cerebral veins and into the adjacent venous sinuses.

VENOUS DRAINAGE OF SPINAL CORD

The veins from the spinal cord drain into about half a dozen longitudinal channels on the surface of the spinal cord. These include the *anterior* and *posterior median veins* and a pair of veins behind the attachment of each of the anterior and posterior nerve roots. These channels drain into the *internal vertebral venous plexus (of Batson),* which in turn drains into the regional veins, corresponding to the regional arteries described above.

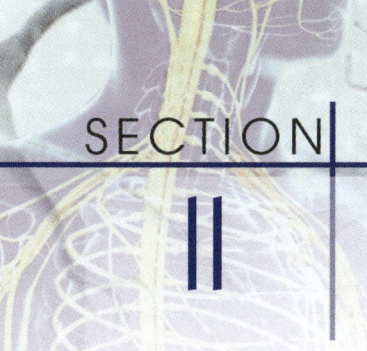

SECTION

II

Peripheral Nervous System

Cranial and Spinal Nerves

CRANIAL NERVES

The cranial nerves are 12 pairs of nerves that arise directly from the brain (including the brainstem). They are: the olfactory **nerve** I, the optic **nerve** II, oculomotor **nerve** III, trochlear **nerve** IV, trigeminal **nerve** V, abducens **nerve** VI, facial **nerve** VII, vestibulocochlear **nerve** VIII, Glossopharyngeal **nerve** IX, vagus **nerve** X, accessory **nerve** XI, and hypoglossal **nerve** XII (Figs 19.1 and 19.2). Depending on definition in humans there are twelve or thirteen cranial nerves pairs, which are assigned Roman numerals I–XII, sometimes also including cranial nerve zero. The numbering of the cranial nerves is based on the order in which they emerge from the brain, front to back (brainstem). The 10 of the 12 cranial nerves originate in the brainstem. Cranial nerves relay information between the brain and parts of the body, primarily to and from regions of the head and neck. The terminal nerves 0, olfactory nerves I and optic nerves II emerge from the cerebrum or forebrain, and the remaining ten pairs arise from the brainstem, which is the lower part of the brain. The cranial nerves are considered components of the peripheral nervous system (PNS), although on a structural level the olfactory I, optic II, and trigeminal V nerves are more accurately considered part of the central nervous system (CNS).

Terminology

Cranial nerves are generally named according to their structure or function. For example, the olfactory nerve I supplies smell, and the facial nerve VII supplies motor innervation to the

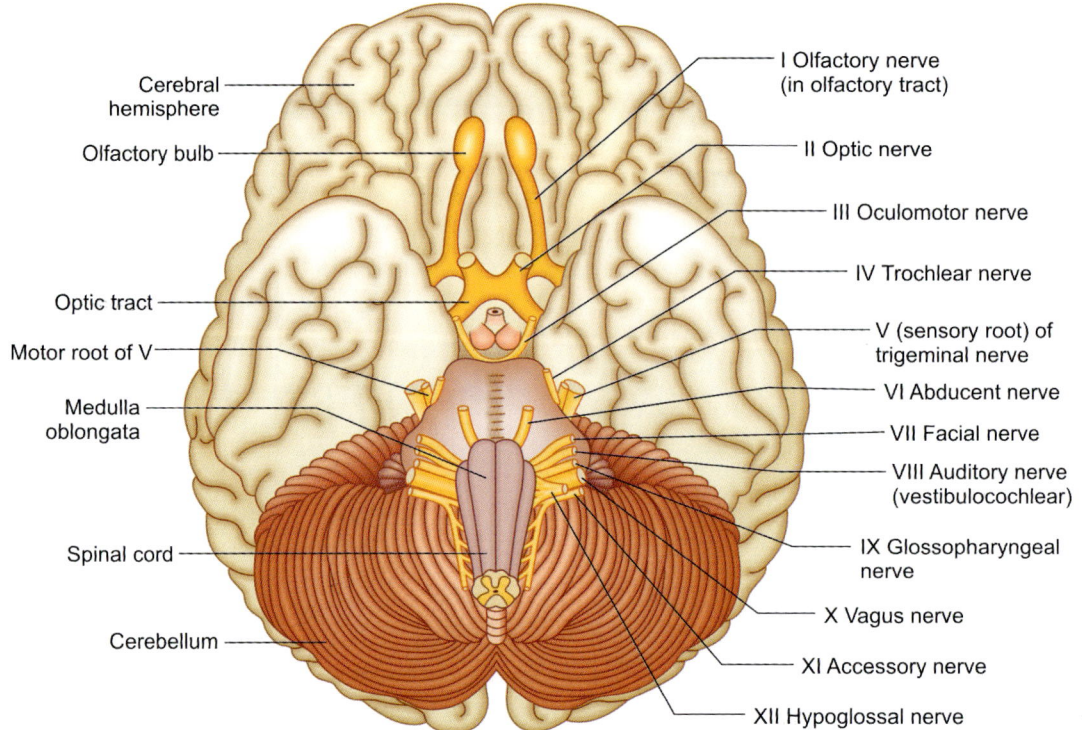

Fig. 19.1: The basal aspect of brain shows the emergence and superficial attachments of the cranial nerves, numbered and listed on the right side

face. Because Latin was the *lingua franca* (common language) of the study of anatomy when the nerves were first documented, recorded, and discussed, many nerves maintain Latin or Greek names, including the trochlear nerve IV, named according to its structure, as it supplies a muscle that attaches to a pulley (Greek: trochlea). The trigeminal nerve V is named in accordance with its three components (Latin: *trigeminus* meaning triplets), and the vagus nerve X is named for its wandering course (Latin: *vagus*).

Emergence on Brain Surface

The cranial nerves are having certain features by which they can be distinguished from the spinal nerves. The main features are listed below, while the remaining are dealt within their functional components (vide infra):

- The first two cranial nerves (I and II) are outgrowths of the brain.
- None of the cranial nerve consists both of an anterior (ventral) and a posterior (dorsal) root. Instead, each cranial nerve is either one of these; which in the region of the head are **never** joined together.
- The III, IV, VI, and XII cranial nerves correspond to the anterior root of the cerebrospinal nerves, while.
- The V, VII, VIII, IX, and X nerves are homologous of with the posterior roots.
- The cranial nerves have nuclei of grey matter.

Classification

The cranial nerves are generally subdivided into *three* subgroups:

i. Related with special senses—**I**, **II**, and **VIII.**
ii. Innervating head muscles—**III**, **IV**, **VI**, and **XII.**
iii. Innervating branchial arch derivatives—**V**, **VII**, **IX**, **X**, and **XI.**

Cranial nerves are numbered based on their rostral-caudal (front-back) position, when viewing the brain. If the brain is carefully removed from the skull the nerves are typically visible in their numeric order, with the exception of the last, CN XII, which appears to emerge rostrally to (above) CN XI.

Cranial nerves have paths within and outside the skull. The paths within the skull are called 'intracranial' and the paths outside the skull are called 'extracranial'. There are many holes in the skull called 'foramina' by which the nerves can exit the skull. All cranial nerves are *paired*, which means that they occur on both the right and left sides of the body. The muscle, skin, or additional function supplied by a nerve on the same side of the body as the side it originates from, is referred to an *ipsilateral* function. If the function is on the opposite side to the origin of the nerve, this is known as a *contralateral* function.

SPINAL NERVES

Spinal nerves emerge from segments of the spinal cord sequentially with the spinal nerve closest to the head (C1) emerging in the space above the first cervical vertebra.

The spinal nerves are located in regular order (*neuromeres*) corresponding to the segmental skeletal muscle pattern called myotomes (*myomeres*) of the trunk and alternate with the segments of the spine; every nerve is attended by a corresponding area of skin (*dermatome*). There are approximately 31 pairs of spinal nerves, named according to their position with respect to associated vertebrae (Fig. 19.2). These are: (i) eight *cervical* nerves C1 to C8; (ii) twelve *thoracic* nerves T1 to T12; (iii) five *lumbar* nerves L1–L5; (iv) five *sacral* nerves S1–S5, and (v) one *coccygeal* nerve C0.

Emergence from Spinal Cord

Every spinal nerve branches off from the spinal cord in two *roots*, a dorsal or posterior *afferent* (or *sensory*) *root*, and a ventral or anterior *efferent* (or *motor*) root. Both roots (Fig. 19.3) traverse the dural sac, penetrate the dura mater, and reach the intervertebral foramen, where the dorsal root swells into the *spinal* (or *intervertebral*) *ganglion* in which the anterior motor root does not participate. Distal to this ganglion, the dorsal and ventral roots unite and emerge from the intervertebral foramen as a mixed spinal nerve trunk, which now contains both sensory and motor fibres. Each of the two nerve-roots is made up of a number of separate rootlets which spread out from one another as they approach their attachment.

Course and Distribution of a Typical Spinal Nerve

A **spinal nerve** is a mixed nerve, which carries motor, sensory, and autonomic signals between the spinal cord and the body. In the human body there are 31 pairs of spinal nerves, one on each side of the vertebral column. Each spinal nerve is formed from the combination of nerve fibres from its posterior and anterior roots (Fig. 19.4). The posterior root is the afferent sensory root and carries sensory information to the brain. The anterior root is the efferent motor root and carries motor information from the brain.

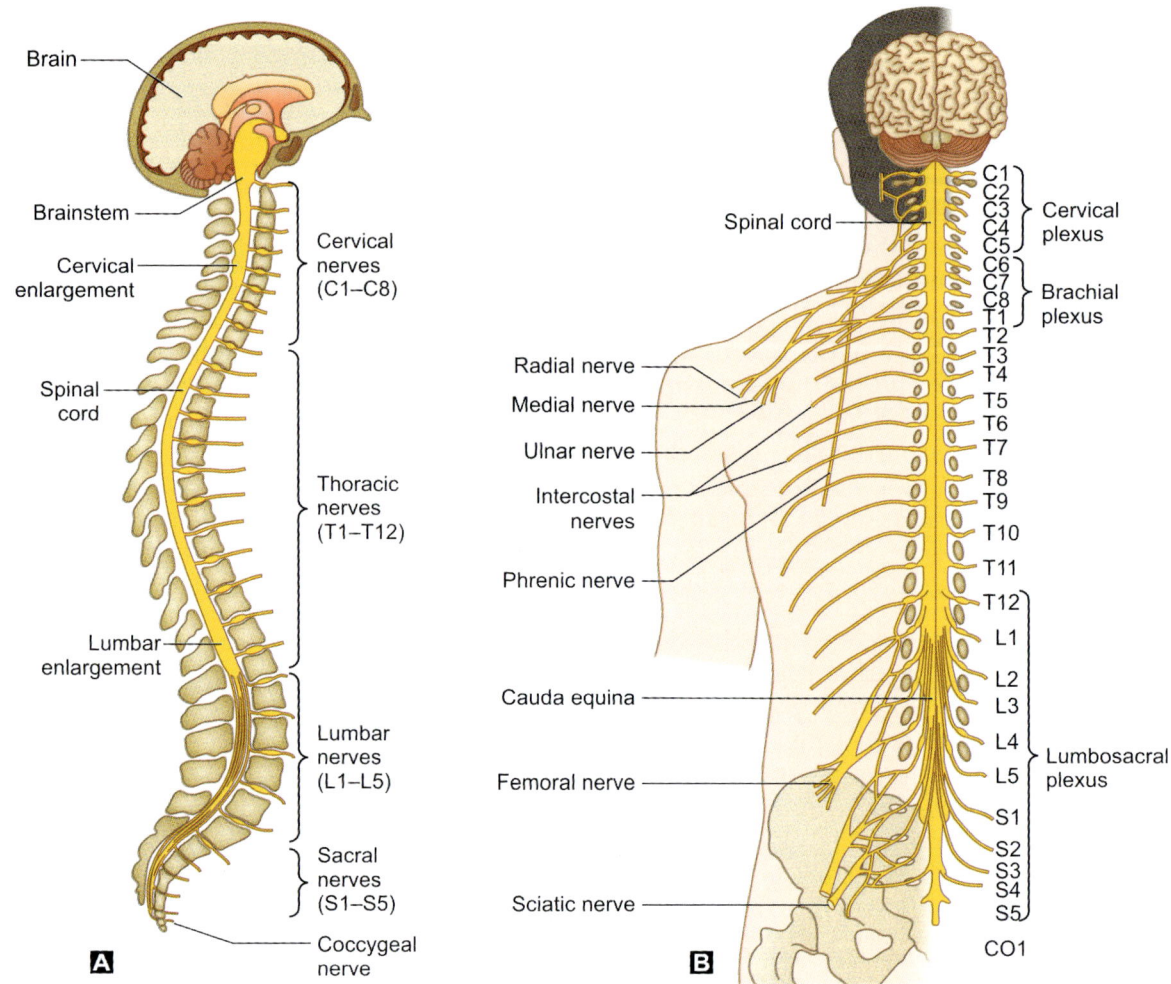

Fig. 19.2: Emergence of spinal nerves from the vertebral canal as viewed from: **A.** the side, and **B.** from posterior aspect

The spinal nerve emerges from the spinal column through an opening (intervertebral foramen) between adjacent vertebrae. This is true for all spinal nerves except for the first spinal nerve pair (C1), which emerges between the occipital bone and the atlas (the first vertebra). Thus, the cervical nerves are numbered by the vertebra below, except spinal nerve C8, which exists below vertebra C7 and above vertebra T1. The thoracic, lumbar, and sacral nerves are then numbered by the vertebra above. In the case of a lumbarised S1 vertebra (aka L6) or a sacralised L5 vertebra, the nerves are typically still counted to L5 and the next nerve is S1.

Outside the vertebral column, the nerve divides into branches. The posterior ramus contains nerves that serve the posterior portions of the trunk carrying visceral motor, somatic motor, and somatic sensory information to and from the skin and muscles of the back (epaxial muscles). The anterior ramus contains nerves that serve the remaining anterior parts of the trunk and the upper and lower limbs (hypaxial muscles) carrying visceral motor, somatic motor, and

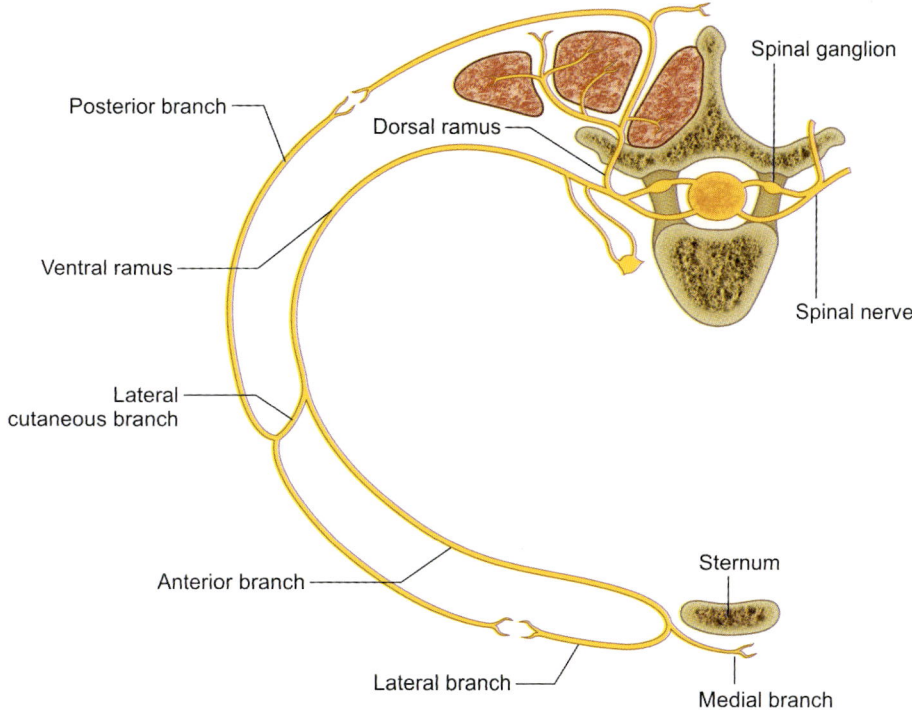

Fig. 19.3: A typical spinal nerve with its branches

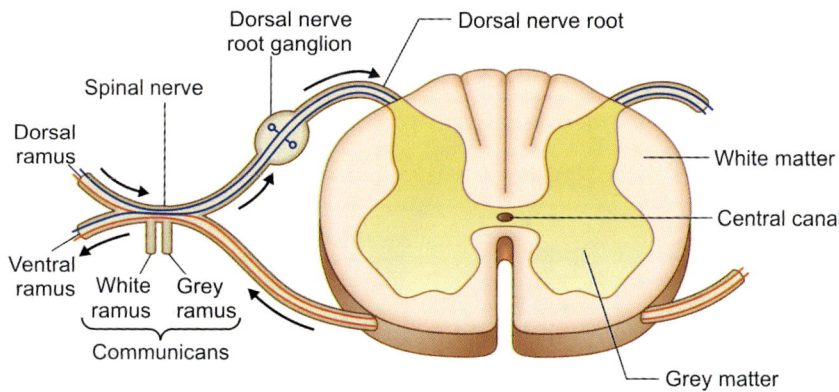

Fig. 19.4: A spinal nerve forms at the intervertebral foramen by the union of a dorsal and a ventral root

sensory information to and from the ventrolateral body surface, structures in the body wall, and the limbs. The meningeal branches (recurrent meningeal or sinuvertebral nerves) branch from the spinal nerve and re-enter the intervertebral foramen to serve the ligaments, dura, blood vessels, intervertebral discs, facet joints, and periosteum of the vertebrae. The rami communicantes contain autonomic nerves that serve visceral functions carrying visceral motor and sensory information to and from the visceral organs.

Some anterior rami merge with adjacent posterior rami to form a nerve plexus, a network of interconnecting nerves. Nerves emerging from a plexus contain fibres from various spinal nerves, which are now carried together to some target location. Major plexuses include the cervical, brachial, lumbar, and sacral plexuses.

Cervical Plexus

The cervical plexus, composed of the anterior rami of C1 to C4 cervical roots, innervates most neck muscles and provides sensory innervation to anterior and lateral neck.

The cervical plexus is formed from the anterior primary rami of C1–C4, deep to the sternocleidomastoid muscle and in front of the scalenus medius and levator scapulae muscles. Sensory branches include the greater and lesser occipital nerves, great auricular nerve, cutaneous cervical nerves, and supraclavicular nerves. The motor branches include the ansa hypoglossi, branches to scalenus medius and levator scapulae muscles, the phrenic nerve, and branches to the spinal accessory nerve. Lesions of the cervical plexus are uncommon, usually resulting from trauma, mass lesions, or as sequelae to surgery such as carotid endartectomy. Involvement of motor branches results in disruption of muscular function, such as shoulder elevation and head rotation and flexion with spinal accessory nerve damage. Involvement of sensory branches results in loss of cutaneous sensation or in pain and paresthesias in regions of the head or neck supplied by these branches.

Hypoglossal Nerve

The hypoglossal **nerve** is the **twelfth cranial nerve**, and innervates all the extrinsic and intrinsic muscles of the tongue, except for the palatoglossus which is innervated by the vagus **nerve**. It is a **nerve** with a solely motor function (Fig. 19.5).

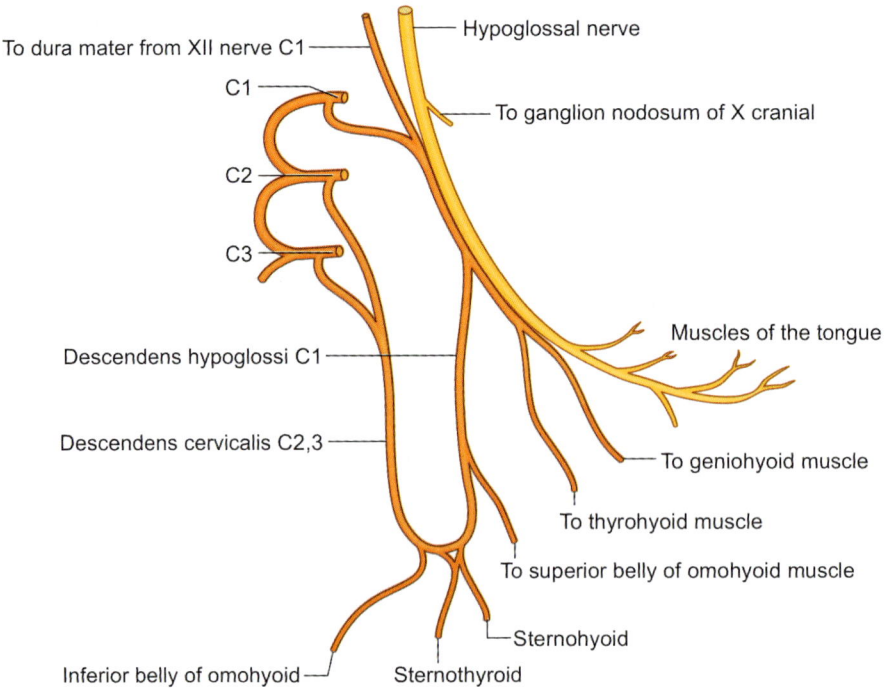

Fig. 19.5: Plan of cervical plexus. Note that C1 fibres travel through the hypoglossal nerve

NERVE IMPULSE AND ITS CONDUCTION

According to Erlanger and Gasser's classification, the nerve fibres are generally classified into three groups: A, B, and C. Group A are heavily myelinated, group B are moderately myelinated, and group C are unmyelinated.

The other classification is a sensory grouping that uses the terms type Ia and type Ib, type II, type III, and type IV, sensory fibres.

Furthermore, there are four subdivisions of group A nerve fibres: alpha (α), beta (β), gamma (γ), and delta (δ). These subdivisions have different amounts of myelination and axon thickness and therefore transmit signals at different speeds. Larger diameter axons and more myelin insulation lead to faster signal propagation (Table 19.1).

Type	Subtype	Fibre diameter (μm)	Conduction velocity (m/sec)	Function Sensory	Motor
Myelinated	α	12–20	70–120	Touch Pressure Proprioceptive	Somatic muscles (extra and intrafusal)
	β	05–12	30–70	—	—
	γ	03–06	15–30	—	—
	δ	02–05	12–30	Pain and temp. (nociceptive)	—
Myelinated	—	<3	03–15	—	Autonomic (preganglionic)
Unmyelinated	—	0.4–1.3	—	Pain and temp. (nociceptive)	Autonomic (postganglionic)

Table 19.1: Nerve fibre types with conduction velocity and functions

The plasma membrane of the dendrites and the cell soma, due to different ionic concentrations on its outer and inner aspects, has a resting potential of about −80 mV. On excitation the resting potential is altered due to differential ionic movements across the membrane. An action potential is set up which spreads to the initial segment of the axon and rapidly sweeps over its surface to reach its terminal. In the myelinated nerve fibres the axonal membrane is exposed only at the nodes of Ranvier and the internodal segments of the nerve fibre are not available for the spread of the action potential. The nerve impulses therefore appear to jump from node to node (*saltatory conduction*) along the nerve fibre. This is much faster mode of impulse conduction compared to the continuous impulse conduction in the non-myelinated nerve fibres. The rate of conduction is directly proportional to the internodal distance as well as the fibre diameter.

20

Functional Components of Spinal and Cranial Nerve Nuclei

- Structure of Cranial Nerve Nucleus
  - Motor and sensory
- Functional Components of Nerves
  - Development of functional components
  - Functional components in spinal nerves
  - Functional components in cranial nerves
- Purely Sensory Cranial Nerves
- Primarily Motor Cranial Nerves
- Mixed Cranial Nerves
- Functional Cranial Nerve Nuclei at a Glance
  - Key to functional columns

A **cranial nerve nucleus** is a collection of neurons (grey matter) in the brainstem that is associated with one or more cranial nerves. Axons carrying information to and from the cranial nerves form a synapse first at these nuclei. Lesions occurring at these nuclei can lead to effects resembling those seen by the severing of nerve(s) they are associated with. All the nuclei except that of the trochlear nerve (CN IV) supply nerves of the same side of the body.

STRUCTURE OF CRANIAL NERVE NUCLEUS

Motor and Sensory

In general, motor nuclei are closer to the front (ventral), and sensory nuclei and neurons are closer to the back (dorsal). This arrangement mirrors the arrangement of tracts in the spinal cord.

- Close to the midline are the **motor efferent nuclei**, such as the oculomotor nucleus, which control skeletal muscle. Just lateral to this are the **autonomic (or visceral) efferent nuclei.**
- There is a separation, called the sulcus limitans, and lateral to this are the **sensory nuclei**. Near the sulcus limitans are the **visceral afferent nuclei**, namely the solitary tract nucleus.
- More lateral, but also less posterior, are the **general somatic afferent nuclei.** This is the trigeminal nucleus. Back at the dorsal surface of the brainstem, and more lateral are the **special somatic afferents**, this handles sensation such as balance.

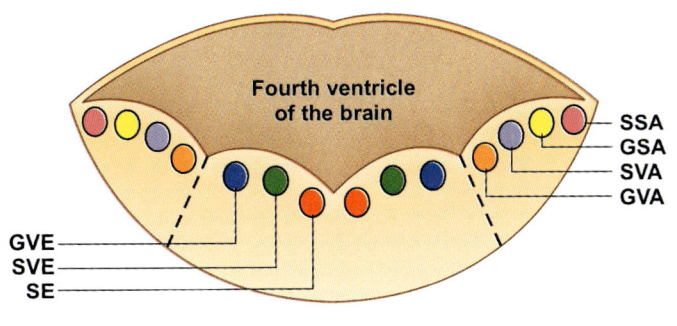

Functional group of cranial nerves:
  I. Olfactory nerve: **Sensory**
  II. Optic nerve: **Sensory**
  III. Oculomotor nerve: **Motor**
  IV. Trochlear nerve: **Motor**
  V. Trigeminal nerve: **Mixed**
     (sensory+motor)
  VI. Abducent nerve: **Motor**
  VII. Facial nerve: **Mixed**
  VIII. Vestibulocochlear nerve: **Sensory**
  IX. Glossopharyngeal nerve: **Mixed**
  X. Vagus nerve: **Mixed**
  XI. Accessory nerve: **Motor**
  XII. Hypoglossal nerve: **Motor**

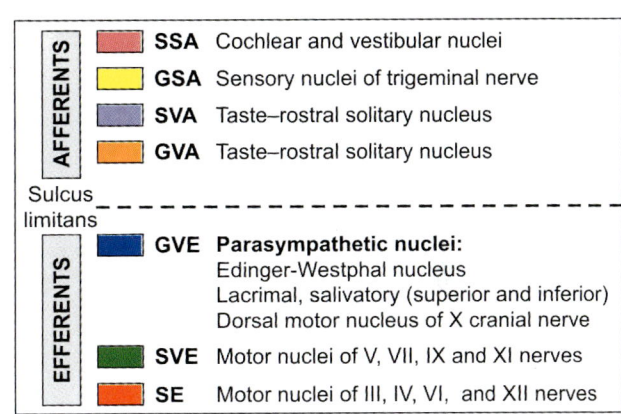

AFFERENTS
  SSA Cochlear and vestibular nuclei
  GSA Sensory nuclei of trigeminal nerve
  SVA Taste–rostral solitary nucleus
  GVA Taste–rostral solitary nucleus

Sulcus limitans

EFFERENTS
  GVE **Parasympathetic nuclei:**
       Edinger-Westphal nucleus
       Lacrimal, salivatory (superior and inferior)
       Dorsal motor nucleus of X cranial nerve
  SVE Motor nuclei of V, VII, IX and XI nerves
  SE   Motor nuclei of III, IV, VI, and XII nerves

Fig. 20.1: Functional groups of cranial nerves listed on the left columns are shown on the right

- Another area, not on the dorsum of the brainstem, is where the **special visceral efferents nuclei** reside. These formed from the pharyngeal arches, in the embryo. This area is a bit below the **autonomic motor nuclei**, and includes the nucleus ambiguus, facial nerve nucleus, as well as the motor part of the trigeminal nerve nucleus (Fig. 20.1).

FUNCTIONAL COMPONENTS OF NERVES

As stated above the nerves arise either from the spinal cord–spinal nerves; or from the brain–cranial nerves. The spinal and cranial nerves both contain *three* kinds of fibers: (i) sensory (*afferent*), (ii) motor (*efferent*), and (iii) a combination of sensory and motor (*mixed*) fibres. All these three kinds of fibres are classified on the basis of their embryological origin or common structural and functional characteristics.

Primary sensory fibers, somatic motor neurons, and pre- and post-ganglionic visceromotor neurons that exhibit, 'like anatomical and physiological characters so that they….act in a common mode' are classified as having a **specific functional component**. For example, fibres conveying sharp pain from widely separated body parts (the foot, hand, and face) have the same functional component is directly applicable to cranial nerves.

Development of Functional Components

In earlier stage of development, the neural tube is oval in outline with a narrow slit-like lumen. Later, the lateral walls of the neural tube (in the caudal portion to form the future spinal cord) thicken due to proliferation of the ependymal cells; the lumen widens in its dorsal part.

Functional Components in Spinal Nerves

A longitudinal groove called **sulcus limitans** develops on the inner aspect of the tube wall on each side. As a result, each lateral wall of the developing neural tube subdivides into a **dorsal** or **alar lamina** and a **ventral** or **basal lamina** (Fig. 20.2A).

Functional Components in Cranial Nerves

A sulcus limitans also develops in the rostral neural tube (the future brainstem—from where the true cranial nerves III–XII arise. The I and II cranial nerves being extension of the brain—hence not actual nerves). But the differentiation of the lateral walls of the neural tube into alar and basal laminae in the region of the developing hindbrain becomes different from that in the spinal cord (Fig. 20.2B). The dorsal edge of the alar lamina gives attachment to the thin expanded roof-plate and is termed the *rhombic lip*.

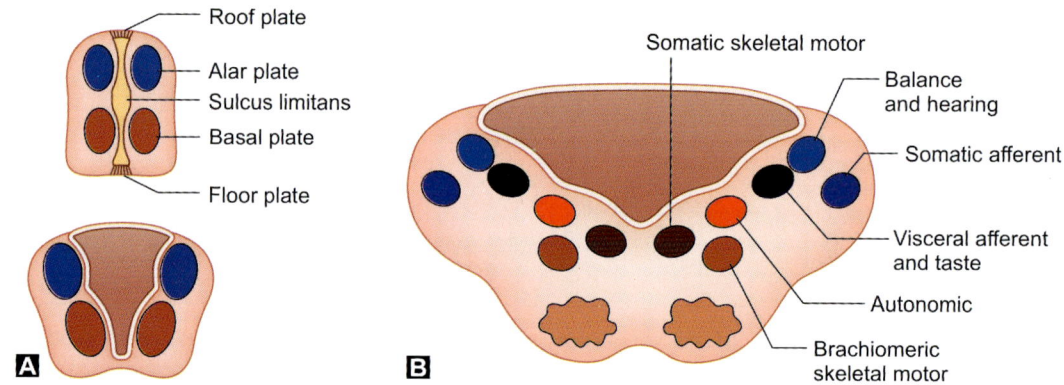

Fig. 20.2: Development of functional columns in: **A.** spinal nerves, and **B.** cranial nerves arising from brainstem

Purely Sensory Cranial Nerves [I, II, and VIII] (Fig. 20.3)

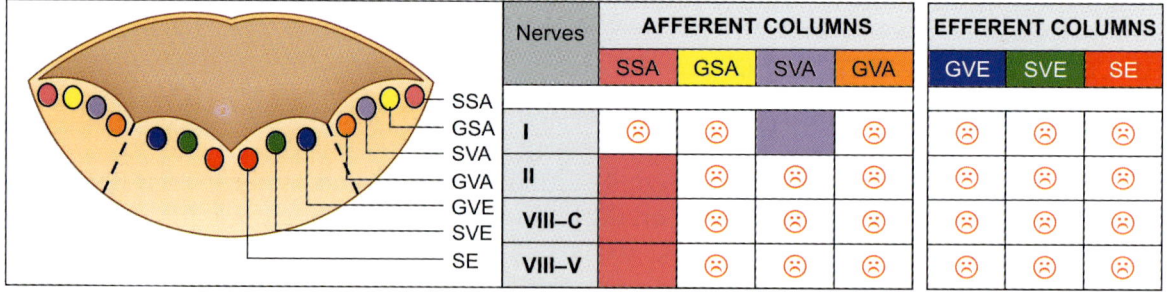

Nerves	AFFERENT COLUMNS				EFFERENT COLUMNS		
	SSA	GSA	SVA	GVA	GVE	SVE	SE
I	☹	☹		☹	☹	☹	☹
II		☹	☹	☹	☹	☹	☹
VIII–C		☹	☹	☹	☹	☹	☹
VIII–V		☹	☹	☹	☹	☹	☹

Notes:

  i. The cranial nerves **I** and **II** both are not attached to brainstem; whereas the first or olfactory carries smell sensations from uppermost olfactory portion of the nasal cavity; the second nerve is regarded as outgrowth from the cerebral hemisphere being actually a collection of axons from the ganglion cells of the retina of the eye

  ii. **VIII–C** = the cochlear division of VIII cranial carrying sensations from the cochlea of the internal ear

  iii. **VIII–V** = the vestibular division of VIII cranial carrying sensations from the vestibule of internal ear. For the dual components, the VIII cranial nerve is termed vestibulocochlear (commonly named incorrectly only auditory) nerve

    The **vestibulocochlear nerve** (auditory **vestibular nerve**), known as the **eighth cranial nerve**, transmits sound and equilibrium (balance) information from the inner ear to the brain.

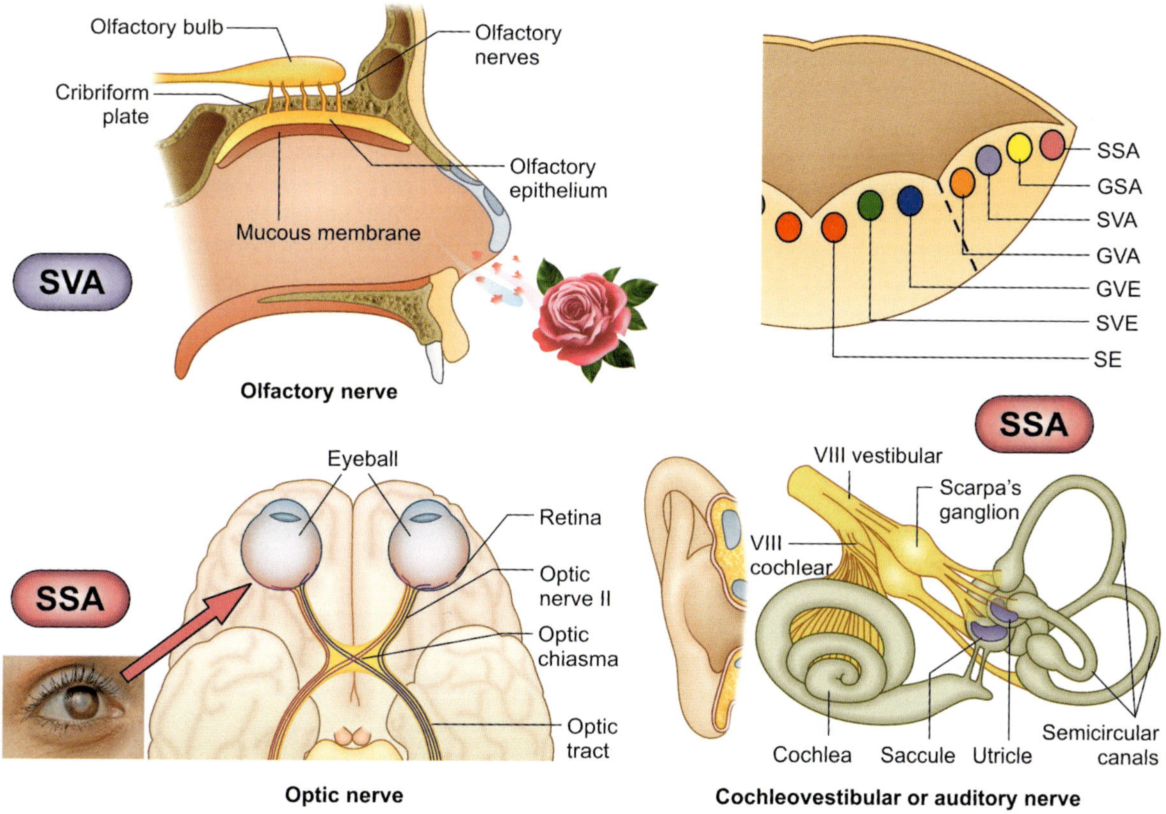

Olfactory bulb
Olfactory nerves
Cribriform plate
Olfactory epithelium
Mucous membrane
SVA
Olfactory nerve

SSA
GSA
SVA
GVA
GVE
SVE
SE

SSA

SSA
Eyeball
Retina
Optic nerve II
Optic chiasma
Optic tract
Optic nerve

SSA
VIII vestibular
Scarpa's ganglion
VIII cochlear
Cochlea   Saccule   Utricle   Semicircular canals
Cochleovestibular or auditory nerve

Fig. 20.3: Functional components in purely sensory nerves: I cranial (SVA: special visceral afferent); II cranial (SSA: special somatic afferent); and VIII cranial (SSA: special somatic afferent)

Primarily Motor Cranial Nerves [III, IV, VI, and XII] (Figs 20.4 and 20.5)

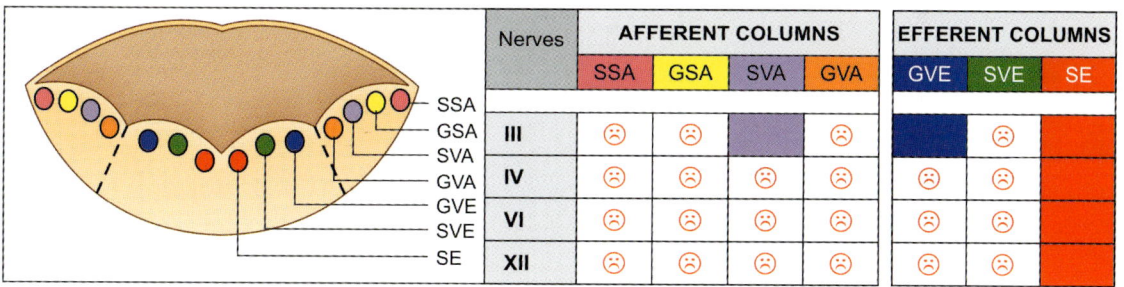

SSA
GSA
SVA
GVA
GVE
SVE
SE

Nerves	AFFERENT COLUMNS				EFFERENT COLUMNS		
	SSA	GSA	SVA	GVA	GVE	SVE	SE
III	☹	☹		☹		☹	
IV	☹	☹	☹	☹	☹	☹	
VI	☹	☹	☹	☹	☹	☹	
XII	☹	☹	☹	☹	☹	☹	

Purely Motor Nerves [III, IV, VI and XII] have only Efferent Column(s)

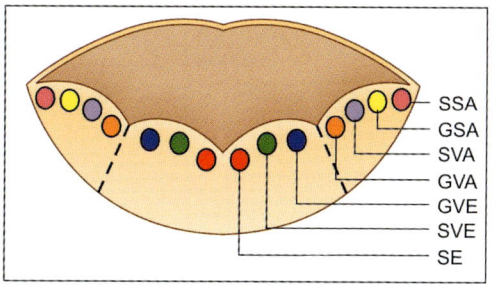

SSA
GSA
SVA
GVA
GVE
SVE
SE

EFFERENT COLUMNS		
GVE	SVE	SE
☹	☹	☹
☹	☹	☹
☹	☹	☹
☹	☹	☹

Notes:

i. All of the four cranial nerves in this category supply skeletal muscles NOT derived from the branchial arch mesoderm. Hence, these are named as somatic efferent (motor) nerves.

ii. The III cranial, the oculomotor, nerve emerges on the medial aspect of the crus cerebri; and is the only nerve out of the four listed in the somatic motor category, which consists of a GVE (general visceral efferent) component from Edinger-Westphal nucleus located in the periaqueductal grey matter and sends preganglionic parasympathetic fibres along the motor branch to the inferior oblique extraocular muscle—as the parasympathetic root of the ciliary (or ophthalmic) ganglion for the motor supply to the constrictor papillae muscle.

iii. The III cranial nerve supplies 5 out of 7 extraocular muscles (2 from the upper division—to the superior rectus and levator palpebrae superioris, and 3 from the lower division of the nerve for the supply of medial and inferior recti and inferior oblique muscle. Thus only 2 extraocular muscles (lateral rectus and superior oblique are not innervated by the third cranial.

iv. Palsy of the nerve to the muscle levator palpebrae (usually congenital) is a major cause of drooping of the upper eyelid resulting into a clinical entity called **ptosis**

v. The IV cranial nerve called trochlear is the only cranial nerve that emerges on the dorsal aspect of the brainstem at the level of the inferior colliculus of the midbrain, encircles the crus cerebri to reach on the ventral aspect, finally supplying only one extraocular muscle—the superior oblique.

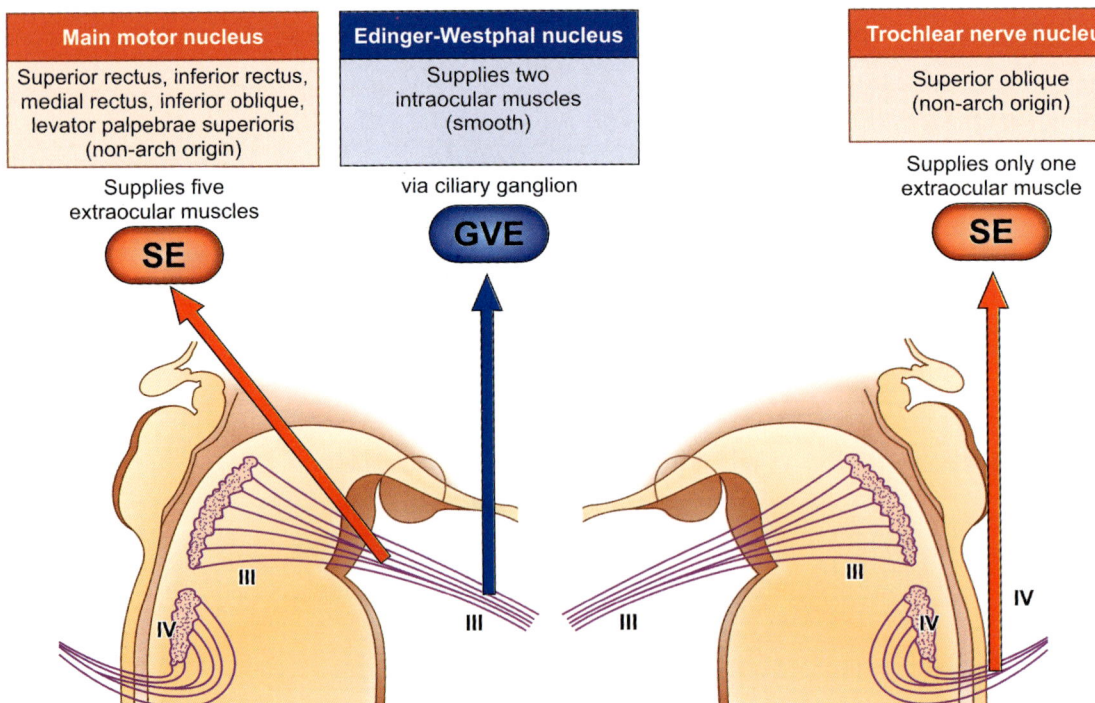

Fig. 20.4: Functional component [SE] of III cranial (oculomotor) and IV cranial (trochlear) nerves

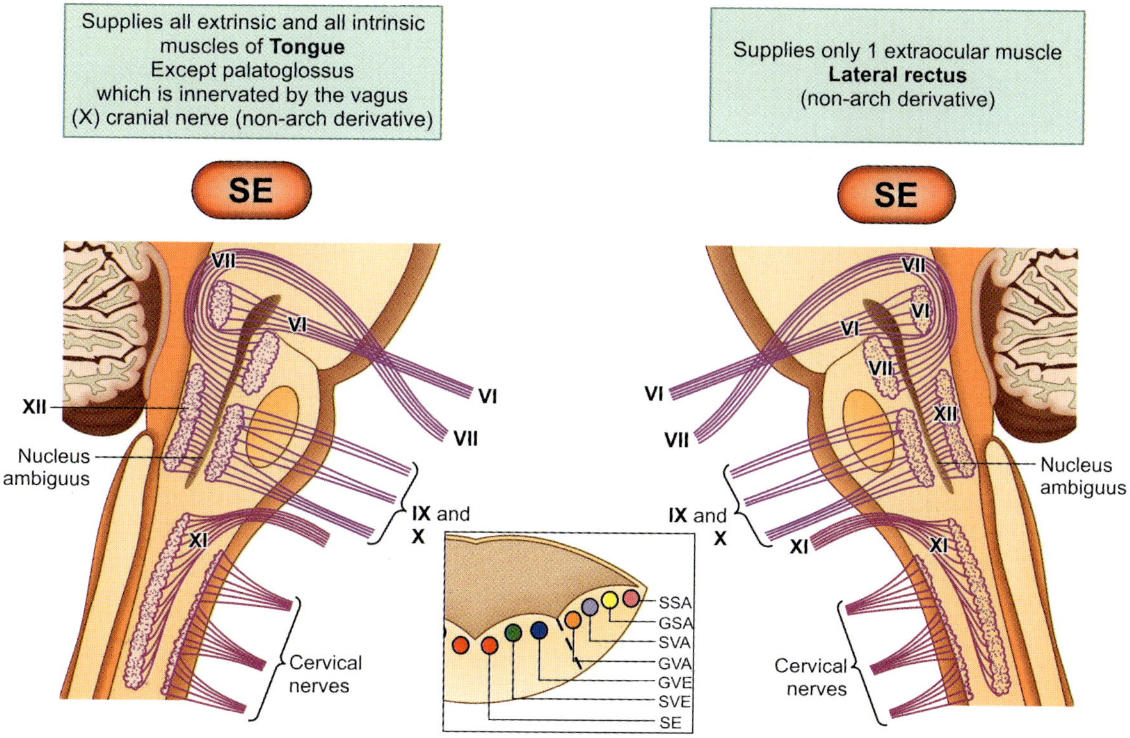

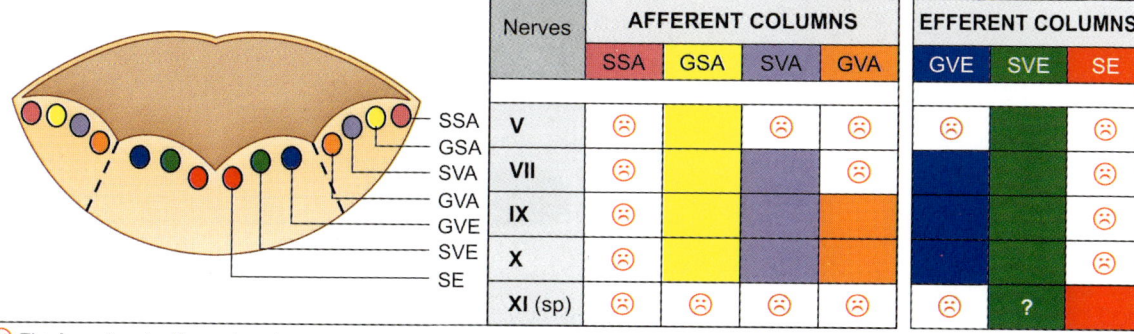

Supplies all extrinsic and all intrinsic muscles of **Tongue**
Except palatoglossus
which is innervated by the vagus (X) cranial nerve (non-arch derivative)
Supplies only 1 extraocular muscle
Lateral rectus
(non-arch derivative)
SE
SE
VII
VI
XII
Nucleus ambiguus
VI
VII
IX and X
XI
Cervical nerves
SSA
GSA
SVA
GVA
GVE
SVE
SE

Fig. 20.5: Functional component of VI cranial (abducens) and XII cranial (hypoglossal) nerve is same and in each nerve only one–somatic efferent (SE) column

Mixed Cranial Nerves (both sensory and motor functions) V, VII, IX, X, and XI Spinal

(Figs 20.6 to 20.10)

Notes:

i. The V cranial nerve (trigeminal) consists of 4 nuclei, out of which 3 are **sensory nuclei** named from rostral to caudal side these are: (a) *mesencephalic nucleus of V*, (b) *main* (or *superior*) *sensory nucleus of V*, and (c) *nucleus of spinal tract of V;* and 1 is a **motor nucleus**

Mixed Cranial Nerves (V, VII, IX, X and XI) have both Afferent and Efferent Column(s)

SSA
GSA
SVA
GVA
GVE
SVE
SE

Nerves	AFFERENT COLUMNS				EFFERENT COLUMNS		
	SSA	GSA	SVA	GVA	GVE	SVE	SE
V	☹		☹	☹	☹		☹
VII	☹			☹			☹
IX	☹						☹
X	☹						☹
XI (sp)	☹	☹	☹	☹	☹	?	

☹ The face sign signifies—absent

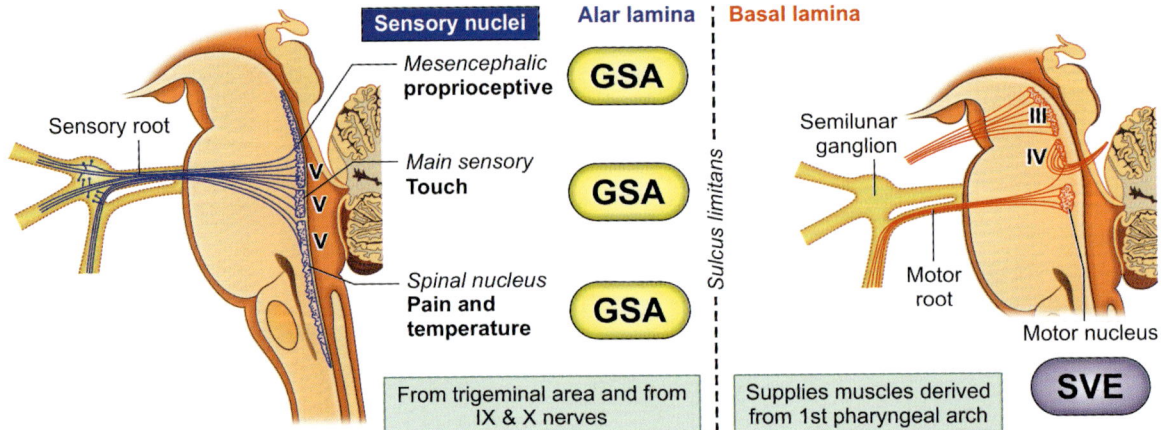

Fig. 20.6: Functional components of V cranial (trigeminal) nerve are both from the alar and basal laminae, because the mandibular division carries fibres for the muscles derived from the 1st pharyngeal arch. The ophthalmic and maxillary divisions are pure sensory. Notice different kinds of sensations are related with the different sensory nuclei described in the text

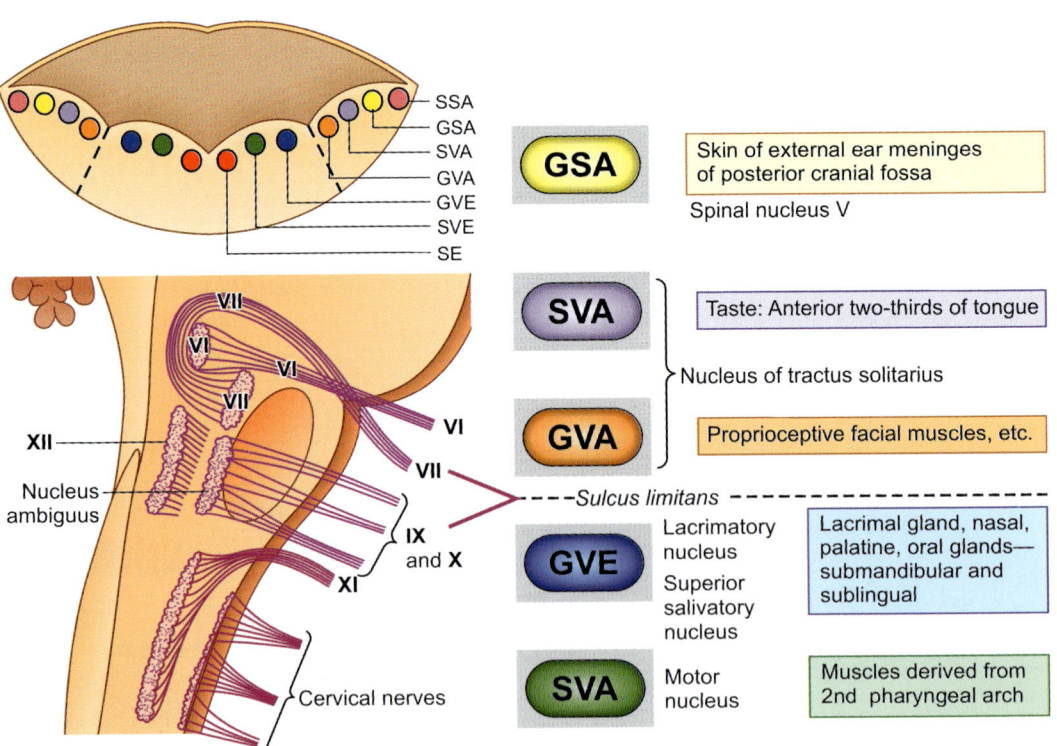

Fig. 20.7: Functional components of VII cranial (facial) nerve are both from the alar (SVA, GVA, and GSA) and basal (GVE and SVE) laminae. The figure details nuclei involved for sensations and supply to muscle and glands of salivary, nasal, and palate and oral region

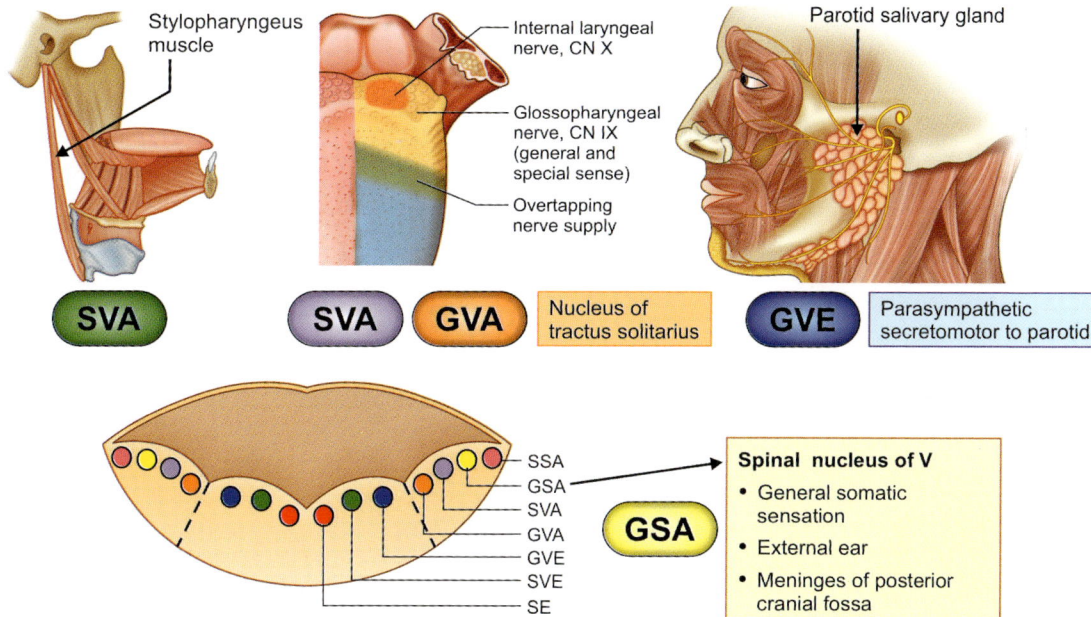

Stylopharyngeus muscle

Internal laryngeal nerve, CN X

Glossopharyngeal nerve, CN IX (general and special sense)

Overlapping nerve supply

Parotid salivary gland

SVA

SVA   **GVA**   Nucleus of tractus solitarius

GVE   Parasympathetic secretomotor to parotid

SSA
GSA
SVA
GVA
GVE
SVE
SE

GSA

Spinal nucleus of V
- General somatic sensation
- External ear
- Meninges of posterior cranial fossa

Fig. 20.8: Functional components of IX cranial (glossopharyngeal) nerve also are both from the alar (SVA, GVA, and GSA) and basal (GVE and SVE) laminae. The IX cranial nerve is the nerve of the 3rd pharyngeal arch and supplies the only muscle—stylopharyngeus derived from this arch

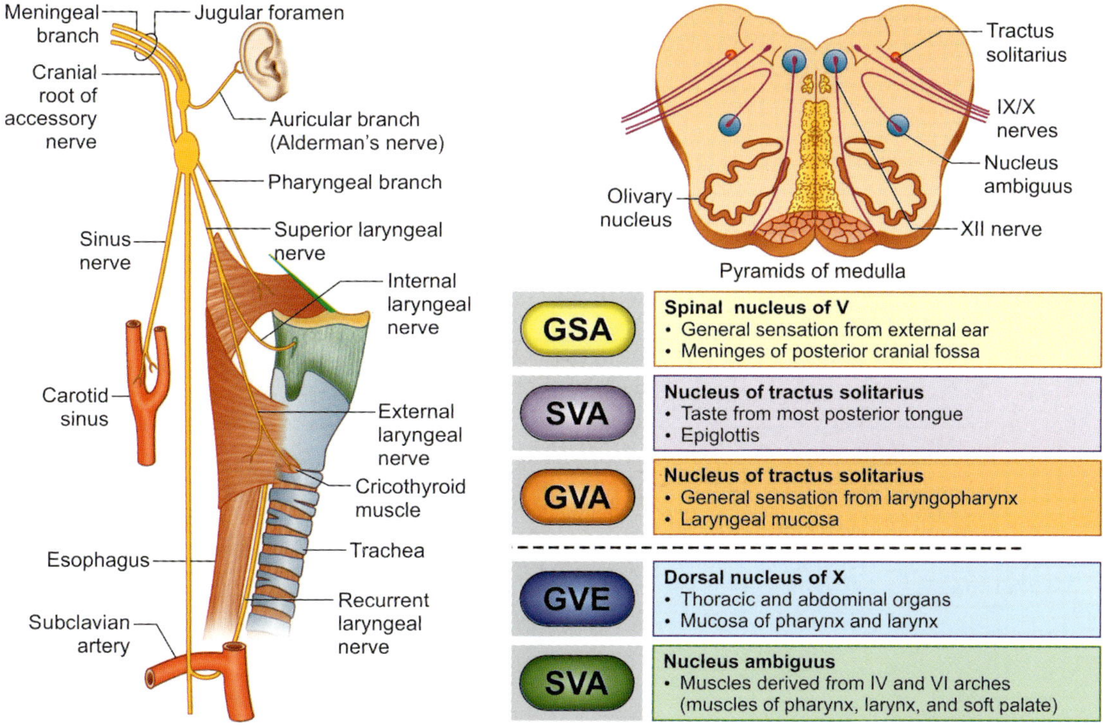

Meningeal branch
Jugular foramen
Cranial root of accessory nerve
Auricular branch (Alderman's nerve)
Pharyngeal branch
Sinus nerve
Superior laryngeal nerve
Internal laryngeal nerve
Carotid sinus
External laryngeal nerve
Cricothyroid muscle
Esophagus
Trachea
Recurrent laryngeal nerve
Subclavian artery

Tractus solitarius
IX/X nerves
Nucleus ambiguus
Olivary nucleus
XII nerve
Pyramids of medulla

GSA   **Spinal nucleus of V**
- General sensation from external ear
- Meninges of posterior cranial fossa

SVA   **Nucleus of tractus solitarius**
- Taste from most posterior tongue
- Epiglottis

GVA   **Nucleus of tractus solitarius**
- General sensation from laryngopharynx
- Laryngeal mucosa

GVE   **Dorsal nucleus of X**
- Thoracic and abdominal organs
- Mucosa of pharynx and larynx

SVA   **Nucleus ambiguus**
- Muscles derived from IV and VI arches (muscles of pharynx, larynx, and soft palate)

Fig. 20.9: Functional components of X cranial (vagus) nerve also are both from the alar (SVA, GVA, and GSA) and basal (GVE and SVE) laminae. These are similar to the five components of the IX cranial nerve

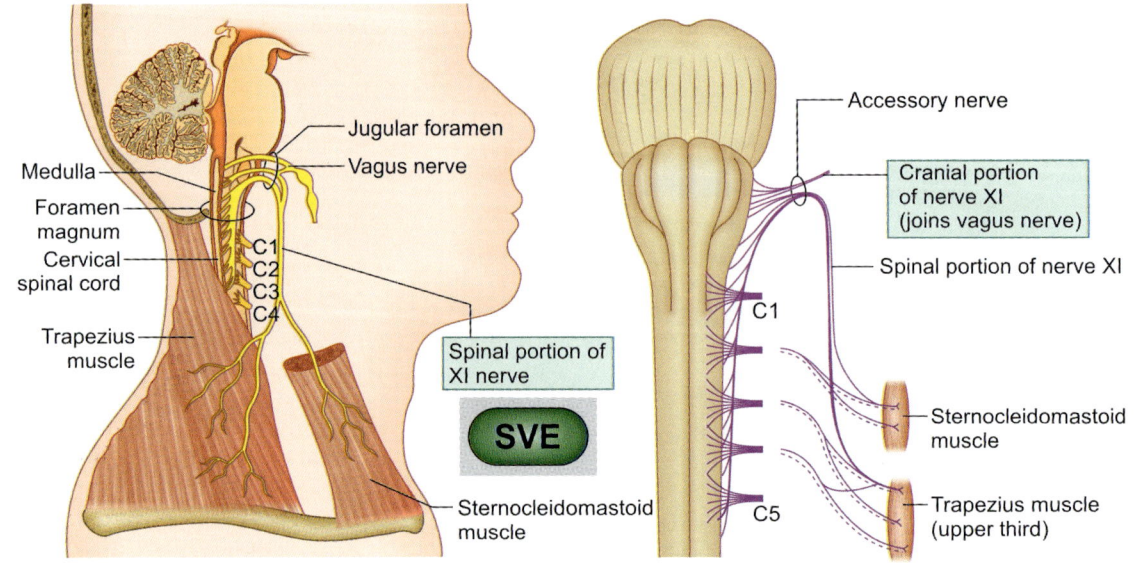

Fig. 20.10: Functional components of XI cranial (accessory) nerve are two: Cranial part supplying muscles of soft palate, pharynx, and larynx—all skeletal muscles of arch origin. The spinal part supplies two skeletal muscles—sternocleidomastoid and trapezius

FUNCTIONAL CRANIAL NERVE NUCLEI AT A GLANCE							
Nerves	**AFFERENT COLUMNS**				**EFFERENT COLUMNS**		
	SSA	GSA	SVA	GVA	GVE	SVE	SE
I			■				
II	■						
III					■		■
IV							
V		■				■	
VI							■
VII			■		■	■	
VIII							
IX			■	■	■	■	
X			■	■	■	■	
XI						?	■
XII							■

SSA	Sensations from special sensory organs: Vision, hearing and equilibrium (balancing)		**GVE**	Autonomic (exclusively parasympathetic): Smooth and cardiac muscles, and glands	
GSA	General sensations: Touch, pain, temperature, pressure, vibration, and proprioception		**SVE**	Skeletal muscles of branchial origin: Jaws, face, larynx and pharynx	
SVA	Special visceral sensation: Smell, and taste		**SE**	Muscles of somatic/myotome origin: Orbits and tongue (except palatoglossus)	
GVA	General sensations from viscera				

Key to functional columns (from dorsolateral to ventrolateral parts separated by sulcus limitans) (Fig. 20.11)

SSA—Special somatic afferent (sensory)—e.g. cranial nerves II for vision and VII (cochlear) nerves (although the II nerve is neither a true cranial nerve nor it is attached to the brainstem)

GSA—General somatic afferent (sensory)—main sensory nucleus of cranial nerve V

SVA—Special visceral afferent (sensory)—special sensations of smell (I) and taste (V, VII, IX, and X)

GVA—General visceral afferent (sensory)—cranial nerves IX an X

GVE—General visceral efferent (motor)—represent preganglionic parasympathetic fibres serving a secretomotor function. Examples are:

- III cranial nerve joined by fibres from ***Edinger-Westphal nucleus*** to supply constrictor papillae muscle
- VII cranial nerve joined by fibres from ***superior salivatory nucleus***
- IX cranial nerve joined with parasympathetic fibres from ***inferior salivatory nucleus***; and
- X cranial nerve having parasympathetic fibres from ***dorsal nucleus of X*** for supply of smooth muscles of thoracic and abdominal organs.

SVE—Special visceral efferent (motor)—always innervate striated muscles (branchial arch derivate of face and neck) represent branchiomotor fibres supplying skeletal muscles derived from pharyngeal (or branchial) arches, Examples are:

- V or trigeminal nerve (muscles derived from first branchial arch: muscles of mastication, anterior belly of digastric, and tensor tympani all of which are supplied by motor nucleus of trigeminal)
- VII or facial nerve (muscles derived from second branchial arch: muscles of facial expression, posterior belly of digastric, and stapedius); and
- IX or glossopharyngeal, X or vagus, and XI or accessory spinal part only (as the cranial part of the nerve travels via branches of vagus).

SE—Somatic efferent (motor)—innervate muscles of somatic origin (involved in locomotion—muscles of limbs, intercostal muscles and of abdominal wall).

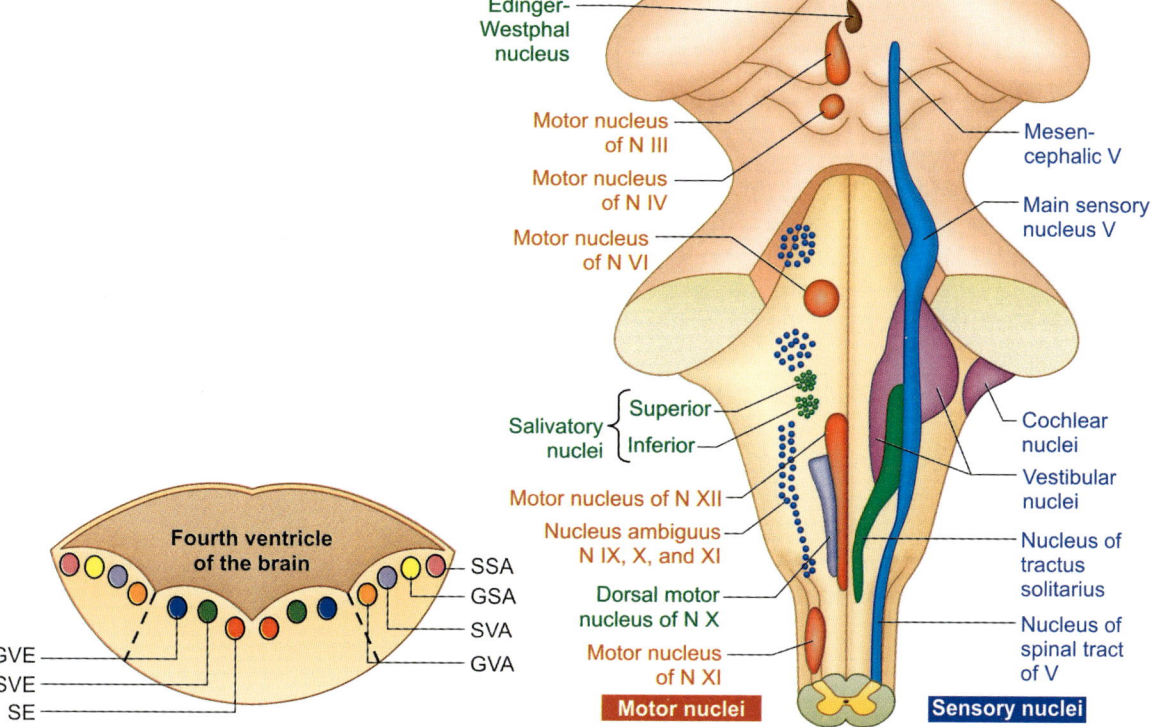

Fig. 20.11: Location of motor (on the left) and sensory (on the right) nuclei of cranial nerves III to XII emerging from the brainstem. Accordingly, the above diagram represents the motor (efferent) and sensory (afferent) functional components in a transverse section of the fourth ventricle

21

Autonomic Nervous System
Overview and Subdivisions

- Introduction to Autonomic Nervous System
- Subdivisions of Autonomic Nervous System
  - Sympathetic nervous system
  - Parasympathetic nervous system
  - Enteric or intrinsic nervous system
- Groups of Autonomic Ganglia
- Transmitters Released at Synapses

INTRODUCTION TO AUTONOMIC NERVOUS SYSTEM

The autonomic nervous system (ANS) is distributed to peripheral tissues and organs by way of **autonomic ganglia**. Its controlling centres are in: (i) hypothalamus, and (ii) brainstem. The *preganglionic neurons* are located in the grey matter of the brainstem and spinal cord. From these neurons **preganglionic fibres** (mostly *myelinated*) project out of the CNS to synapse upon multipolar neurons in the autonomic ganglia. The **postganglionic fibres** (mostly *unmyelinated*) emerge from the autonomic ganglia and form terminal networks in the target tissues.

The *first neuron* or the **preganglionic neuron** is located in:
i. The nuclei of III, VII, IX, and X cranial nerves—**cranial portion** of the craniosacral (parasympathetic) outflow in the brainstem.
ii. The lateral grey horn cells of T1 to L2 segments of the spinal cord—**thoracolumbar** (sympathetic) outflow of the autonomic nervous system.
iii. The lateral grey horn cells of S2, 3, 4 segments of the spinal cord—**sacral portion** of the craniosacral (parasympathetic) outflow in the brainstem.

The *second neuron* or the **postganglionic neuron** is located outside the CNS and forms the autonomic (motor) ganglion.

SUBDIVISIONS OF AUTONOMIC NERVOUS SYSTEM

Both anatomically and functionally, the ANS is composed of three divisions: sympathetic, parasympathetic, and enteric or intrinsic (Fig. 21.1 and Table 21.1).

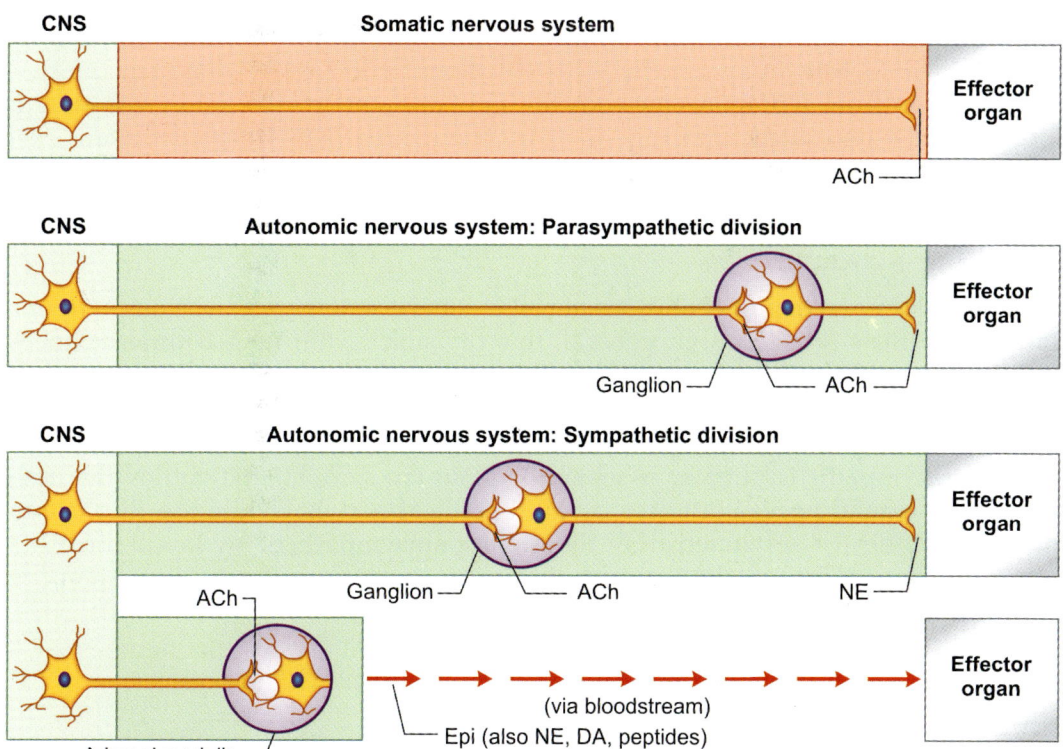

Fig. 21.1: Chemically, the fibres are named according to the transmitter substances released at the synapse between the postganglionic fibres and the target organs. Also notice that the length of postganglionic fibre is greater in sympathetic system than that of the preganglionic fibres; the reverse occurs in parasympathetic innervations where the preganglionic fibres are much longer than the postganglionic ones

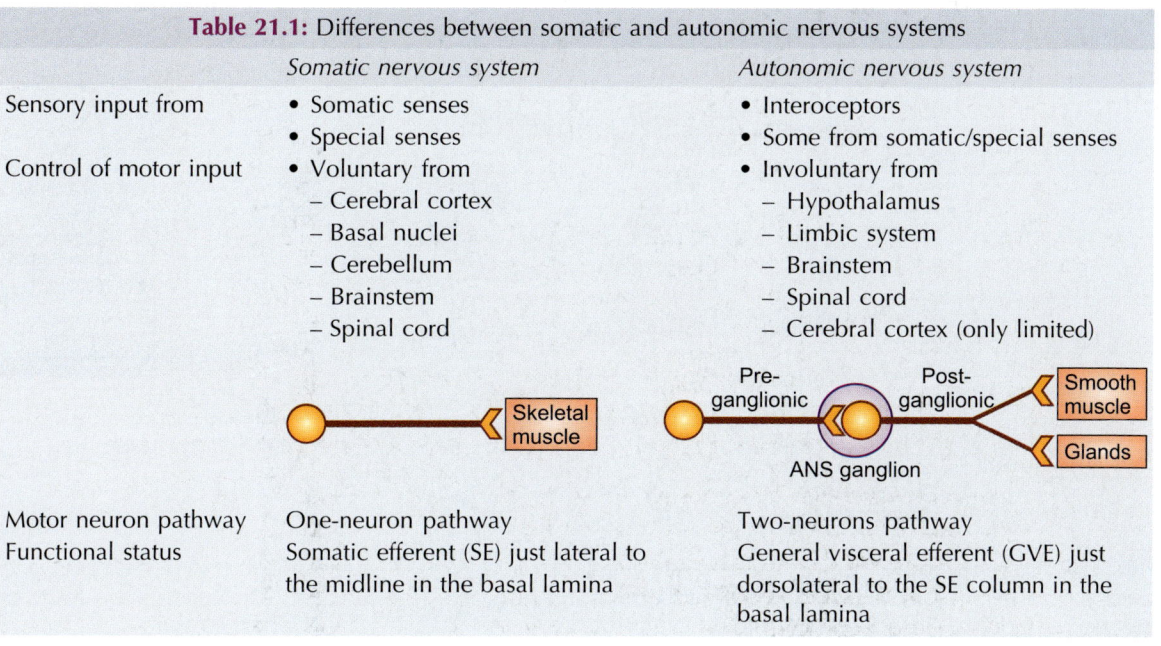

Table 21.1: Differences between somatic and autonomic nervous systems		
	Somatic nervous system	*Autonomic nervous system*
Sensory input from	• Somatic senses • Special senses	• Interoceptors • Some from somatic/special senses

Control of motor input	• Voluntary from
	  – Cerebral cortex
	  – Basal nuclei
	  – Cerebellum
	  – Brainstem
	  – Spinal cord
		• Involuntary from
		  – Hypothalamus
		  – Limbic system
		  – Brainstem
		  – Spinal cord
		  – Cerebral cortex (only limited)

Motor neuron pathway	One-neuron pathway	Two-neurons pathway
Functional status	Somatic efferent (SE) just lateral to the midline in the basal lamina	General visceral efferent (GVE) just dorsolateral to the SE column in the basal lamina

Sympathetic Nervous System

The sympathetic (acting in sympathy with emotions) nervous system (Fig. 21.2) has a **thoracolumbar outflow**. It prepares the body for 'fight or flight' in association with emergency situations usually associated with rage or fear. The sympathetic nervous system exerts a continuous constrictor control on blood vessels in the limbs, closes sphincters of the alimentary and urinary tracts, increases the heart rate, and dilates the pupils.

Parasympathetic Nervous System

The parasympathetic (acting in conditions at rest—with no emergency) nervous system has a **craniosacral outflow** (Fig. 21.2). In general, this division of the ANS counterbalances the sympathetic system. The preganglionic fibres emerge from the brainstem in four cranial nerves (III, VII, IX, and X) forming the **cranial** part of the outflow—and from middle three sacral segments (S2–4) forming the **sacral** part of the outflow.

Cranial parasympathetic outflow is separated from the sympathetic outflow by not only the XI and XII cranial nerves but also by all 8 cervical nerves. While the thoracolumbar (sympathetic) outflow is separated from the sacral parasympathetic by lower three lumbar and first sacral nerves. So actually there are *three* parts in autonomic nervous system.

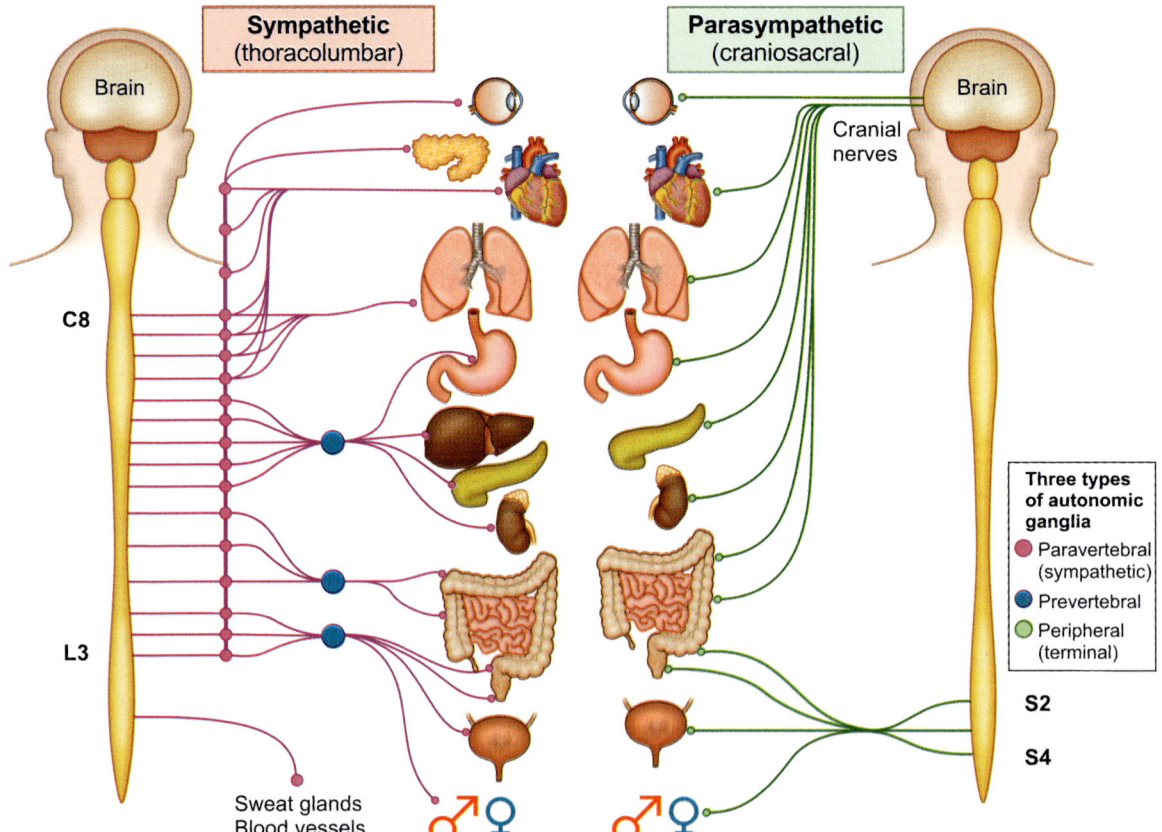

Fig. 21.2: The autonomic nervous system has two major subdivisions—sympathetic (thoracolumbar) and parasympathetic (craniosacral). The cranial part is not shown here (see Chapter 23). Notice three types of autonomic ganglia described in the text

Enteric or Intrinsic Nervous System

The enteric nervous system (ENS) controls: (i) peristaltic activity, (ii) glandular secretion, and (iii) water and ion transfer. It consists of a network of **intrinsic neurons** in the wall of the alimentary tract (from the mid-region of the oesophagus all the way to the anal canal). For this reason ENS is sometimes referred to as the 'gut brain' or 'second brain'.

GROUPS OF AUTONOMIC GANGLIA

There are **three kinds of autonomic ganglia** (Fig. 21.2):
1. *Vertebral ganglia:* These constitute the **sympathetic trunk** or **chain** with sympathetic ganglia possessing a distinct capsule; and are located on either side of the vertebral column along its entire length. Hence, such ganglia are also termed **paravertebral ganglia**.
2. *Collateral ganglia* called **prevertebral ganglia** these surround abdominal aorta and its larger visceral branches.
3. *Terminal or peripheral ganglia* are close or within the structures they innervate.

TRANSMITTERS RELEASED AT SYNAPSES

1. Between preganglionic fibres and postganglionic neuron in all the three outflows mentioned above the transmitter substance released is **Acetylcholine** (ACh)—hence the fibres are referred as **cholinergic.**
2. At the termination of the postganglionic fibres in the viscera and the craniosacral outflow are **cholinergic**, but the thoracolumbar outflow releases adrenaline or norepinehrine and hence termed **adrenergic** (Fig. 21.3)

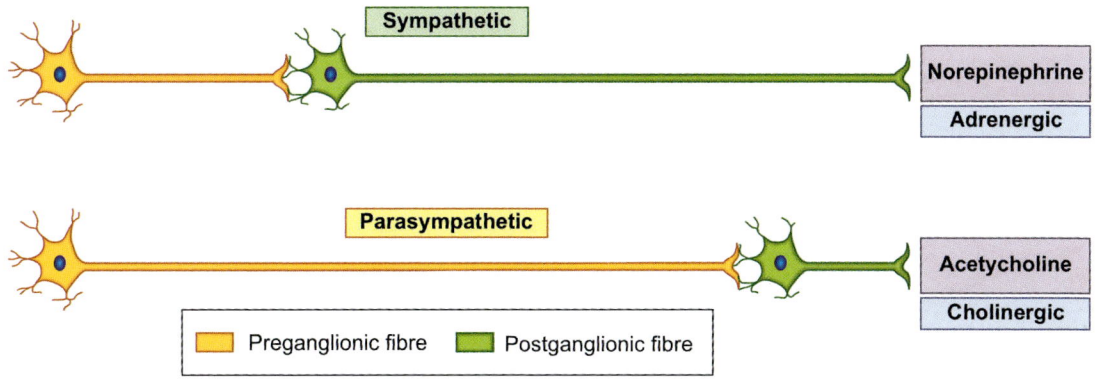

Fig. 21.3: Chemically, the fibres are named according to the transmitter substances released at the synapse between the postganglionic fibres and the target organs. Also notice that the length of postganglionic fibre is greater in sympathetic system than that of the preganglionic fibres; the reverse occurs in parasympathetic innervations where the preganglionic fibres are much longer than the postganglionic ones

22

Sympathetic Division of ANS
Thoracolumbar Outflow

INTRODUCTION

The **sympathetic nervous system** is division of the **autonomic nervous system** (ANS) that activates what is often termed the fight or flight response mainly under emergencies that cause stress and require a person to *fight*, *fright* and *flight*. **Fight** means to defend oneself against an attack; **fright** means a sudden intense feeling of fear and **flight** means to run away. It originates in the spinal cord. The sympathetic part is mainly concerned with **trophic functions** responsible for intensification of oxidation processes, nutrient consumption and respiration and increases the rate of cardiac activity and supply of oxygen to the muscles.

Three more facts about the sympathetic nervous system are as follows:
i. The synapse in the sympathetic ganglion uses acetylcholine as a neurotransmitter
ii. The synapse of the postganglionic neuron with the target organ uses the neurotransmitter called norepinephrine. Of course, there is one exception: the sympathetic postganglionic neuron that terminates on the sweat glands uses acetylcholine.
iii. The sympathetic and parasympathetic systems are contrasting subdivisions of the ANS. In general, it may be said that sympathetic reactions tend to be 'mass reactions', widely diffuse in their effect, and that they are directed towards the mobilisation of the resources of the body for the expenditure of energy in dealing with emergencies or emotion crises.

PREGANGLIONIC AND POSTGANGLIONIC EFFERENT FIBRES

Specifically, the cell bodies of the first neuron (the *preganglionic* neuron) are located in the thoracic and lumbar spinal cord. Cell bodies of the preganglionic neuron of this division are located in the intermediolateral horn of the spinal cord.

- The axons of the myelinated **preganglionic sympathetic neurons** leave the spinal cord *via* the ventral roots of the spinal cord at the level of T1–L2 (thoracolumbar). The preganglionic neurons then make synapses with **postganglionic neurons** in the paravertebral sympathetic chain ganglia: (the upper 8 chain ganglia merge into superior, middle and inferior cervical ganglia) or in the *prevertebral collateral ganglia* (celiac, superior and inferior mesenteric ganglia). The nonmyelinated axons of the postganglionic neurons travel from these chain and collateral ganglia to the tissues that they innervate.

Axons of the sympathetic preganglionic neurons leave the spinal cord via the ventral roots and end in the sympathetic ganglion chain or in the collateral ganglia where cell bodies of the **postganglionic neuron** are located.

As the sympathetic system promotes a fight-or-flight response, it corresponds with arousal and energy generation, and inhibits digestion:

- **Diverts blood flow away from the gastrointestinal** (GI) tract and **skin via vasoconstriction**
- **Blood flow to skeletal muscles and the lungs is enhanced** (by as much as 1200% in the case of skeletal muscles).
- **Dilates bronchioles** of the lung through circulating epinephrine, which allows for **greater alveolar oxygen exchange.**
- **Increases heart rate** and the contractility of cardiac cells (myocytes), thereby providing a mechanism for **enhanced blood flow** to skeletal muscles.
- **Dilates pupils** and **relaxes the ciliary muscle** to the lens, allowing more light to enter the eye and enhances far vision.
- Provides **vasodilation** for the **coronary vessels of the heart.**
- **Constricts all the intestinal sphincters** and the urinary sphincter.
- Inhibits **peristalsis.**
- Stimulates **orgasm.**

GANGLIA IN SYMPATHETIC OUTFLOW

The ganglia are seen in two ganglionated cords symmetrically placed along the anterolateral aspect of the vertebral column. Various body organs receive sympathetic outflow from the different spinal segments as indicated in Fig. 22.1.

Sympathetic Chain (Trunk)

Sympathetic trunks are two long ganglionated nerve strands, one on each side of the vertebral column, extending from the base of the skull to the coccyx. The preganglionic fibres arise from the corresponding spinal segments for supply of different body organs. They synapse in the paravertebral ganglia of the sympathetic system: (i) either at the same level, or (ii) at levels higher or below, or (iii) in distant prevertebral collateral ganglia (Figs 22.2 and 22.3) to continue with the postganglionic fibres.

For simplicity in description, the ganglia in the sympathetic trunk may be classified in the anatomical regions:

Cervical Portion of Sympathetic Trunk

The cervical portion of the sympathetic trunk is placed behind the carotid sheath and in front of the transverse processes of the cervical vertebrae. This part of the trunk contains three

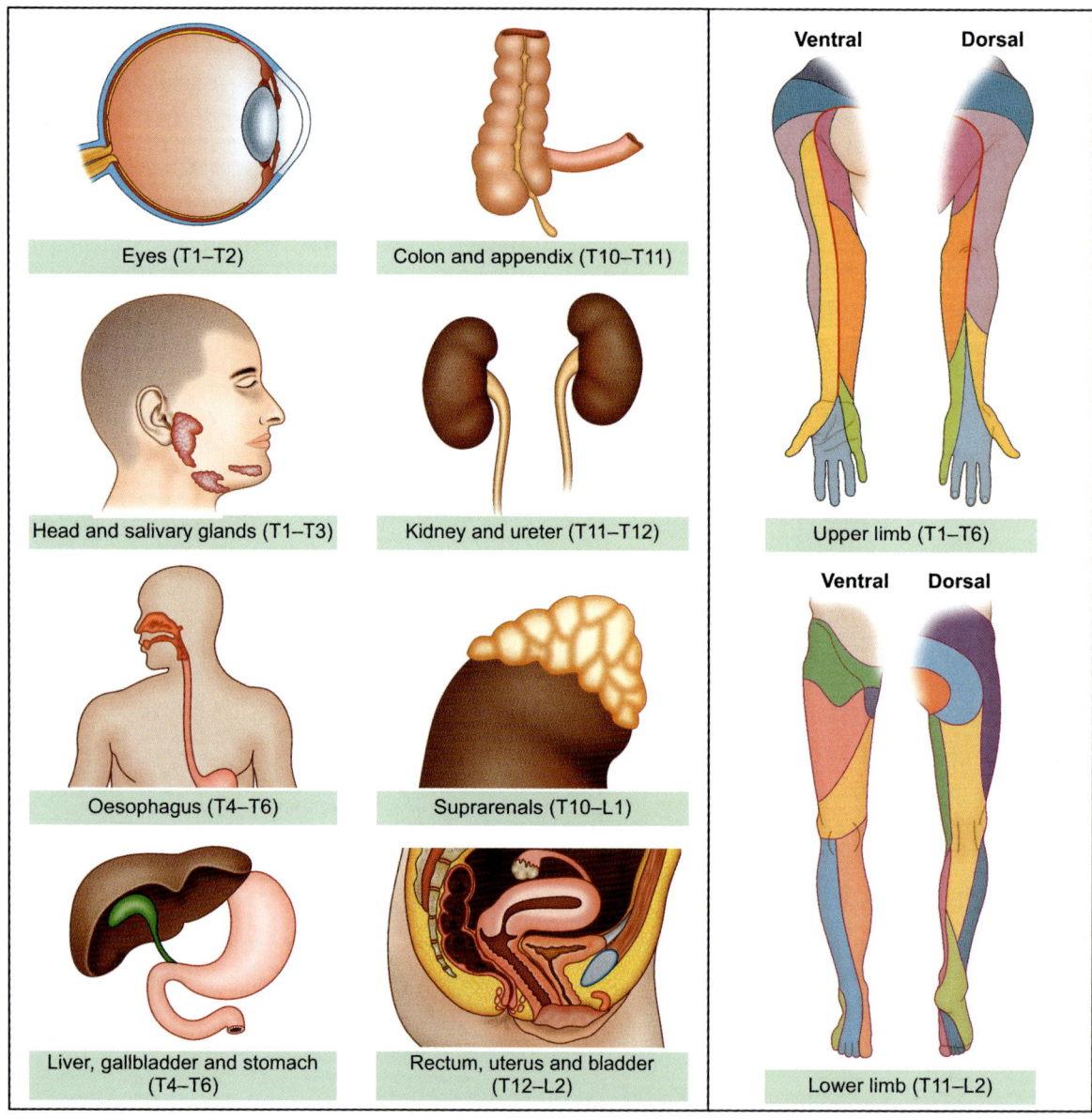

Fig. 22.1: Diagrammatic representation of spinal level of sympathetic connector cells

ganglia connected by intervening cords. These ganglia are probably formed by fusion of the original eight segmental ganglia:

Superior Cervical Ganglion

It is the largest of the three cervical ganglia (believed to be formed by fusion of four ganglia), and is placed opposite the C2 and C3 vertebrae (Figs 22.4–22.6). The following are three sets of branches:

1. **Anterior branches** ramify over:
   - Common carotid artery.

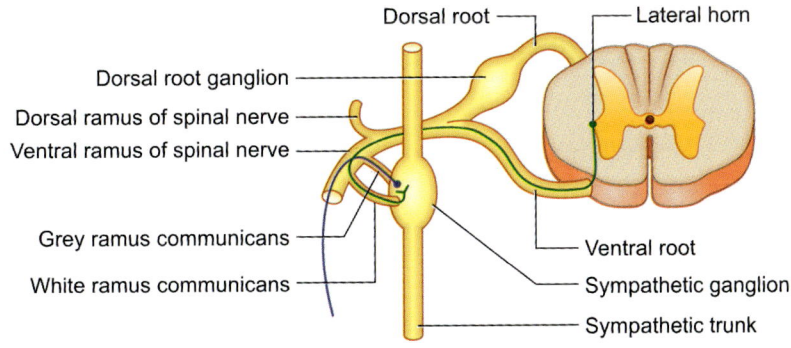

Dorsal root — — Lateral horn

Dorsal root ganglion — —

Dorsal ramus of spinal nerve — —

Ventral ramus of spinal nerve — —

Grey ramus communicans — —

White ramus communicans — —

— Ventral root

— Sympathetic ganglion

— Sympathetic trunk

1. Synapse at the same level

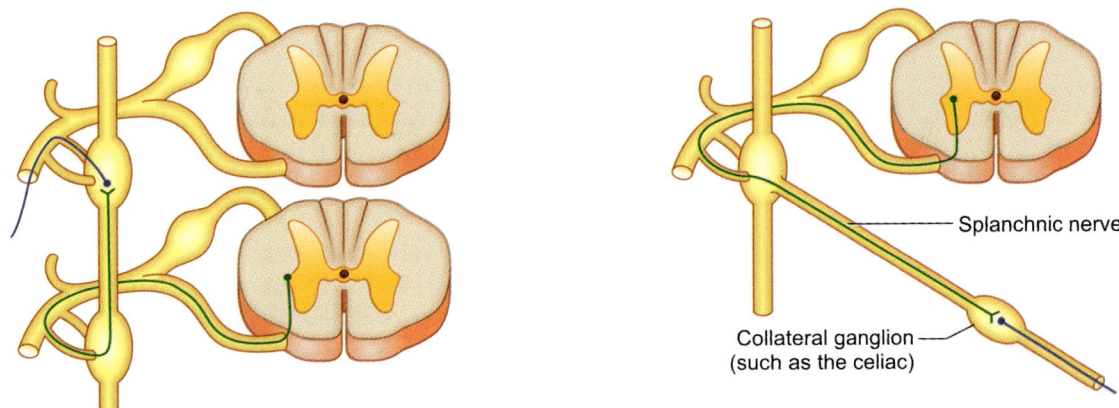

— Splanchnic nerve

Collateral ganglion — —
(such as the celiac)

2. Synapse at a higher or lower level

3. Synapse in a distant collateral ganglion anterior to the vertebral column

Fig. 22.2: Three pathways of sympathetic innervation: Notice that synapses between the preganglionic sympathetic fibres (green) and postganglionic sympathetic fibres (blue) are present: 1. at same level, 2. higher or lower level, and 3. in a distant collateral prevertebral ganglion

- External carotid and its branches, the plexus on the middle meningeal artery (given from the first part of the maxillary artery) gives a nerve called *external petrosal nerve*, to the ganglion of the facial nerve.

2. **Medial branches:**
   - *Larygopharyngeal nerve*—to carotid body
   - *Cardiac branch.*

3. **Lateral branches:**
   - Grey rami communicantes—to upper four cervical nerves.
   - Inferior ganglion of X cranial nerve.
   - XII cranial nerve.
   - **Jugular nerve**—ascends to the base of skull and divides into two twigs: One for the inferior ganglion of IX cranial, and the second to superior ganglion of X cranial.

Middle Cervical Ganglion

It is the smallest of the three cervical ganglia, and placed opposite the sixth cervical vertebra. It is formed by the coalescence of ganglion corresponding with fifth and sixth cervical spinal nerves.

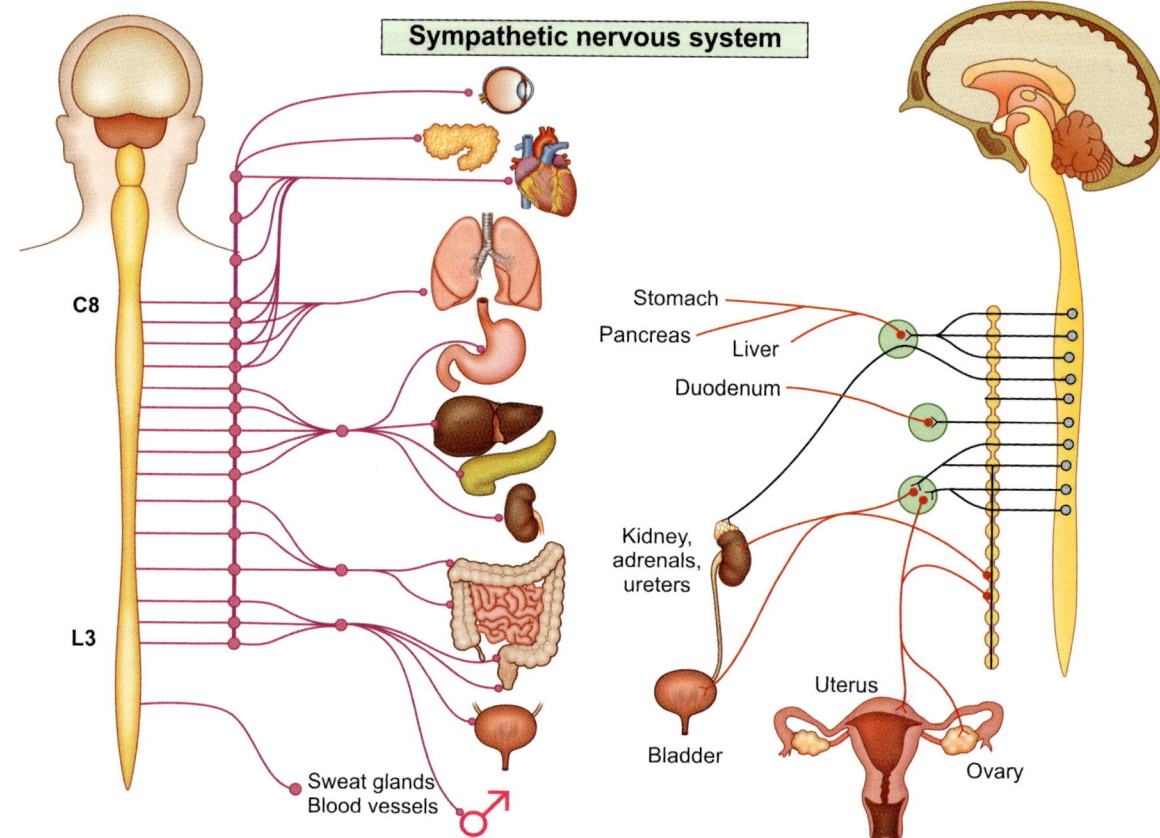

Fig. 22.3: The distribution of pathways of sympathetic nervous system

Following branches are given from this ganglion:
- Grey rami communicantes—to C_5 and C_6 nerves.
- **Ansa subclavia**—a loop passing in front of and then below the first part of the subclavian artery.
- **Cardiac branch**—to the deep cardiac plexus.
- Branches to trachea.
- Branches to oesophagus.

Inferior Cervical Ganglion

It is placed between C7 transverse process and neck of first rib behind the vertebral vessels. This ganglion, formed by coalescence of C7 and C8 ganglia, gives following branches:
- Grey rami communicantes—to C7 and C8 nerves.
- Cardiac branch—to join deep part of the cardiac plexus.

Thoracic Portion of Sympathetic Trunk

The thoracic part of the sympathetic system (Fig. 22.7) consists of a series of ganglia usually corresponding in number to that of the thoracic spinal nerves. The first thoracic ganglion may be fused with the inferior cervical ganglion and the twelfth thoracic ganglion may be fused with the first lumbar ganglion.

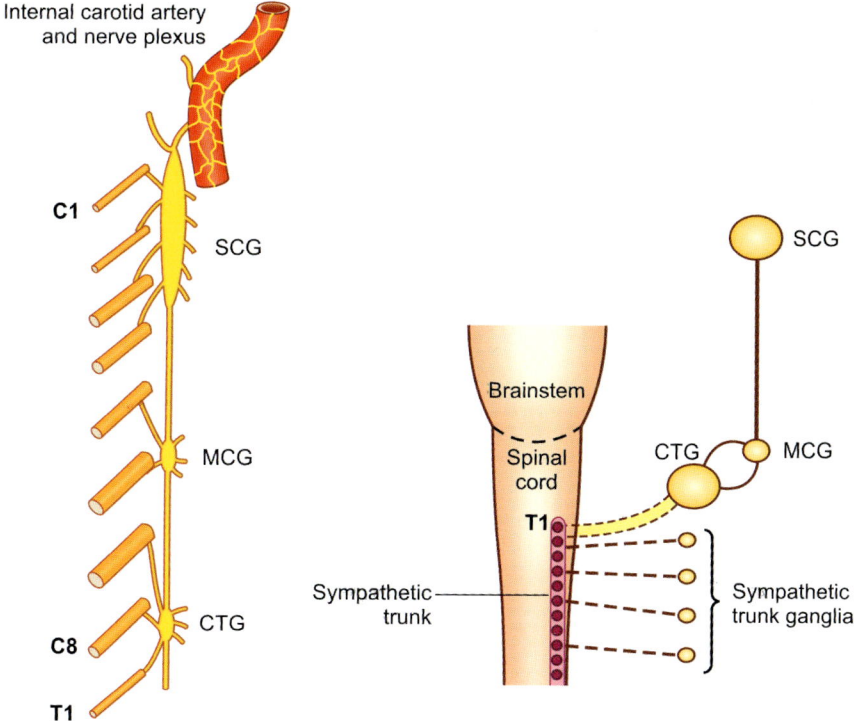

Fig. 22.4: The cervical part of sympathetic nervous system. SCG—superior cervical sympathetic ganglion, MCG—middle cervical sympathetic ganglion, and CTG—cervicothoracic or stellate ganglion formed by fusion of the inferior cervical sympathetic ganglion with first thoracic sympathetic ganglion

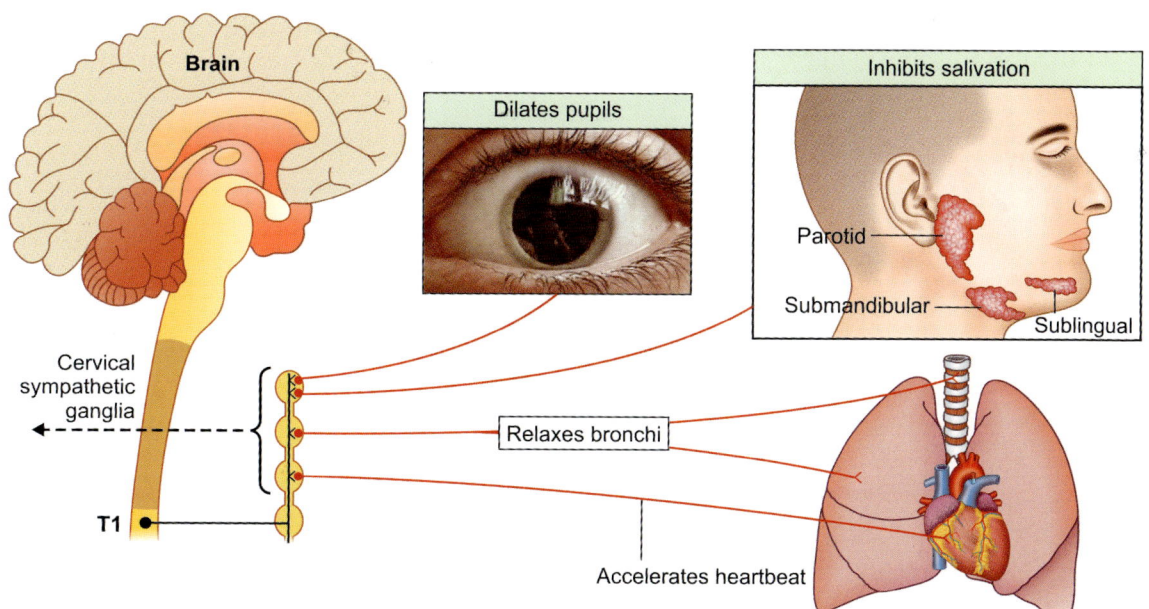

Fig. 22.5: Functional details of cervical sympathetic fibres on main body parts

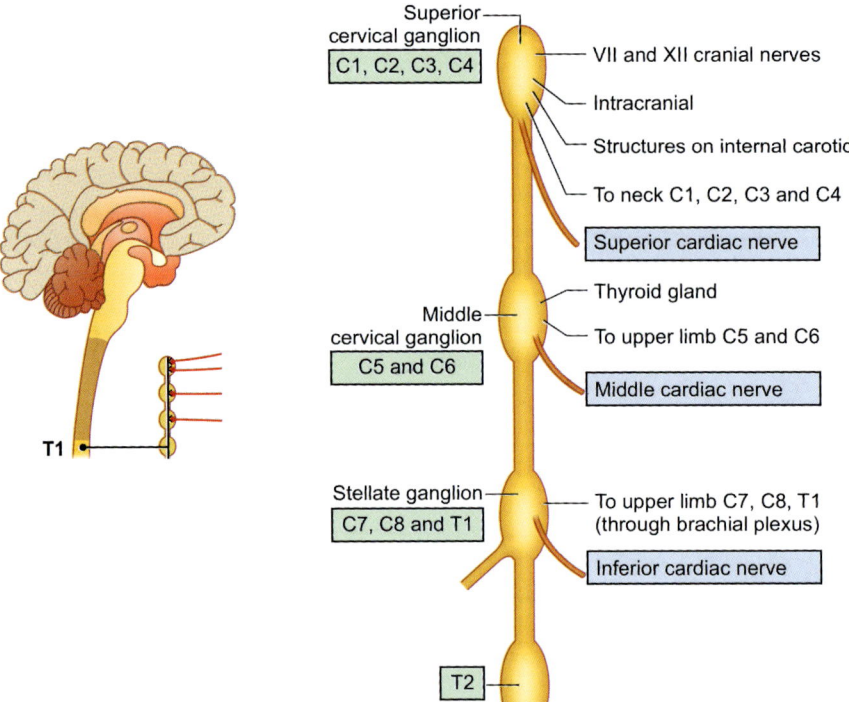

Fig. 22.6: The formation and branches of distribution of the three sympathetic ganglia in the neck. Notice that each cervical ganglion gives a cardiac branch for supply of heart. For details *see* Chapter 24

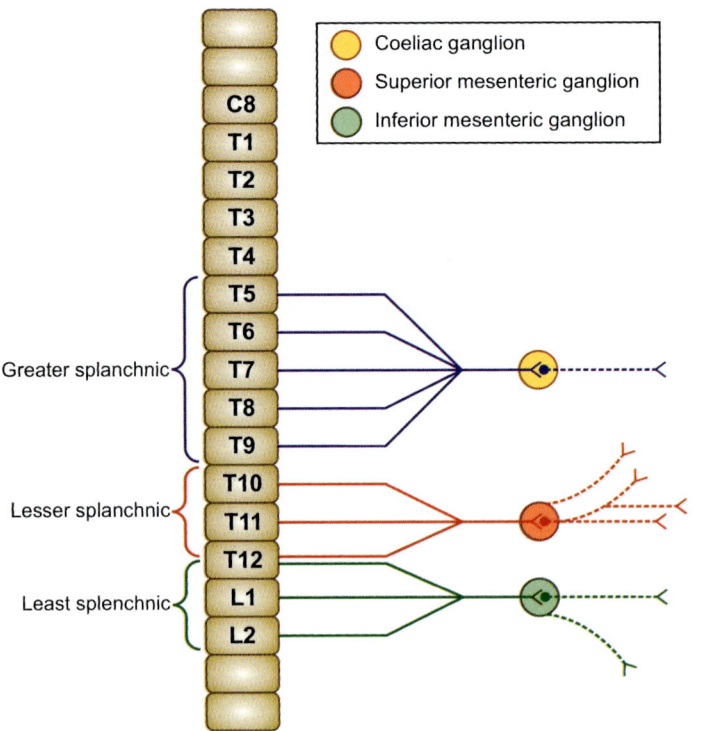

Fig. 22.7: Diagrammatic sketch of thoracic segment shows splanchnic nerves

Branches from Thoracic Ganglia

- The medial branches from the upper 5 thoracic ganglia are very small and send filaments to the thoracic aorta and its branches.
- The medial branches of lower 7 thoracic ganglia are large, distribute filaments to the abdominal aorta.
- These branches from T5 –T12 thoracic ganglia unite to form—**splanchnic nerves**, which are *three* in number namely: greater, lesser, and lowest (or least) splanchnic nerves (Fig. 22.7).
  - *Greater splanchnic nerve*—formed by branches from T5–T9 ganglia. It perforates the crus of the diaphragm, and ends mainly in the **coeliac ganglion** but partly in the suprarenal gland.
  - *Lesser splanchnic nerve*—formed by filaments from T10, and sometimes T11 or T12 and follows the greater splanchnic nerve to end in the **aorticorenal ganglion**.
  - *Lowest or least splanchnic nerve*—arises from T12 ganglion (also L1, and L2), and accompanies the sympathetic trunk to enter the abdomen.

23

Parasympathetic Division of ANS

Craniosacral Outflow

- Introduction
- Parasympathetic Outflow
  - Cranial nerves
  - Spinal nerves
- Cranial Parasympathetic Ganglia
- Relationship to Sympathetic Nervous System

INTRODUCTION

The parasympathetic nervous system (PSNS) is one of *three* divisions of the autonomic nervous system (ANS)—a division of the peripheral nervous system (PNS), the other being the sympathetic nervous system. Sometimes called the 'rest and digest' or 'feed and breed' system, because of the activities that occur when the body is at rest, especially after eating, including sexual arousal, salivation, lacrimation (tears), urination, digestion and defecation. Its action is described as being complementary to that of the sympathetic nervous system, which is responsible for stimulating activities associated with the fight-or-flight response. Owing to its location, the parasympathetic system (Fig. 23.1) is commonly referred to as having 'craniosacral outflow', which stands in contrast to the sympathetic nervous system, which is said to have 'thoracolumbar outflow'.

The ***parasympathetic system*** conserves energy as it slows the heart rate, increases intestinal and gland activity, and relaxes sphincter muscles in the gastrointestinal tract. Formerly, the enteric nervous system (ENS) was considered as the third division of ANS, but ENS is now usually referred to as separate from the autonomic nervous system since it has its own independent reflex activity. Functions of nerves within the parasympathetic nervous system include:

- Dilating blood vessels leading to the GI tract, increasing the blood flow.
- Constricting the bronchiolar diameter when the need for oxygen has diminished.
- Dedicated cardiac branches of the vagus and thoracic spinal accessory nerves impart parasympathetic control of the heart (myocardium).

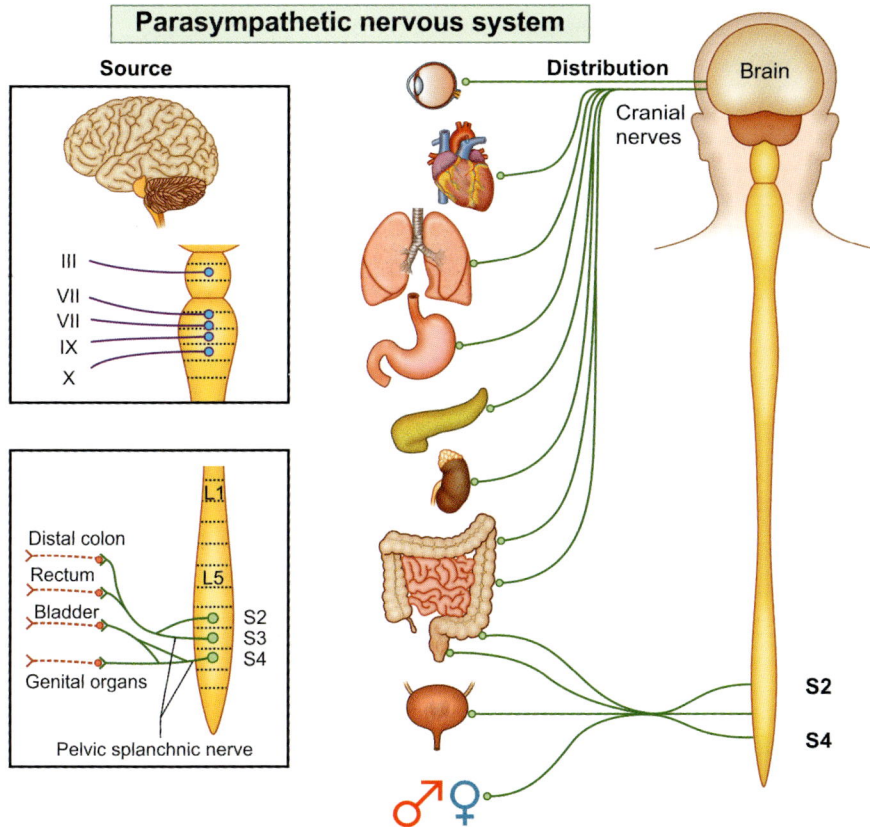

Fig. 23.1: Parasympathetic nervous system consists of a cranial and a sacral outflow. The cranial parasympathetic fibres leave through cranial nerves III, VII, IX, and X. The sacral parasympathetic fibres leave through the pelvic splanchnic nerves from S2 to S4 spinal segments. For distribution refer to Fig. 23.2

- Constriction of the pupil and contraction of the ciliary muscles, facilitating accommodation and allowing for closer vision.
- Stimulating salivary gland secretion, and accelerates peristalsis, mediating digestion of food and, indirectly, the absorption of nutrients.

PARASYMPATHETIC OUTFLOW

Cranial Nerves

The only **cranial nerves** that transmit **parasympathetic** fibres are the oculomotor, facial, glossopharyngeal, and vagus **nerves** (Fig. 23.2). Nerve fibres of the parasympathetic nervous system arise from the central nervous system. Specific nerves include several cranial nerves, specifically the oculomotor nerve, facial nerve, glossopharyngeal nerve, and vagus nerve. Like the sympathetic nervous system, each effector cell is influenced by two neurons in series. The cell bodies of *preganglionic neurons* of this division are located in the cranial portion of the brainstem and in the sacral segments of the spinal cord (craniosacral). Unlike the sympathetic system, the preganglionic neuron is long and terminates close to the effector organ, making synapses with the *postganglionic neuron* that is present close to or within the organ.

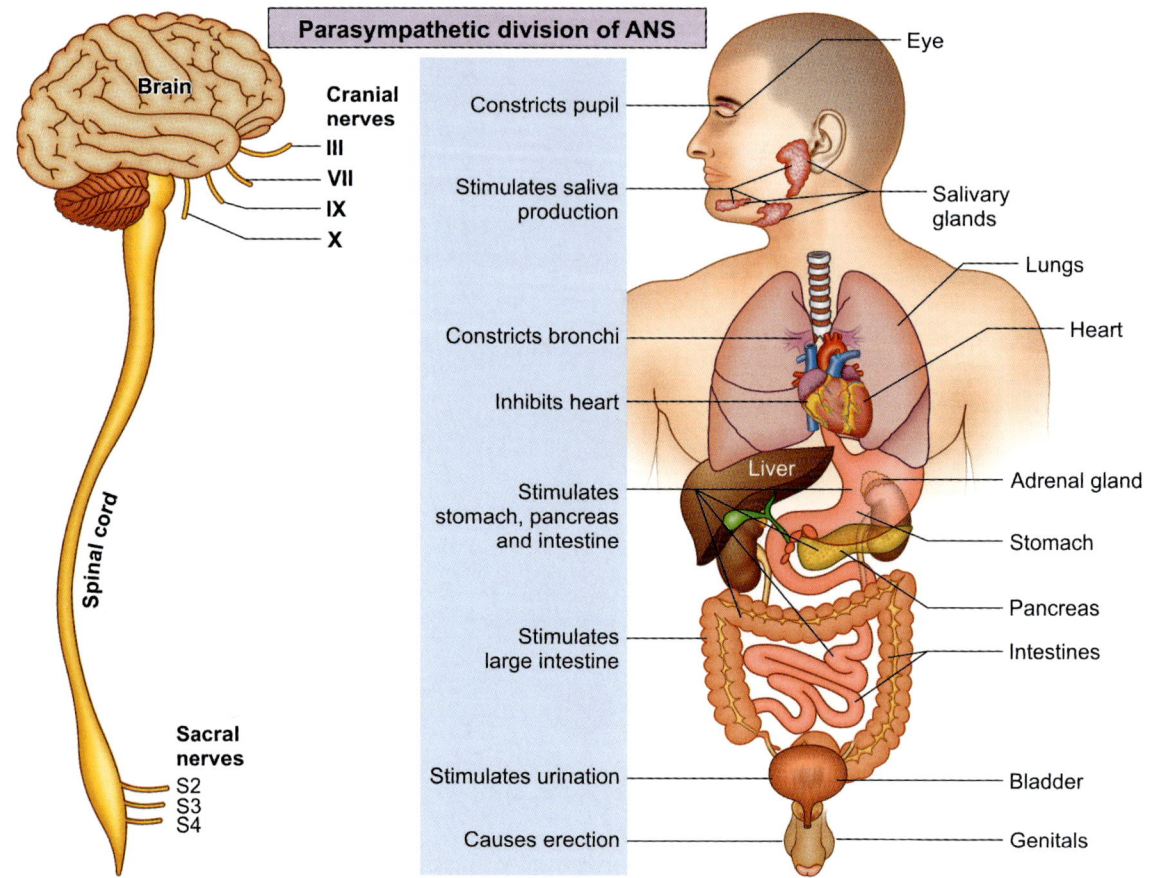

Fig. 23.2: Parasympathetic nervous system consists of a cranial and a sacral outflow. The functional components are summarised for each component

1. The **oculomotor nerve** is responsible for a number of parasympathetic functions related to the eye. The oculomotor PNS fibres originate in the Edinger-Westphal nucleus in the central nervous system and travel through the superior orbital fissure to synapse in the ciliary ganglion located just behind the orbit (eye). From the ciliary ganglion the *postganglionic parasympathetic fibres* leave via short ciliary nerve fibres, a continuation of the nasociliary nerve (a branch of ophthalmic division of the trigeminal nerve). The short ciliary nerves innervate the orbit to control the ciliary muscle (responsible for accommodation) and the iris sphincter muscle, which is responsible for miosis or constriction of the pupil (in response to light or accommodation).

2. The **parasympathetic aspect of the facial nerve** controls secretion of the sublingual and submandibular salivary glands, the lacrimal gland, and the glands associated with the nasal cavity. The *preganglionic fibres* originate within the CNS in the superior salivatory nucleus and leave as the intermediate nerve (which some consider a separate cranial nerve altogether) to connect with the facial nerve just distal (further out) to it surfacing the central nervous system. Just after the facial nerve geniculate ganglion (general sensory ganglion) in the temporal bone, the facial nerve gives off **two separate parasympathetic nerves**. The *first* is the **greater petrosal nerve** and the second is the **chorda tympani**.

The greater petrosal nerve travels through the middle ear and eventually combines with the *deep petrosal nerve* (sympathetic fibres) to form the **nerve of the pterygoid canal**. The parasympathetic fibres of the nerve of the pterygoid canal synapse at the pterygopalatine ganglion, which is closely associated with the maxillary division of the trigeminal nerve (CN V2). The *postganglionic parasympathetic fibres* leave the **pterygopalatine ganglion** (Fig. 23.3 and Table 23.1) in several directions. One division leaves on the zygomatic division

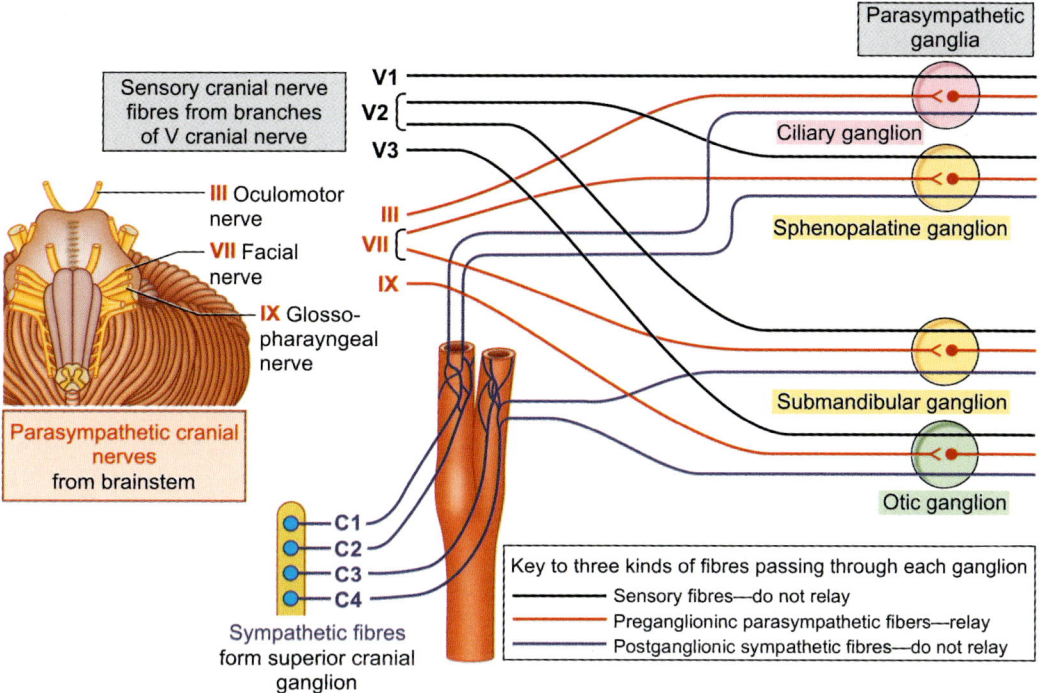

Fig. 23.3: Diagram shows a summary of cranial nerves that carry parasympathetic fibres to four parasympathetic ganglia. Despite three kinds of afferent fibres (sensory, sympathetic, and parasympathetic) to each ganglion, only the last type (i.e. parasympathetic fibres) relay, the remaining two only pass but are not relayed in parasympathetic ganglia. See text Tables 23.1 and 23.2 for detail

Ganglion	Parasympathetic or 'motor' root		Sensory root	Sympathetic root (postganglionic)
	Connector cells located in	Brainstem	Trigeminal ganglion	Upper 3 thoracic segments
Ciliary		Edinger-Westphal nucleus	Ophthalmic division of V cranial nerve	Plexus around internal carotid artery
Sphenopalatine		Superior salivary nucleus	Maxillary division of V cranial nerve	Plexus around internal carotid artery
Submandibular		Superior salivary nucleus	Maxillary division of V cranial nerve	Plexus around external carotid artery
Otic		Inferior salivary nucleus	Mandibular division of V cranial nerve	Plexus around external carotid artery

Table 23.1: Connector cell source and 'roots' of cranial parasympathetic ganglia

of CN V2 and travels on a communicating branch to unite with the lacrimal nerve (branch of the ophthalmic nerve of CN V1) before synapsing at the lacrimal gland. These parasympathetic fibres to the lacrimal gland control tear production.

A separate group of parasympathetic leaving from the pterygopalatine ganglion are the descending palatine nerves (CN V2 branch), which include the *greater* and *lesser palatine nerves*. The greater palatine parasympathetic synapses on the hard palate and regulate mucus glands located there. The lesser palatine nerve synapses at the soft palate and controls sparse taste receptors and mucus glands. Yet another set of divisions from the pterygopalatine ganglion are the posterior, superior, and inferior lateral nasal nerves; and the nasopalatine nerves (all branches of CN V2, maxillary division of the trigeminal nerve) that bring parasympathetic innervation to glands of the nasal mucosa. The second parasympathetic branch that leaves the facial nerve is the chorda tympani. The chorda tympani nerve travels through the middle ear and attaches to the lingual nerve. It carries **secretomotor fibres** to the **submandibular and sublingual glands**. After joining the lingual nerve, the preganglionic fibres synapse at the submandibular ganglion and send postganglionic fibres to the sublingual and submandibular salivary glands.

3. The IX cranial or **glossopharyngeal nerve** has parasympathetic fibres that innervate the *parotid salivary gland*. The preganglionic fibres depart CN IX as the tympanic nerve and continue to the middle ear where they make up a tympanic plexus on the cochlear promontory of the mesotympanum. The tympanic plexus of nerves rejoin and form the lesser petrosal nerve and exit through the foramen ovale to synapse at the otic ganglion. From the otic ganglion postganglionic parasympathetic fibres travel with the auriculotemporal nerve (mandibular branch of trigeminal, CN V3) to the parotid salivary gland.

4. The vagus nerve, named after the Latin word *vagus* (because the nerve controls such a broad range of target tissues—*vagus* in Latin literally means 'wandering'), has parasympathetic that originate in the **dorsal nucleus of the vagus nerve** and the **nucleus ambiguous** in the CNS.

The vagus nerve is an unusual cranial parasympathetic in that it does not join the trigeminal nerve in order to get to its target tissues. Another peculiarity is that the vagus has an autonomic ganglion associated with it at approximately the level of C1 vertebra. *The vagus gives no parasympathetic to the cranium.* Several parasympathetic nerves come off the vagus nerve as it enters the thorax. One nerve is the **recurrent laryngeal nerve**, which becomes the inferior laryngeal nerve. From the left vagus nerve the recurrent laryngeal nerve hooks around the aorta to travel back up to the larynx and proximal oesophagus while, from the right vagus nerve, the recurrent laryngeal nerve hooks around the right subclavian artery to travel back up to the same location as its counterpart. Each recurrent laryngeal nerve supplies the trachea and the oesophagus with parasympathetic secretomotor innervation for glands associated with them (and other fibres that are not PN).

Spinal Nerves

Three spinal nerves in the sacrum (S2–S4), commonly referred to as the pelvic splanchnic nerves, also act as parasympathetic nerves to innervate the pelvic viscera. Unlike in the cranium, where one parasympathetic is incharge of one particular tissue or region, for the most part the pelvic splanchnics each contribute fibres to pelvic viscera by travelling to one or more plexuses before being dispersed to the target tissue. These plexuses are composed of mixed autonomic nerve fibres (parasympathetic and sympathetic) and include the vesical, prostatic, rectal, uterovaginal, and inferior hypogastric plexuses. The **preganglionic neurons in the pathway do not synapse in a ganglion as in the cranium** but rather in the walls of the tissues or organs that they innervate. Nerves of the peripheral nervous system are involved in the erection of genital tissues via the pelvic splanchnic nerves 2–4. They are also responsible for stimulating sexual arousal.

CRANIAL PARASYMPATHETIC GANGLIA

There are four parasympathetic ganglia (Fig. 23.3) associated with three cranial nerves (III, VII, and IX) that carry parasympathetic fibres for supplying the structures in the head and neck regions. Each of these ganglia consists of three 'roots' (Table 23.1): (i) a parasympathetic 'motor root', which carries the preganglionic filament that relays in the concerned ganglion and leaves the ganglion as its 'branch'(es) as postganglionic nerve filament, (ii) a sympathetic, and (iii) a sensory 'root' both containing postganglionic fibres bound for similar destinations enter the concerned ganglion, and both roots without relay leave the ganglion.

Key to fibres traversing through parasympathetic ganglia in Table 23.2

Table 23.2: Cranial parasympathetic ganglia (colour as in Fig. 23.3) and their branches of distribution

Ganglion	Cranial nerve associated	Fibres passing through ganglion	Branches of distribution to
Ciliary	III cranial oculomotor nerve	V1 / III / Ophth	• Sphincter papillae • Ciliary muscle
Sphenopalatine (pterygopalatine)	VII cranial facial nerve	V2 / VII / ICA	• Lacrimal gland • Nasal mucosa • Nasopharynx • Paranasal air sinuses • Palate • Submandibular gland • Sublingual gland
Submandibular		V2 / VII / ECA	
Otic	IX cranial glossopharyngeal nerve	V3 / IX / ECA	• Parotid salivary gland

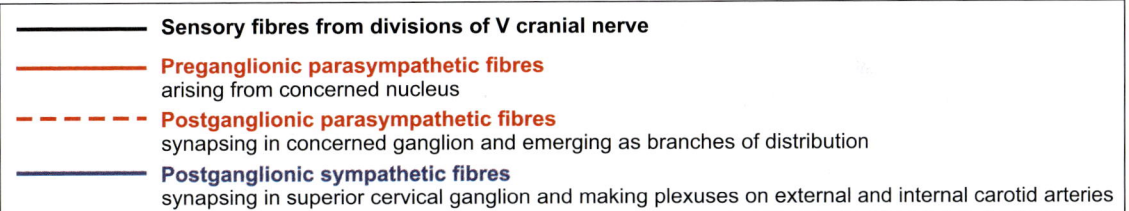

———————— Sensory fibres from divisions of V cranial nerve

———————— **Preganglionic parasympathetic fibres**
arising from concerned nucleus

– – – – – – **Postganglionic parasympathetic fibres**
synapsing in concerned ganglion and emerging as branches of distribution

———————— **Postganglionic sympathetic fibres**
synapsing in superior cervical ganglion and making plexuses on external and internal carotid arteries

RELATIONSHIP TO SYMPATHETIC NERVOUS SYSTEM

Sympathetic and parasympathetic divisions of ANS typically function in opposition to each other. The sympathetic division typically functions in actions requiring quick responses. The parasympathetic part of the ANS works at rest. It is an 'antagonist' to the sympathetic system. The normal function of our body is ensured by the coordinated action of these two parts of the ANS. This coordination and regulation of functions is brought about by the cerebral cortex. The parasympathetic division calls for 'rest and digest' responses. It, thus, saves energy—blood pressure decreases, heart beats slower and digestion can start. The parasympathetic division functions with actions that do not require immediate reaction. A useful mnemonic to summarise the functions of the parasympathetic nervous system is **SSLUDD** (**s**exual arousal, **s**alivation, **l**acrimation, **u**rination, **d**igestion and **d**efecation).

The cranial part of the parasympathetic nervous system is supplied by the four cranial nerves [cranial nerve III = **oculomotor** (pupillary constriction and accommodation), VII = **facial** (lacrimation and salivation), IX = **glossopharyngeal** (salivation) and X = **vagus** (input to thoracic and abdominal viscera)]. These nerves innervate the head, thoracic viscera and most of the abdominal viscera. Axons of the parasympathetic preganglionic neurons leave the brainstem (cranial outflow) and end near the visceral structures in the head, thorax and upper abdomen. Another group of axons of the parasympathetic preganglionic neuron leave the S2-S4 of the spinal cord and end near the viscera in the lower abdominal and pelvic region.

- The sympathetic part of the autonomic system (or the thoracolumbar division) prepares the body for emergency situations, also known as fight-or-flight reactions. It increases the heart rate, constricts blood flow to the most peripheral arteries, and raises blood pressure. The point is to supply more blood to the brain, heart, and muscles by reducing blood flow to the skin and to the digestive system.
- The parasympathetic part (or the craniosacral division) of the autonomic system is active during times of rest and normal conditions by decreasing the heart rate and stimulating the digestive system. This part of the autonomic system helps you rest and digest.

24

Autonomic Innervations of Important Vital Body Organs

- Autonomic Distribution
  - Branches to cranial and spinal nerves
  - Branches to nerve plexuses
  - Branches to skin
- Innervations of the Heart
  - Thoracolumbar (sympathetic)
  - Craniosacral (parasympathetic)
  - Sensory innervation of heart
- Cardiac Plexuses
  - Superficial cardiac plexus
  - Deep cardiac plexus

- Innervations of the Lungs
  - Pulmonary plexuses
- Innervations of the Internal Organs
  - Branches to blood vessels
  - Branches to stomach and intestine
  - Branches to liver
  - Branches to kidneys
  - Branches to urinary bladder
  - Branches to genital organs

AUTONOMIC DISTRIBUTION

Branches to Cranial and Spinal Nerves

- All peripheral nerves receive postganglionic fibres from the sympathetic trunk except:
  - I cranial (olfactory) nerve.
  - II cranial (optic) nerve.
  - VIII cranial (vestibulocochlear) nerve.
- Direct and indirect branches are given to different cranial nerves (*see* Chapter 20).
- From all thoracic and all lumbar ganglia branches are given through thoracic and abdominal aortic plexuses.

Branches to Nerve Plexuses

The great plexuses of the abdomen, although associated with the blood vessels, are however, of a different character, being mainly concerned with the innervation of the viscera. They are joined by:

1. Parasympathetic fibres from vagus (X cranial) nerve.
2. Thoracic splanchnic nerves.

Branches to Skin

The autonomic distribution to the skin (Fig. 24.1) follows the pattern of peripheral nerves—not those of blood vessels—and the sensory defects after injury to a peripheral nerve are coincident with the trophic changes in the skin (thin, translucent, shiny, pink or bluish, lacking in sweat secretion, the hairs becoming grey or getting lost). The innervation of the skin is **wholly from the thoracolumbar (sympathetic)** outflow. It is important to note that while the other postganglionic sympathetic fibres are adrenergic, those supplying the sweat glands are cholinergic.

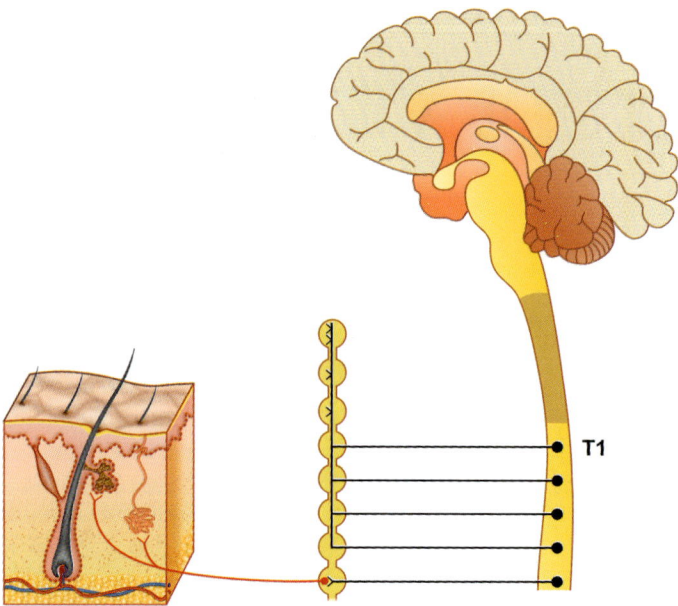

Fig. 24.1: Autonomic supply to skin

INNERVATIONS OF THE HEART

The main autonomic control of the heart resides with the **medulla oblongata** (Fig. 24.2). There is an area called the **cardioacceleratory centre**, or **pressor centre**, in the upper part of the medulla oblongata, and an area called the **cardioinhibitory centre**, or **depressor centre**, in the lower part. Together they are called the **cardioregulatory centre**, since they interact to control heart rate, etc. The nervous supply to the heart is **autonomic**, consisting of both sympathetic and parasympathetic parts. The sympathetic fibres arise from the pressor centre, while the parasympathetic fibres arise in the depressor centre.

Thoracolumbar (Sympathetic)

The **sympathetic nervous system** acts on the **sinoatrial (SA) node**, increasing the heart rate. The sympathetic fibres arise from the superior, middle, and inferior cervical ganglia (but originating in the medulla oblongata).
- *Preganglionic fibres*—arise in the lateral cell column in upper 4 thoracic segments of the spinal cord under the influence of the posterior region of hypothalamus; these fibres are

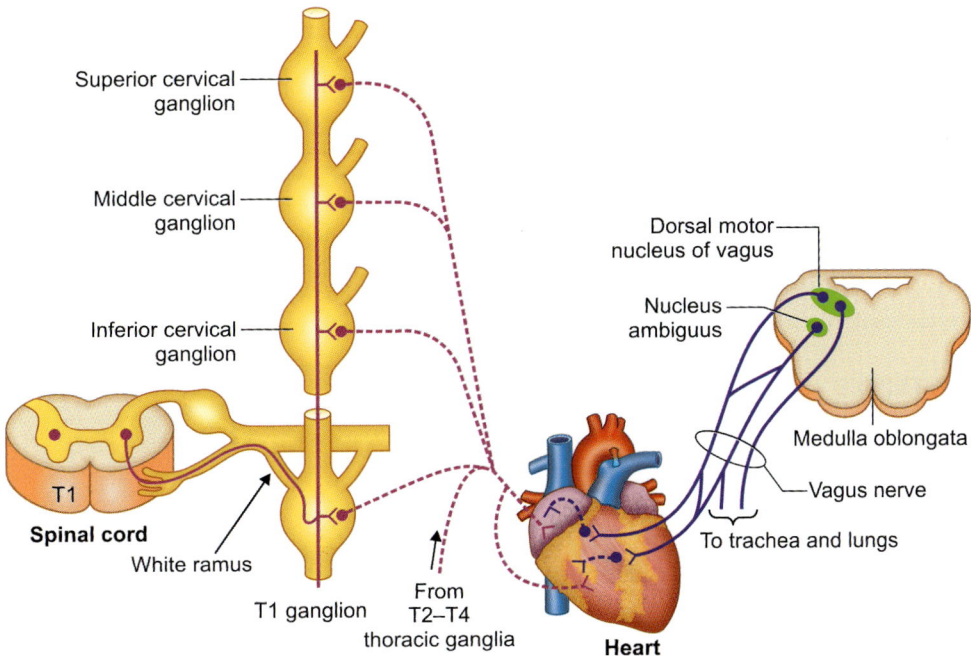

Fig. 24.2: Autonomic supply to the heart: sympathetic (purple) and parasympathetic (blue). In both cases, solid lines represent preganglionic fibres, and interrupted lines postganglionic fibres. Notice that the vagus nerve sends parasympathetic preganglionic fibres to trachea and lungs

relayed in the superior cervical ganglion of the sympathetic trunk; and they have an accelerator action upon the heart.

- *Postganglionic fibres*—run through the **cardiac nerves** to be distributed through the cardiac plexuses.

Craniosacral (Parasympathetic)

The **parasympathetic system** works in reverse in order to slow the heart rate down. The parasympathetic fibres, which originate in the medulla oblongata, and pass down by way of the vagus nerve, join in the cardiac plexus (which has superficial and deep parts). From here they enter the heart.

- *Preganglionic fibres*—arise in the dorsal nucleus of X nerve in medulla oblongata; pass through the vagus nerve, and have a continuous braking or depressor action.
- *Postganglionic fibres* are very short lying on the surface of heart.

Sensory Innervation of Heart

Sensory impulses from the heart travel through the **carotid sinus nerve** formed by:
- Twigs from the inferior ganglion of vagus (X cranial) nerves.
- Branch of glossopharyngeal (IX cranial) nerves directly or through its pharyngeal branch.
- Filament from the superior cervical ganglion of sympathetic trunks.

Clinical Significance

The heart itself has a natural pacemaker, the sinoatrial node, which does not need a nervous supply to function. If you sever all the nerves to the heart, then it will continue to beat. In fact, it will beat faster than normal, since there is normally a parasympathetic supply slowing the heart down. The sensory component of the sympathetic supply to the heart passes to the same sensory root as these, hence feeling a band of pain across the chest when having a heart attack. T1 is dragged into the upper limb, hence the referred pain in the arm during a heart attack. The pain is more usually felt in the left arm (since the heart is more to the left than the right), but it is not impossible to get pain in the right arm during a heart attack. The pain is not carried by the vagus nerve; instead it goes through the fibres in the posterior roots of T1 – T4 (intercostal nerves) to reach the sympathetic trunks mainly through the inferior cervical cardiac nerve and to a lesser extent through the middle cervical and thoracic cardiac nerves. The treatment is to remove inferior cervical ganglion but also at least upper four thoracic ganglia.

CARDIAC PLEXUSES

The cardiac plexus is situated at the base of the heart, and is divided into a *superficial* and a *deep part*, which are closely connected with each other.

Superficial Cardiac Plexus (Fig. 24.3)

- Lies below aortic arch, in front of right pulmonary artery between phrenic and vagus nerves. It is formed by:
  - Cardiac branch of the superior cervical ganglion of the left sympathetic trunk.
  - Lower cervical cardiac branch of the left vagus nerve.
- Branches are given to:
  - Deep cardiac plexus.
  - Right coronary plexus.
  - Left anterior pulmonary plexus.
- A small **cardiac ganglion** is present immediately below the arch of aorta, on the right side of the ligamentum arteriosum.

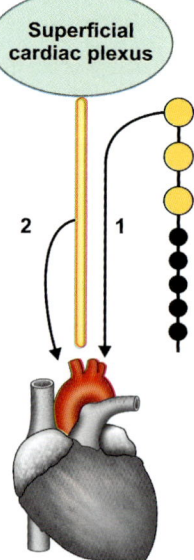

Fig. 24.3: Formation of superficial cardiac plexus is by two nerves only: 1. cardiac branch of left superior cervical sympathetic ganglion, and 2. inferior cardiac branch of the left vagus (parasympathetic)

Deep Cardiac Plexus

- Lies in front of the bifurcation of trachea, above the point of division of the pulmonary trunk, and below and medial to the arch of aorta (Fig. 24.4). It is formed by:
  - Cardiac branches of the cervical and upper 4 thoracic ganglia of both sympathetic trunks. The neural regulation of the heart is depicted in Fig. 24.5.

INNERVATIONS OF THE LUNGS

The **lung** is innervated by both components of the **autonomic nervous** system (Fig. 24.6). **Parasympathetic nerves** arise from the vagus **nerve**, and **sympathetic nerves** are derived from the upper thoracic and cervical ganglia of the **sympathetic** trunk.

The sympathetic neurons **to Lungs and Bronchi** are located in the intermediolateral nucleus in cord segments T1–T5. These traverse through inferior cervical and thoracic T1–T5 sympathetic ganglia. The *preganglionic* **parasympathetic** neurons are located in the dorsal motor nucleus of vagus nerve. The *postganglionic* fibres synapse in the ganglia of pulmonary plexus.

Pulmonary Plexuses

The pulmonary plexuses are located on the front and back of the bronchial and vascular structures in the roots of the lungs. There are two pulmonary plexuses: an *anterior* much smaller than the *posterior* pulmonary plexus. The formation of these plexuses is summarised as follows (Table 24.1):

From the plexuses, nerves pass into the lung around the branches of the bronchi and pulmonary arteries, extending as far as the visceral pleura. The *afferent* parasympathetic vagal fibres are concerned in the cough-reflex. The *efferent* parasympathetic fibres (from vagus) are bronchoconstrictor, secretomotor to the mucous glands of bronchi and vasodilator in function.

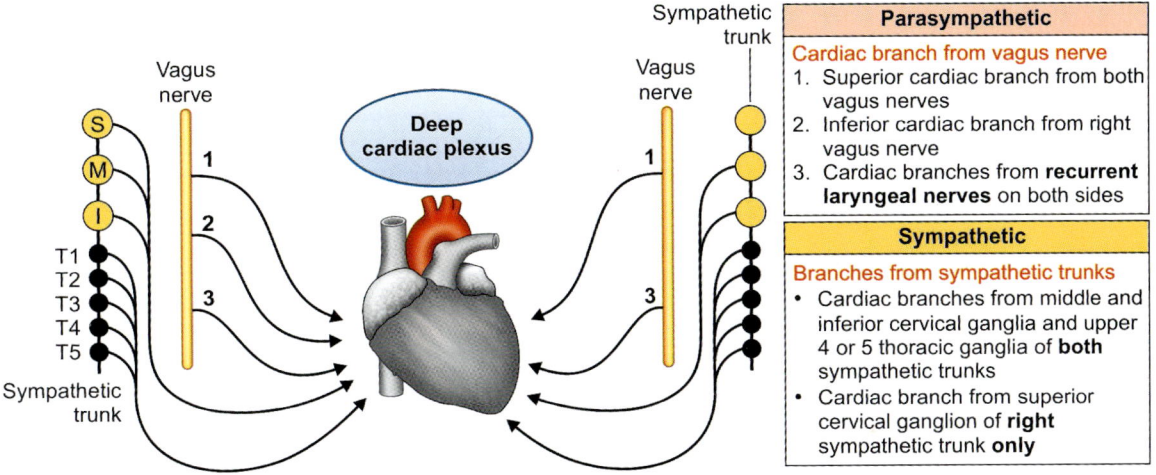

Fig. 24.4: Formation of deep cardiac plexus is except by two nerves only forming the superficial cardiac plexus shown in Fig. 24.3. The parasympathetic fibres derived by both X cranial nerves and the sympathetic fibres from the two sympathetic trunks are listed in detail on the right part of the figure

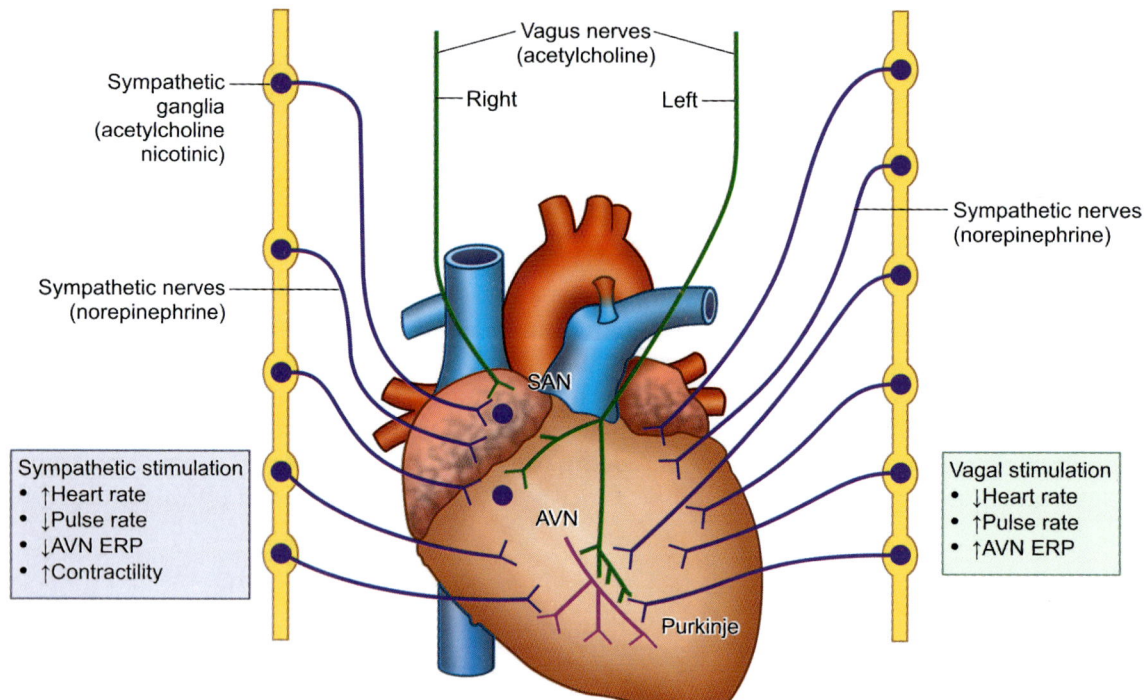

Fig. 24.5: Neural regulation of the heart

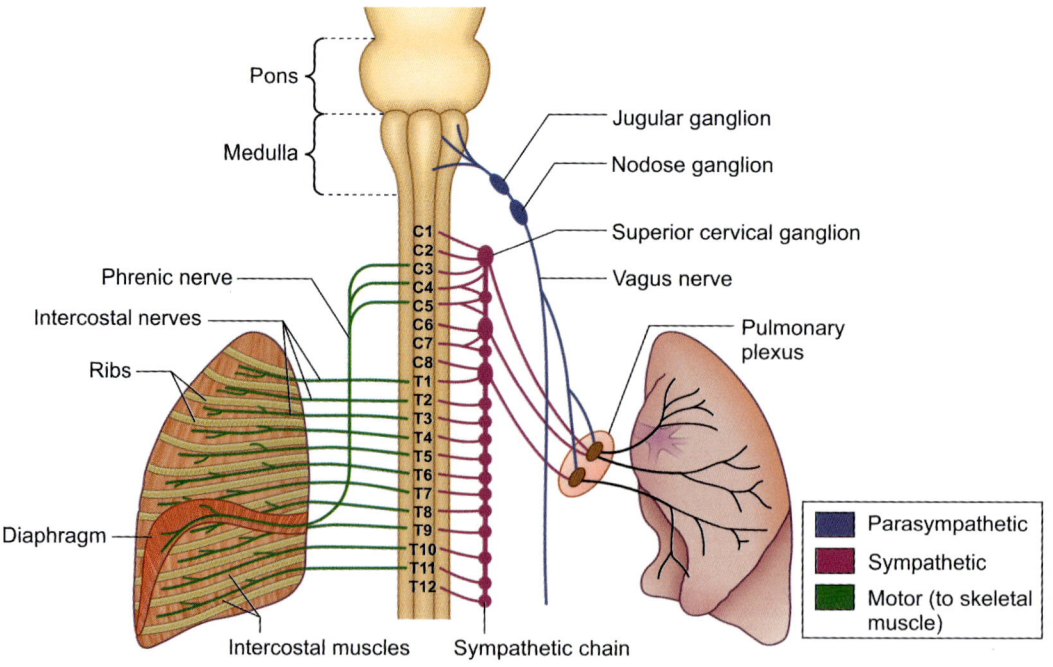

Fig. 24.6: Autonomic innervations of the lungs

Table 24.1: Contributions in the formation of pulmonary plexuses	
Anterior pulmonary plexus	*Posterior pulmonary plexus*
• Branches from the vagus (parasympathetic) • Branches from deep cardiac plexus • Additional branches from superficial cardiac plexus *for left anterior plexus* only	• Branches from the vagus (parasympathetic) • Branches from deep cardiac plexus • T2–T5 sympathetic ganglia • Additional branches from left recurrent laryngeal nerve for *left posterior plexus* only

INNERVATIONS OF THE INTERNAL ORGANS

Branches to Blood Vessels

Smooth muscle present in the walls of the blood vessels (arteries, arterioles, venules, and veins) receives branches from the sympathetic, required for the muscle, and its stimulation causes muscle contraction, hence of independent action (Fig. 24.7). This causes vasoconstriction, which results in: *generalised effect* by raising the blood pressure; and local effect—whereby the blood is shunted to other regions in urgent need.

Sympathetic branches of ANS use vasomotor fibres to supply smooth muscle in artery and arteriole walls. Vasomotor impulses stimulate contraction causing vasoconstriction—which reduces diameter of vessel. When the vasomotor impulses are inhibited, muscle fibres relax and diameter of vessel increases. The changes in diameter of vessels greatly influence blood flow and pressure.

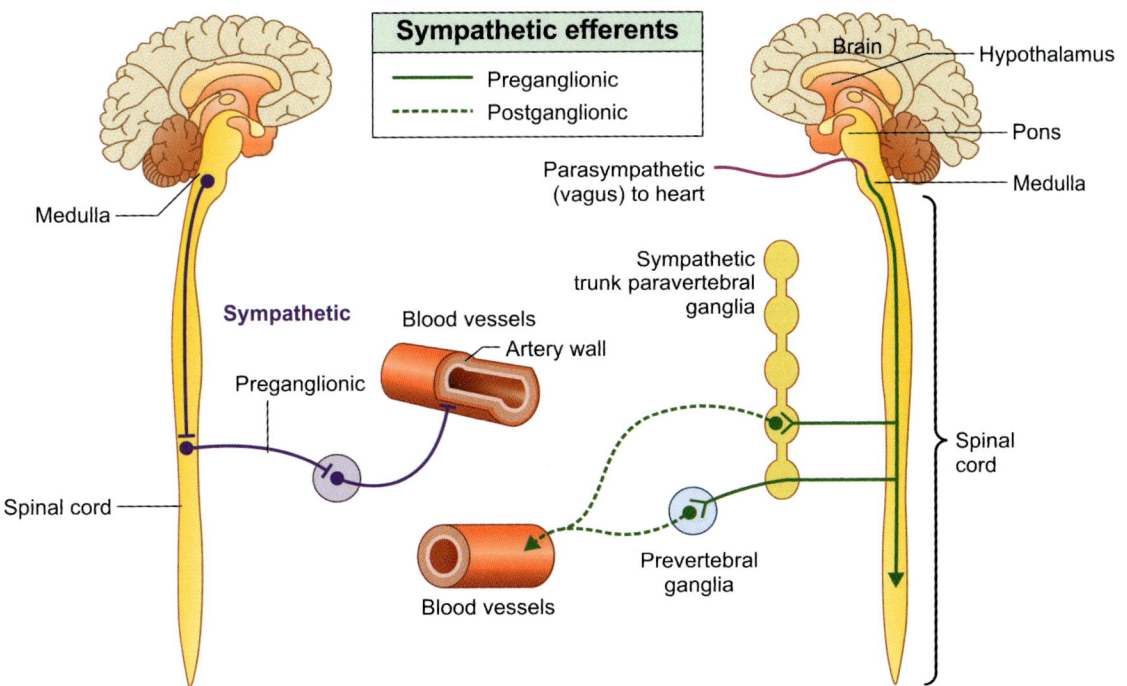

Fig. 24.7: Autonomic nerve supply to blood vessels

Control of Vessel Tone

The control of vessel tone is caused by two parts of the brain:
- Medulla oblongata.
- Posterior part of hypothalamus.

These parts of the brain are influenced by:
- Somatic and visceral sources.
- Cold.
- Cerebral cortex.
- Emotion.

From higher centres influence reaches the intermediolateral cell column in T1 – L2 segments of the spinal cord. From here the *preganglionic fibres* start. They pass via white rami communicantes to relay in the **paravertebral ganglia** of the sympathetic trunk. Each fibre relays with as many as 20 ganglion cells. The *postganglionic fibres* pass from here through grey rami communicantes to:

1. Large vessels—periarterial plexuses
2. Small vessels—through a nerve

Direct arterial branches from the sympathetic trunk are given for large vessels; and run through a branch of a spinal nerve.

Branches to Stomach and Intestine

The stomach has *four* main anatomical divisions; the cardia, fundus, body, and pylorus (Fig. 24.8):
- **Cardia**—Surrounds the superior opening of the stomach at the T11 level.
- **Fundus**—The rounded, often gas filled portion superior to and left of the cardia.
- **Body**—The large central portion inferior to the fundus.
- **Pylorus**—This area connects the stomach to the duodenum. It is divided into the pyloric antrum, pyloric canal and pyloric sphincter. The pyloric sphincter demarcates the transpyloric plane at the level of L1.

Stomach

The stomach is supplied by both the parasympathetic and sympathetic parts of the ANS:

1. **Parasympathetic** 90% *preganglionic fibres* come from right (posterior vagal trunk) and left (anterior vagal trunk) vagus nerves. The *postganglionic fibres* are very short and lie within the wall of the stomach (Fig. 24.8B).
2. **Sympathetic** *preganglionic fibres* are mainly derived from spinal segments T5–T10—the thoracic splanchnic nerves. The *postganglionic* fibres arise in the ganglia of the celiac plexus.

Duodenum

The duodenum receives both sympathetic and parasympathetic innervation. The vagus nerve (CN X), provides parasympathetic fibres via the celiac and superior mesenteric plexuses, while the sympathetic trunk also gives fibres to the intestinal plexuses that travel along the pancreaticoduodenal arteries.

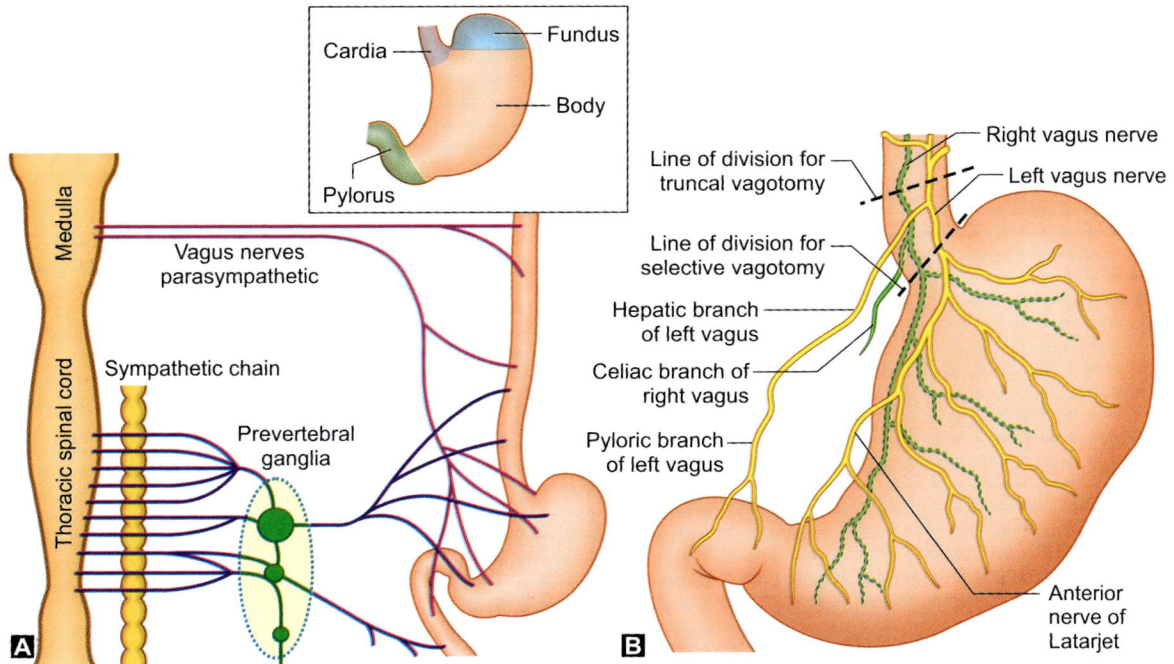

Fig. 24.8: A. Autonomic nerve supply to oesophagus, stomach, and duodenum part of small intestine. Parasympathetics shown in violet are derived from vagus nerves; the sympathetic fibres are shown in blue arising from the thoracic segments of the spinal cord—traverse through prevertebral ganglia to be relayed in coeliac ganglia for supply of distal oesophagus, stomach, and initial part of the duodenum. The inset on the top shows the four parts of the stomach described in the text. **B.** Two vagal trunks and their branches supplying the stomach

Branches to Liver

The autonomic innervations to liver are via the **hepatic plexus**—largest subdivision of the celiac plexus, which also receives filaments from: *both vagus nerves* and *the right phrenic nerve*. In the liver, the nerves are confined to the vicinity of hepatic artery and portal vein. From the plexus branches are also given to the pylorus and first part of the duodenum.

The **liver** is **innervated** by both the **sympathetic** and the **parasympathetic** nerve systems. These nerves are derived from the splanchnic and vagal nerves that surround the portal vein, **hepatic** artery, and bile duct ... Furthermore, **liver innervation** has been associated with **hepatic** fibrosis, regeneration, and circadian rhythm.

Branches to Kidneys

The **parasympathetic** supply—to kidneys is through the renal branches, which arise from both vagus nerves and join the renal plexus. The **sympathetic** supply is derived from the branches of celiac plexus—**called renal plexus** formed by filaments from:

  i. Celiac ganglion and celiac plexus.
 ii. Lowest thoracic splanchnic nerve.
iii. First lumbar splanchnic nerve.
iv. Aortic plexus.

The renal plexus is continued into the kidney around the branches of the renal artery to supply the vessels and renal glomeruli and tubules particularly in the cortex of the kidney. Input from the **sympathetic nervous** system triggers vasoconstriction in the **kidney**, thereby reducing **renal** blood **flow**.

Branches to Urinary Bladder

Autonomic regulation **of the bladder** (Fig. 24.9) is by both parasympathetic and sympathetic divisions of the autonomic nervous system. **The parasympathetic** control **of the bladder** musculature, **the** contraction **of** which causes **bladder** emptying, originates with neurons **in the** sacral spinal cord segments (S2–S4) that innervate visceral motor neurons **in parasympathetic** ganglia **in** or near **the bladder** wall.

The **vesical plexus** arises from the anterior part of the inferior hypogastric plexus. Numerous nerves which accompany the vesical arteries (supplying the urinary bladder) form the vesical plexus. The sympathetic preganglionic efferent fibres in the vesical plexus arise from T11 and T12 and L1 and L2 segments of the spinal cord.

Sensory fibres pass from the bladder in both parasympathetic and sympathetic nerves. Sensations aroused by distension are mediated by the afferent sympathetic nerves. The efferent parasympathetic nerves convey motor fibres to the muscular coats. However, it is believed that the sympathetic fibres are mainly vasomotor in function and that filling and emptying of the urinary bladder are normally controlled exclusively by the parasympathetic nerves.

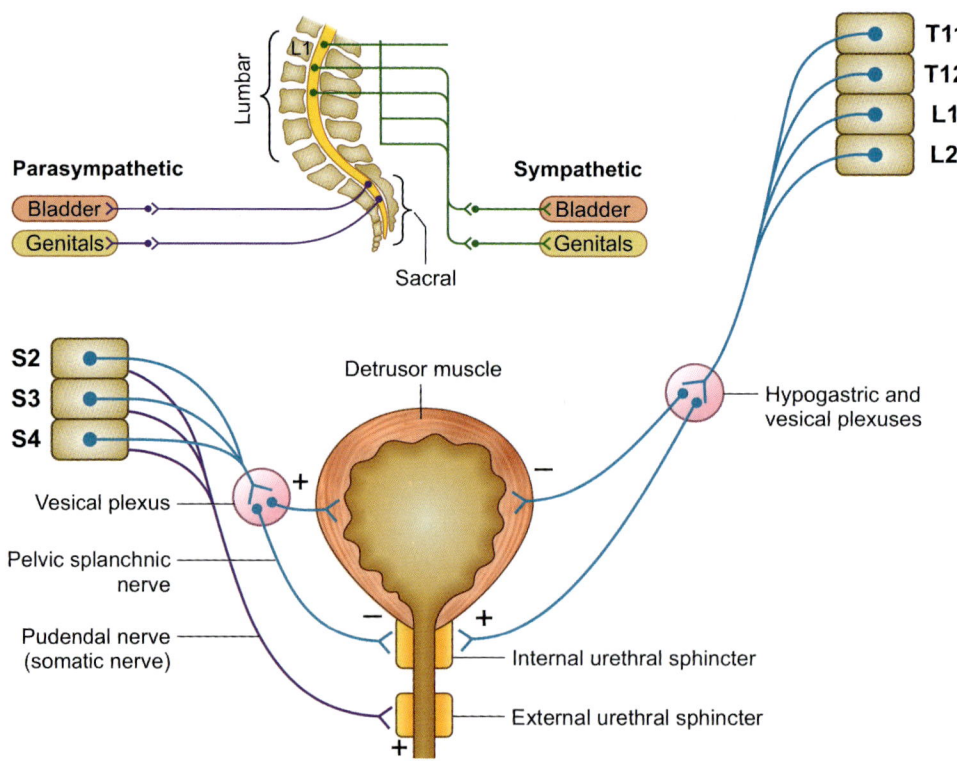

Fig. 24.9: Autonomic nerve supply to urinary bladder and genitals

Branches to Genital Organs

Much like control of the bladder, sexual responses are mediated by the coordinated activity of sympathetic, parasympathetic, and somatic innervation. The reflexes differ in detail in human males and females, basic similarities allow the two sexes to be considered together. The important autonomic effects include:

i. Mediation of vascular dilation, which causes penile or clitoral erection.
ii. Stimulation of prostatic or vaginal secretions.
iii. Smooth muscle contraction of the vas deferens during ejaculation or rhythmic vaginal contractions during orgasm in females.
iv. Contractions of the somatic pelvic muscles that accompany orgasm in both sexes.

Like the urinary tract, the reproductive organs receive preganglionic parasympathetic innervation from the sacral spinal cord, preganglionic sympathetic innervation from the outflow of the lower thoracic and upper lumbar spinal cord segments, and somatic motor innervation from motor neurons in the ventral horn of the lower spinal cord segments (Fig. 24.10). The sacral parasympathetic pathway controlling the sexual organs in both males and females originates in the sacral segments S2–S4 and reaches the target organs via the pelvic nerves. Activity of the postganglionic neurons in the relevant parasympathetic ganglia causes dilation of penile or clitoral arteries, and a corresponding relaxation of the smooth muscles of the venous (cavernous) sinusoids, which leads to expansion of the sinusoidal spaces. As a result, the amount of blood in the tissue is increased, leading to a sharp rise in the pressure and an expansion of the cavernous spaces (i.e. erection).

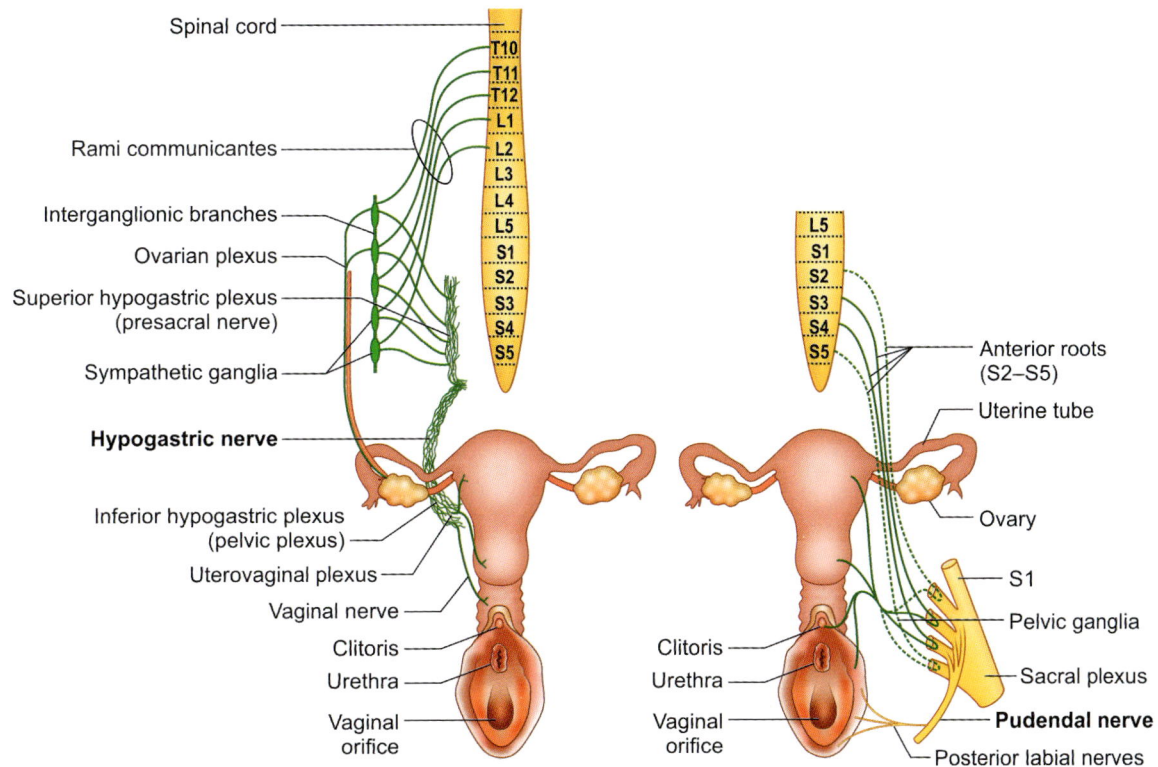

Fig. 24.10: Autonomic nerve supply to female reproductive organs and genitals

Male genital organs		Female genital organs	
Part	Supply	Part	Supply
• Prostate • Seminal vesicles • Prostatic urethra • Ejaculatory ducts • Corpora cavernosa • Corpus spongiosum • Membranous and cavernous parts of urethra • Bulbourethral glands	**Prostatic plexus** from lower part of inferior hypogastric plexus	• Uterus • Cervix • Vagina	**Inferior hypogastric** and **uterovaginal plexus**

Enteric (Intrinsic) Nervous System
Second or *GIT* Brain

- Introduction to Enteric Nervous System
  - Development
  - Extent and location
- Autonomic Components in Intrinsic Plexuses
  - Parasympathetic
  - Sympathetic

INTRODUCTION TO ENTERIC NERVOUS SYSTEM

The **enteric nervous system** (ENS) or **intrinsic nervous system**, often referred to as our body's second brain, is one of the main divisions of the **autonomic nervous system** (ANS) and consists of a **mesh-like system** of neurons that governs the function of the gastrointestinal system. These neurons are located in sheaths of tissue lining the oesophagus, stomach, small intestine, and colon. There are hundreds of millions of neurons connecting the brain to the enteric nervous system, the part of the nervous system that is tasked with controlling the gastrointestinal system—a complex organ system that performs a range of functions that are essential for life including mixing, segmentation, digestion, absorption, secretion, propulsive movements (peristalsis, migrating motor complexes), excretion, and defense. Many of these gut functions are controlled by intrinsic neurons of the enteric nervous system (ENS) and/or by extrinsic sympathetic, parasympathetic (via the vagus and pelvic nerves), and sensory neurons (in the vagal and spinal pathways).

However, the central nervous system plays an essential role in controlling esophageal and gastric motility, and in regulating gut function in different emotional states, while extrinsic peripheral nerve pathways coordinate activity between distant regions of the gastrointestinal tract.

Development

The development of the ENS involves a number of processes. Early processes include: (i) invasion of the foregut by ENS precursors derived from *vagal neural crest cells* (*vagal NCCs*), (ii) subsequent rostral-to-caudal migration of these vagal NCC-derived ENS precursors to colonize the myenteric (outer) region of the gut, and (iii) later processes include colonisation

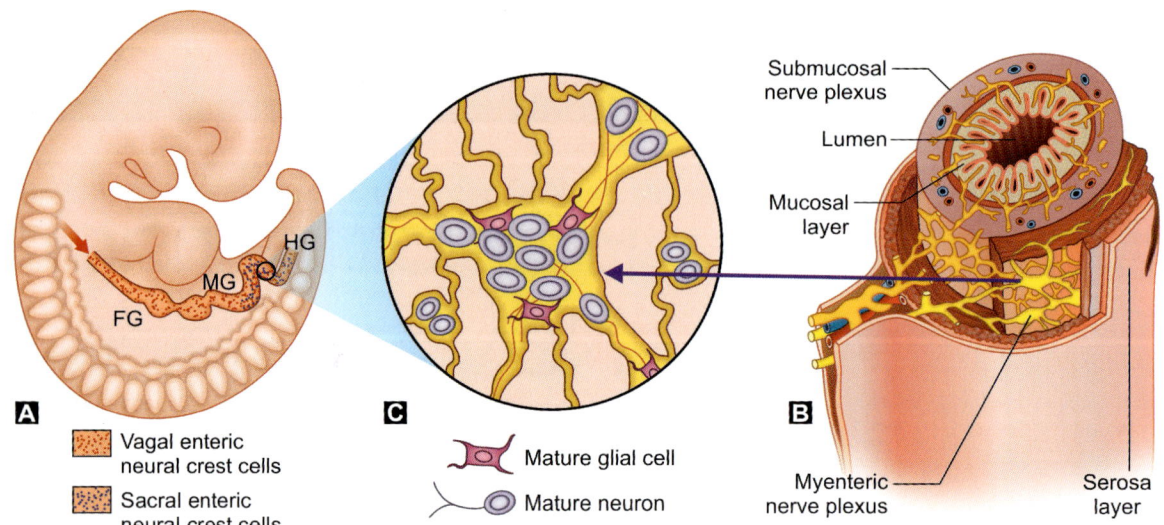

Fig. 25.1: **A.** Developing mouse embryo shows migration of vagal and sacral innervations into the gut, **B.** a transverse section of the hindgut region showing typical four distinct layers in its wall with two intramural nerve plexuses in gastrointestinal tract, **C.** scheme depicts postnatal myenteric plexus with mature glial and neuronal cells

of the submucosal (inner) region of the gut by ENS precursors, entry of sacral NCC-derived ENS precursors into the hindgut, and the projection of fibres from extrinsic sensory and visceromotor neurons (from vagal, dorsal root, sympathetic and pelvic ganglia) to the gut. Neuronal and glial differentiation is detectable during early ENS development and continues postnatally (Fig. 25.1). Many of these developmental processes overlap in time.

Extent and Location

The **enteric nervous system** (ENS) extends from the midregion of the oesophagus all the way to the anal canal. The enteric nervous comprises a network of neurons spread throughout two layers of gut tissue, the submucosal plexus and the myenteric plexus. The intrinsic neurons of the gut are mainly located in two intramural plexuses (Fig. 25.1):

1. *Myenteric plexus (of Auerbach)*—present between longitudinal and circular layers of muscularis externa coat of the gut wall. Layer contains the neurons responsible for regulating the enzyme output of adjacent organs.

2. *Submucosal plexus (of Meissner)*—present in the submucosal layer outside the muscularis mucosae of the innermost mucosa layer of the gut. The submucosal layer contains sensory cells that communicate with the myenteric plexus and the motor fibres that stimulate the secretion of fluids into the lumen.

The lumen has no nerves actually entering this area. The brains in the head and gut have to monitor conditions in the lumen across the lining of the bowel. The serosa forms mesentery that attaches the gut to the body wall and contains major arteries, veins, lymphatics, and external nerves.

AUTONOMIC COMPONENTS IN INTRINSIC PLEXUSES

Parasympathetic

The principal 'drivers' of the muscle and glands belong to the parasympathetic division of the autonomic nervous system. The dorsal motor nucleus of the vagus nerve provides the preganglionic parasympathetic supply to all parts of the gut with the exception of the **distal colon** and **rectum** (Fig. 25.2), which receive their preganglionic supply from the *pelvic splanchnic nerves* having parent neurons in the intermediolateral cell column of the spinal cord segments (S2, S3, and S4). The 'drivers' throughout are intramural ganglion cells located in both intramural plexuses (Fig. 25.3).

The postganglionic fibres of the myenteric plexus initiate peristaltic waves by simultaneously causing the gut to contract in their own location and to relax distally by activating inhibitory neurons. Parasympathetic ganglion cells in the wall of the gallbladder cause expulsion of bile. The ganglion cells in the submucosal plexus, and in the pancreas, cause glandular secretion.

Sympathetic

The **preganglionic** sympathetic nerve supply originates in the lateral horn cells of the spinal cord (T5–T11). The visceral afferents reaching the CNS have their unipolar somas in a nodose ganglion of the vagus nerve and in posterior root-ganglia at spinal levels T5–T11. These fibres traverse the sympathetic ganglion of the sympathetic trunk **without synapsing** here (Fig. 25.4) and terminate in the *prevertebral splanchnic ganglia* within the abdomen (celiac, superior

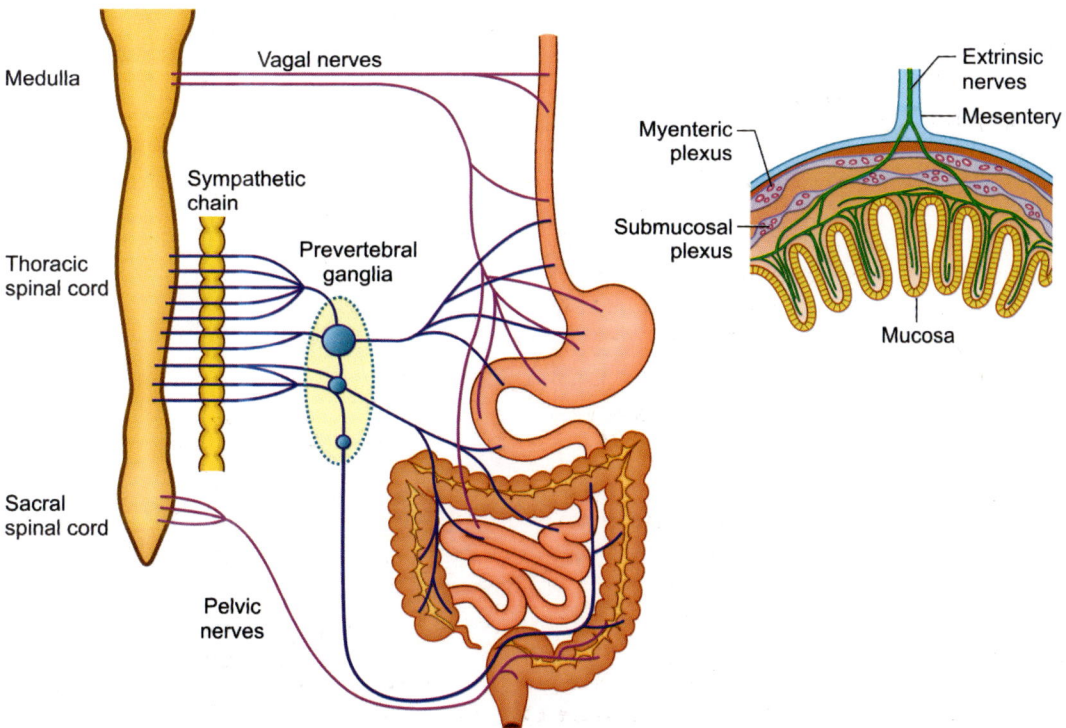

Fig. 25.2: Sympathetic (blue) and parasympathetic (violet) innervations of the gastrointestinal tract through vagal, sympathetic pelvic pathways

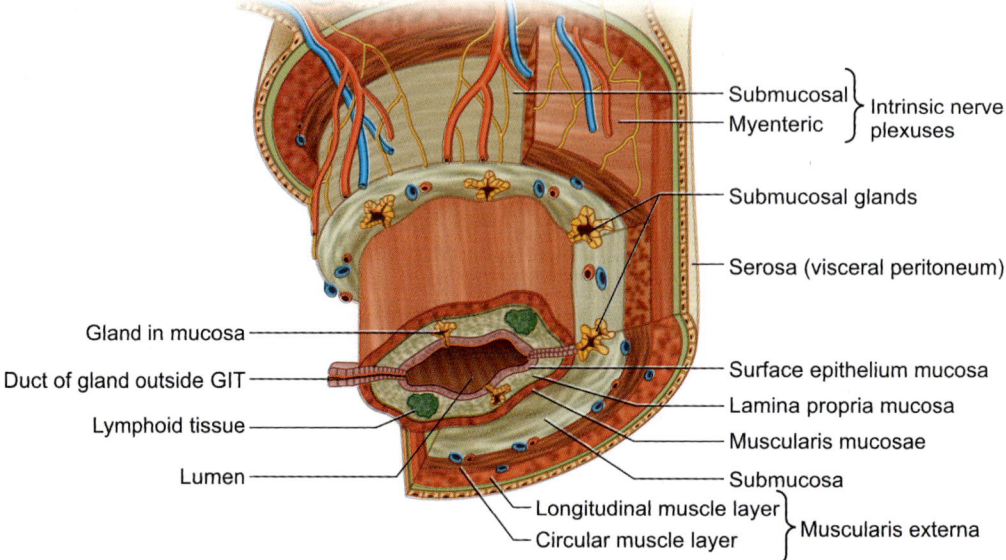

Fig. 25.3: A 3-D diagram of the gut wall showing different histological layers and location of two intrinsic nerve plexuses described earlier

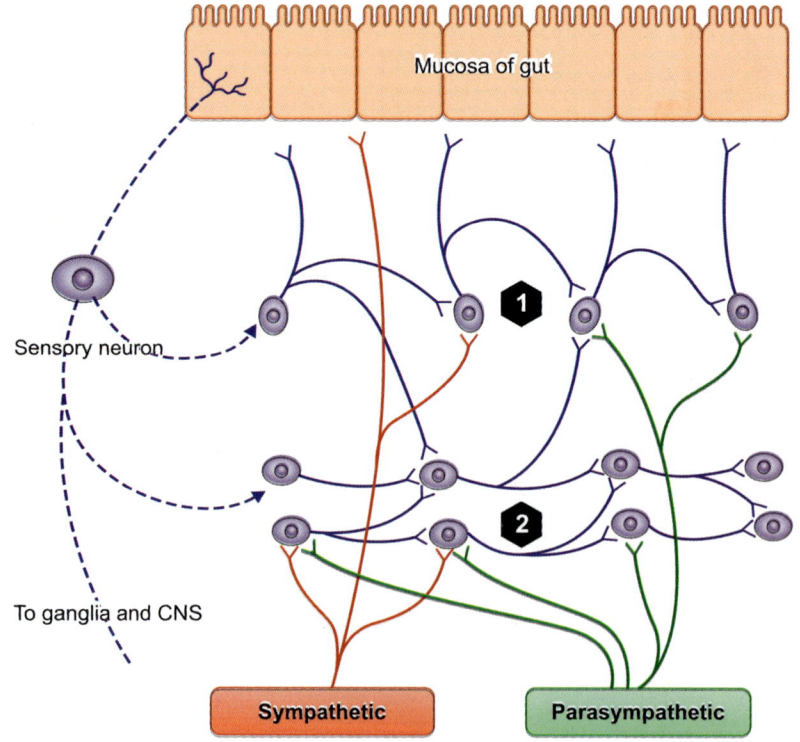

Fig. 25.4: A schematic illustration of neural control of the gut wall by the autonomic nervous system through network of neurons at two sites: 1. submucosal (Meissner's) plexus, 2. myenteric (Auerbach's) plexus

mesenteric, and inferior mesenteric). The **postganglionic** fibres supply the smooth muscle of the intestine and blood vessels, which they relax via β_2 receptors.

In most animals the brain is located near to the entrance to the gut which suggests that the brain arose as the gut's way of controlling its intake by accepting nutritious foods and rejecting toxins. There are several families of genes that govern both brain and gut development. There is strong evidence that the brain and the gut compete for metabolic energy in the organism and that gut size limits brain size. The following box lists some similarities and difference between the brain and the gut brain (or second brain).

Brain	Second brain
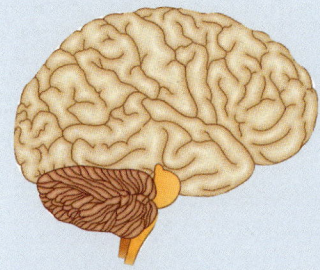	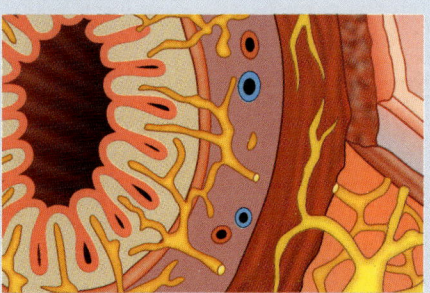
Glial cells support	Glial cells support
85 billion neurons	500 billion neurons
100 neurotransmitters identified	40 neurotransmitters identified
Produces 50% of all dopamine	Produces 50% of all dopamine
Produces 5% of all serotonin	Produces 95% of all serotonin
Barrier restrict blood flow to brain	Barrier restricts blood flow to second brain

Glossary of Neuroanatomical Terms

Neuroanatomy, like other aspects of anatomy, uses specific terminology to describe anatomical structures. This terminology helps ensure that a structure is described accurately, with minimal ambiguity. Terms also help ensure that structures are described consistently, depending on their structure or function. Terms are often derived from Latin and Greek, and like other areas of anatomy are generally standardised based on internationally accepted lexicons such as Terminologia Anatomica. To help with consistency, humans and other species are assumed when described to be in *standard anatomical position*, with the body standing erect and facing observer, arms at sides, palms forward. Standard terms used throughout anatomy include *anterior/posterior* for the front and back of a structure, *superior/inferior* for above and below, *medial/lateral* for structures close to and away from the midline respectively, and *proximal/distal* for structures close to and far away from a set point. Some terms are used more commonly in neuroanatomy, particularly: Rostral and caudal: the term rostral (from the Latin **rostrum**, meaning 'beak') is synonymous with anterior and the term caudal (from the Latin cauda, meaning 'tail') is synonymous with posterior.

Due to humans having an upright posture, however, their nervous system is considered to bend about 90° (Fig. G.1). This is considered to occur at the junction of the midbrain and diencephalon (the **midbrain-diencephalic junction**). Thus, the terminology changes at either side of the midbrain-diencephalic junction. Superior to the junction, the terminology is the same as in animals with linear nervous systems; *rostral* is synonymous with *anterior* and *caudal* is synonymous with posterior. Inferior to the midbrain-diencephalic junction the term *rostral* is synonymous with *superior* and *caudal* is synonymous with *inferior*. In humans, however the terminology differs on either side of the midbrain-diencephalic junction. Superior to the junction, the terminology is the same as in animals with linear nervous systems; *dorsal* is synonymous with *superior* and *ventral* is synonymous with *inferior*. However, inferior to the midbrain-diencephalic junction the term *dorsal* is synonymous with *posterior* and *ventral* is synonymous with *anterior*.

1. **Adiadochokinesia (or dysdiadochokinesia):** Inability to perform rapidly alternating movements (*a* = negative; *diadocho* = succeeding; and *kinesia* = movement).

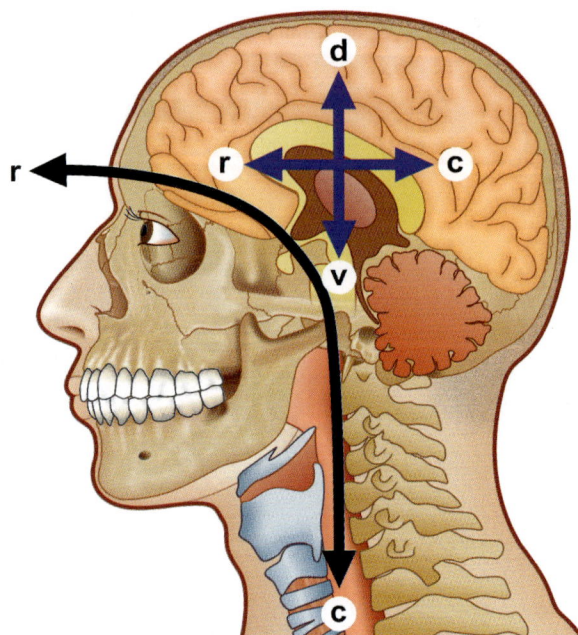

Fig. G.1: The anatomical axes of orientation of the human brain are at odds with the anatomical axes of the human body in the standard anatomical position. Black axes show how the head bent forward as the back pointed upwards; c: caudal; r: rostral. Blue axes show the conventions for naming directions in the brain itself: c: caudal (though not tail direction), d: dorsal, r: rostral (effectively unchanged); v: ventral (though not belly direction)

2. **Afferent fibres:** Nerve fibres that take messages from the periphery to the brain; afferent fibres are almost always sensory fibres.

3. **Agnosia:** Agnosia is a complex, receptive perceptual cerebral disorder and may involve any of the sensory input systems, i.e. visual, auditory, somesthetic, etc. There are following *three* types of agnosias:
   a. Tactile agnosia—failure to recognise objects by means of tactile and proprioceptive sensibilities when both are normal. This leads to **astereognosis**—lesions are of the left supramarginal gyrus.
   b. Visual agnosia (also called *word blindness* or alexia)–failure to recognise objects that cannot be attributed to a defect of visual acuity or to intellectual impairment. The patient is unable to recognise an object by sight, the disability usually is limited to small objects. Lesions are in the lateral visual association areas in the dominant cerebral hemisphere.
   c. Auditory agnosia (also called *word deafness*)—patients with unimpaired hearing fail to detect objects.

4. **Alexia with agraphia:** Difficulties with reading and writing; may be the result of damage to the angular gyrus in the hemisphere dominant for speech and language.

5. **Alpha cells:** The principle lower motor neurons of the spinal cord (they are located on the ventral aspect of the cord); they form the main part of the final common pathway and conduct rapid motor impulses; each alpha cell innervated approximately 200 muscle fibres.

6. **Allocheiria:** Disturbance of sensibility; concerns false localisation; i.e. if one extremity is stimulated, the sensation is referred to the other side.
7. **Alternating hemiplegia:** Paralysis of different structures on each side of the body; this condition may be the result of a lesion in the brainstem that damages both the nucleus of a cranial nerve and one side of the upper motor neurons of the pyramidal tract.
8. **Amygdala:** A structure which is attached to the tail of the caudate nucleus; it is considered to be a part of the limbic system and is involved in emotion.
9. **Anastomosis:** Communication or connection between the separate components of a branching system; as in the circle of Willis, anastomosis allows blood carried by different arterial branches to come together and be redistributed.
10. **Angular gyrus:** The gyrus that lies near the superior edge of the temporal lobe, and immediately posterior to the supramarginal gyrus; it is involved in the recognition of visual symbols (Geschwind referred to it as the 'association cortex for association cortices' and 'the most important cortical areas of speech and language').
11. **Anomia:** Difficulty with word-finding or naming; anomia may be the result of damage to the angular gyrus in the hemisphere dominant for speech and language.
12. **Anopsia:** A defect of vision—see ophthalmic register.
13. **Anosmia:** A loss of the sense of smells; may be a result of a lesion on the olfactory pathway.
14. **Anterior cerebral artery:** A branch of the internal carotid artery; the anterior cerebral artery supplies blood to the medial cortex, some areas of the frontal lobe, and the corpus striatum.
15. **Anterior commissure:** One of the three major groups of commissural fibres; the anterior commissure connects the temporal lobes, as well as connecting the temporal lobe to the amygdala and to the opposite occipital lobe; it is also connected to the corpus callosum.
16. **Anterior communicating artery:** An artery which arises from the internal carotids; it joins together the anterior cerebral arteries of each hemisphere.
17. **Aorta:** The main artery supplying blood to the body (with the **exception of the lungs**); it ascends from the heart then forms an arch, from which two subclavian arteries arise.
18. **Aphasia:** A defect of the power of expression by speech or of comprehending spoken or written language; the characteristic features of different types of aphasias and the site of their lesions is summarised in Table G.1:

Table G.1	
Types of aphasia with features	*Lesion site*
Motor aphasia (expressive):	
a. Inability in verbal expression. Patient is aware what to say, and may also produce sounds, but unable to produce meaningful sentences	Area 44 (Broca's)
b. Inability to write (agraphia): Even though general motor coordination is unimpaired	Area 9 (part)
Sensory aphasia (receptive)	
a. *Word deafness (confused speech or auditory agnosia):* Patient unable to understand the spoken word even though general hearing is unaffected	Area 22 (part)
Types of aphasia–with features	*Lesion site*
b. *Word blindness (alexia or visual agnosia):* Patient unable to recognise the printed or written word and/or sentences. He is unable to read. May also manifest agraphia because he is unable to read what he has just written	Area 39 (angular gyrus)

19. **Apical dendrites:** A type of dendrite which has a stalk that is filled with cytoplasm, these appear to be part of the soma of the neuron to which they are attached; the majority of apical dendrites are found in the cerebral cortex.

20. **Apraxia:** Apraxia is a motor disorder caused by damage to the brain (specifically the posterior parietal cortex) in which the individual has difficulty with the motor planning to perform learned, complex purposeful movements or tasks when asked, provided that the request or command is understood and he/she is willing to perform the task. The nature of the brain damage determines the severity, and the absence of sensory loss or paralysis helps to explain the level of difficulty. The term comes from the Greek words: *a-* ('without') and *praxis* ('action'). For example, the patient may refuse to open his mouth when asked to, but will open it spontaneously to eat or yawn, suggesting that the peripheral muscles are intact, and that the lesion is central.

    The condition of apraxia, which is normal in young child, may be met within later life in pathological lesions in the neighbourhood of area 6. Usually such patients are unable to perform coordinated movements (such as lighting a pipe) despite their ability to carry out individual movements without difficulty.

21. **Aqueduct of Sylvius (cerebral aqueduct):** An opening which connects the third and fourth ventricles.

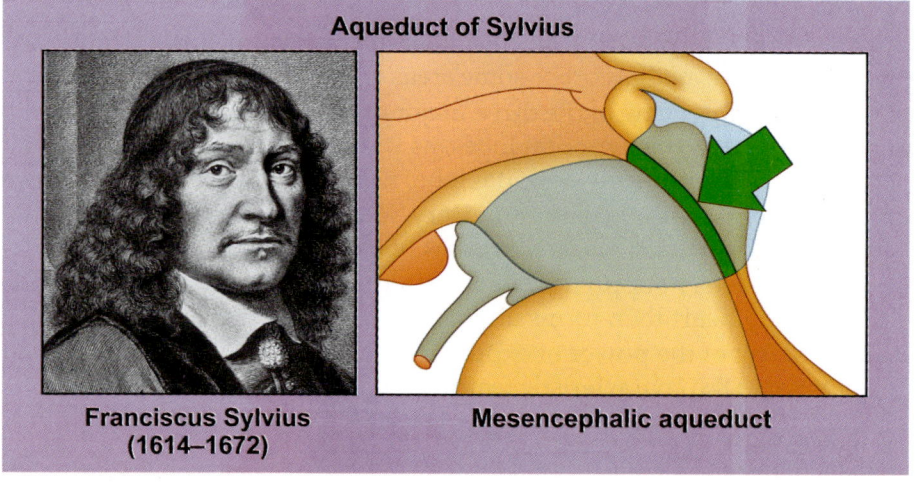

Aqueduct of Sylvius

Franciscus Sylvius
(1614–1672)

Mesencephalic aqueduct

22. **Arachnoid mater:** The middle layer of the meninges; in some areas it has projections (arachnoid granulations or villi) into the sinuses formed by the dura mater.

23. **Arachnoid villi (arachnoid granulations):** Projections of the arachnoid mater into the sinuses formed by the dura mater that transfer cerebrospinal fluid back into the bloodstream.

24. **Arcuate fasciculus:** The groups of fibres that connect Broca's area with Wernicke's area (these fibres pass through the area of the angular gyrus).

25. **Argyll Robertson pupil:** The pupil does not respond to light but reacts to accommodation. It is classically seen in neurosyphilis. Douglas Argyll Robertson (1837–1909), ophthalmic surgeon, Edinburgh.

26. **Arnold-Chiari malformation:** This malformation is characterised by descent of cerebellar tonsils and sometimes inferior vermis of the cerebellum into the cervical canal more

than 5 mm below the line joining basion and opisthion. There is also a change in the shape of the cerebellar tonsils, so that their inferior margin becomes pointed.

27. **Arteriosclerosis:** Hardening of the arteries.

28. **Ascending reticular formation (reticular activating system):** The component of the reticular formation that is responsible for the sleep-wake cycle; it mediates various levels of alertness.

29. **Association fibres:** Nerve fibres that connect areas within the same hemisphere; the most prevalent type of neuron found in the cortex.

30. **Asynergia:** Disturbance of that proper association in the contraction of muscles which assures that the different components of an act follow in proper sequence, at the proper moment, and of the proper degree, so that the act is executed accurately.

31. **Astereognosis:** Loss of ability to recognise objects or to appreciate their form by touching or feeling them; owing to sensory impairment at a cortical level; with the eyes closed.

32. **Ataxia:** An in coordination of motor movement with irregularity of muscle action; ataxia results from cerebellar lesions; the term may also be used to describe the unsteady walk and unusual postures seen in patients who have suffered injury to the cerebellum.

33. **Athetosis:** Bizzare, writhing (*twist in pain*) movements of the extremeties and neck musculature, especially of fingers and toes.

34. **Autonomic nervous system:** One of the three main functional divisions of the nervous system that is responsible for homeostatic reflexes that coordinate control of cardiac and smooth muscle, as well as glandular tissue. It innervates the involuntary structures of the body (e.g. heart, smooth muscles, glands) and is involved in control of automatic and glandular functions. It is divided into two parts, the sympathetic and parasympathetic divisions.

35. **Autonomic tone:** Tendency of an organ system to be governed by one division of the autonomic nervous system over the other, such as heart rate being lowered by parasympathetic input at rest.

36. **Auerbach's plexus:** Nerve plexus between the circular and longitudinal muscle coats of intestine.

37. **Axon:** The part of the neuron that allows it to send messages to other nerve cells; although each neuron can have only one axon, the axon itself can have many branches which connects it to many others. It is responsible for homeostatic reflexes that coordinate control of cardiac and smooth muscles, as well as glandular tissue.

38. **Ballismus:** Large, flailing movements of one or more extremeties. Violent forceful flinging movements affect proximal and appendicular muscles.

39. **Baroreceptor:** A mechanoreceptor that senses the stretch of blood vessels to indicate changes in blood pressure.

40. **Basal ganglia:** The largest subcortical structure of the brain; it is made up of the caudate nucleus and the lenticular nucleus; it is located at the level of the thalamus.

41. **Basal ganglionic disease:** In approximately two-thirds cases of basal nuclei disorders—involvement of one limb is the initial feature; the commonest sequence of limb involvement is from one upper limb to ipsilateral lower limb within 1 year, followed by contralateral limb within 3 years. A 'pill-rolling' movement of index and middle fingers against the thumb pad is characteristic. Typically, the tremor involves muscle groups that are 'at rest'.

42. **Blood–brain barrier (BBB):** It is a diffusion barrier essential for the normal function of the central nervous system. The BBB endothelial cells differ from endothelial cells in the rest of the body by the absence of fenestrations, more extensive tight junctions (TJs), and sparse pinocytic vesicular transport. Endothelial cell tight junctions limit the paracellular flux of hydrophilic molecules across the BBB. In contrast, small lipophilic substances such as O_2 and CO_2 diffuse freely across plasma membranes.

In addition to endothelial cells, the BBB is composed of the capillary basement membrane (BM), astrocyte end-feet ensheathing the vessels, and pericytes (PCs) embedded within the BM.

The blood–brain barrier (BBB) is a multicellular structure at the interface of circulation and central nervous system (CNS). The morphological basis of the BBB is formed by cerebral endothelial cells ensheathing the vessels of the brain. Important role in the formation of the barrier play pericytes.

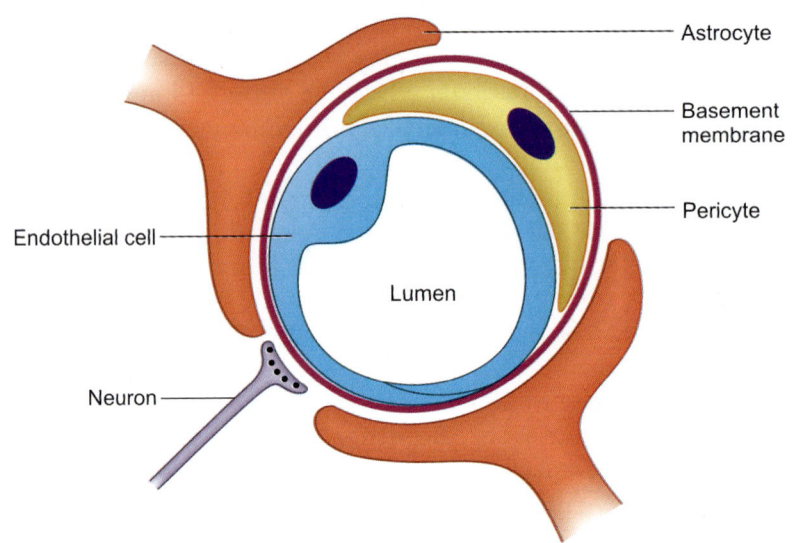

43. **Basilar artery (vertebral basilar artery):** The artery that is formed when the two vertebral arteries join together at the lower border of the pons; the basilar artery again divides at the superior border of the pons to form the posterior cerebral arteries (other arteries that arise from the basilar prior to this division include the anterior cerebellar arteries, inferior cerebellar arteries, posterior cerebellar arteries, and the pontine branches).

44. **Basilar dendrites:** A type of dendrite that does not have a stalk; these are more numerous than apical dendrites.

45. **Brain:** The large organ of the central nervous system composed of white and grey matter, contained within the cranium and continuous with the spinal cord.

46. **Brainstem:** The part of the brain consisting of midbrains, pons, and medulla oblongata.

47. **Broad-based gait:** A term used to describe the way in which some patients compensate for problems related to cerebellar injury by walking with their feet far apart.

48. **Broca's area:** The area of the brain involved in the programming of motor movements for the production of speech sounds; it is also involved in syntax; Broca's area is located on the inferior third frontal gyrus in the hemisphere dominant for language; injuries here may result in apraxia or Broca's aphasia. **Broca's area**—The anterior portion of the

inferior frontal gyrus; on the dominant side it is the **motor area of speech**. Pierre Broca (1824–1880), Professor of Clinical Surgery in Paris.

49. **Brown-Sequard syndrome:** Produced by hemisection of the spinal cord. Charles Edouard Brown-Sequard (1817–1894).

50. **Brodmann's classification system:** A map of the cortex developed by neurologist Korbinian Brodmann that classifies the different areas of the brain by number.

51. **Bulbar lesions:** Injuries to the nuclei of the cranial nerves located in the brainstem; they are considered to be lesions of the final common pathway.

52. **Bulbar palsy:** The paralysis produced by bulbar lesions.

53. **Cauda equina:** The part of the vertebral column that lies below the spinal cord; cauda equina is Latin for 'horse's tail'.

54. **Caudate nucleus:** One of the two structures that make up the basal ganglia; it is divided into a head, body, and tail and is bounded on one side by the lateral ventricle.

55. **Central canal:** The space in the middle of the grey matter of the spinal cord; it contains cerebrospinal fluid.

56. **Central sulcus (fissure of Rolando):** The deep sulcus that separates the frontal and parietal lobes.

57. **Cerebellum:** One of the parts of the brai; it is involved in the coordination and production of speech, the organisation of muscle movement, coordination of fine motor movement, and balance; it is the centre of a feedback loop involving motor and sensory information; 'cerebellum' means 'little brain' in Latin.

58. **Cerebellum (deep nuclei of):** Four different nuclei (the dentate nucleus, the emboliform nucleus, the globose nucleus, and the fastigial nucleus) located deep within each cerebellar hemisphere that have axons to the brainstem and thus send messages out to be conveyed to other parts of the central nervous system; these nuclei are regulated by Purkinje cells.

59. **Cerebellar disease:** In diseases involving neocerebellar cortex, dentate nucleus, and superior cerebellar peduncle, there occur in-coordination of voluntary movements, particularly in the upper limb. When fine purposive movements are attempted (e.g. grasping a glass, using a key) an **intention tremor** (also called **action tremor**) develops. There are faulty muscle synergies around the elbow and wrist.
    a. The hand may travel past the target—'overshoot'.
    b. Dysdiodochokinesia—quite irregular rapid alternating movements (e.g. pronation/supination).
    c. The 'finger-to-nose' and 'heel-to-knee' tests are performed with equal irregularity whether the eyes are open or closed—in contrast to performance in posterior column disease, where performance is adequate when the eyes are open.

60. **Cerebellar peduncles:** Three pairs of fibre bundles (the superior cerebellar peduncle, the middle cerebellar peduncle, and the inferior cerebellar peduncle) which connect the cerebellum to the brainstem; information passes on these tracts in both directions, every message that is sent or received by the cerebellum travels on the cerebellar peduncles.

61. **Cerebellar dysarthria (ataxic dysarthria):** A disorder that results in jerky, uncoordinated movements of the speech musculature; it is caused by lesions in the cerebellum.

62. **Cerebral peduncles:** Fibre bundles that are located in the midbrain; the cerebral peduncles connect the pons to the cerebrum.

63. **Cerebrospinal fluid (CSF):** A clear liquid produced within the ventricles and found in the ventricles, inside the subarachnoid space (surrounding the brain and spinal cord), and inside the central canal of the spinal cord; it functions as a protective cushion for, brings nutrients to, and removes waste from, the neuraxis.
64. **Chorea:** Quick, repeated, involuntary movements of the distal extremity muscles, and muscles of face and tongue that are brisk graceful series of successive involuntary movements of distal portions of extremities and muscles of facial expression.
65. **Choreo-athetoid movements:** Involuntary, course, irregular (at times jerky) movements, of distal portions of the extremeties.
    Site of lesion—caudate nucleus or corpus striatum (caudate nucleus + putamen).
    Relieved/abolished by—anterior chordotomy (without injury to lateral corticospinal tract.
66. **Choroid plexes:** Structures that produce cerebrospinal fluid by allowing certain components of blood to enter the ventricles; formed by a fusing of the pia mater and the ependyma.
67. **Cingulate gyrus:** A cortical area (a gyrus) considered to be a part of the limbic system; it is located immediately superior to the corpus callosum.
68. **Circle of Willis (circulus arteriosus):** The main arterial anastomatic trunk of the brain; the Circle of Willis is a point where the blood carried by the two internal carotids and the basilar system comes together and is subsequently redistributed by the anterior, middle, and posterior cerebral arteries.
69. **Claustrum:** A structure considered by some anatomists to be a part of the basal ganglia.
70. **Collateral circulation:** A safety mechanism of the arterial system of the brain; collateral circulation involves the circulation of blood through a route that is different than normal; it can be crucial when blockages occur.
71. **Column of Goll:** Medial tract of the posterior column of the spinal cord (fasciculus gracilis). Friedrich Goll (1829–1903).
72. **Commissural fibres:** Nerve fibres that connect the hemispheres of the brain; the corpus callosum, anterior commissure, and the posterior commissure are composed of commissural fibres.
73. **Commissurectomy:** An operation that severs the corpus callosum; commissurectomies have been used as a treatment for severe epileptic seizures.
74. **Conduction aphasia:** A type of aphasia that may be the result of a lesion to the arcuate fasciculus.
75. **Contralateral innervation:** When a cranial nerve, or a portion of it, receives information only from fibres on the opposite side of the brain.
76. **Conus medularis:** The point at which the spinal cord ends, just above the small of the back.
77. **Convolution:** Includes both gyri and sulci.
78. **Coronal cut:** A cut that separates brain into front and back portions; a cut that runs from ear to ear.
79. **Corpora quadrigemina:** Consists of the tectum and the four colliculi which are bumps on the tectum (two superior colliculi and two inferior colliculi) located on the posterior surface of the midbrain.
80. **Corpus callosum:** Latin for 'large body', the corpus callosum is the major group of commissural fibres; is located some distance down inside the longitudinal cerebral fissure; it connects the hemispheres it and mainly connects mirror image sites.

81. **Corpus striatum:** The group of structures that includes the basal ganglia and internal capsule; it is called the 'striped body' because the internal capsule runs between the caudate nucleus and lenticular nucleus of the basal ganglia, creating a striped appearance.
82. **Cortex:** The layer of cells that cover the two hemispheres of the brain; its surface is composed of gyri and sulci.
83. **Corticobulbar tract:** The fibres of the pyramidal tract that synapse with the cranial nerves located in the brainstem.
84. **Corticopontine tract:** Fibres sent from the corticospinal and corticobulbar tracts to the pontine nuclei of the pons (the fibres of the corticopontine tract end in the pons); this portion of the pyramidal tract (although it may also be considered to be a part of the extrapyramidal system) carries information about the type and strength of motor impulses generated in the cortex to the cerebellum, by synapsing with second order neurons that carry this information via the middle cerebellar peduncle.
85. **Corticopontocerebellar tract:** A fibre tract that brings a copy of the motor information (including information about the nature, destination, strength, and speed of the motor impulse being sent by the precentral gyrus) to the cerebellum from the frontal lobe; the information travels on this tract from the precentral gyrus, descending in the internal capsule, then synapsing with cells in the pons; the pontine nuclei then send second order neurons to the cerebellum on the middle cerebellar peduncle.
86. **Corticospinal tract:** The fibres of the pyramidal tract that synapse with spinal nerves; these fibres carry information about voluntary movement to the skeletal muscles; as they descend they form part of the posterior limb of the internal capsule.
87. **Corpus striatum:** The group of structures that includes the basal ganglia and internal capsule; it is called the 'striped body' because the internal capsule runs between the caudate nucleus and lenticular nucleus of the basal ganglia, creating a striped appearance.
88. **Cranial:** A synonym of superior; cranial refers to the upper parts of the nervous system.
89. **Crossed paralysis** or **hemiplegia alternans:** Paralysis of one or more ipsilateral cranial nerve(s) and contralateral paralysis of the arm and leg.
90. **Dendrite:** The part of the neuron that receives messages from the axons of other nerve cells; the two types of dendrites are apical dendrites and basilar dendrites.
91. **Descending reticular formation:** The component of the reticular formation that is involved in autonomic nervous system activity; it receives information from the thalamus; the descending reticular formation also plays a role in motor movement.
92. **Diencephalon:** The thalamus and hypothalamus—the median part of the forebrain vesicle.
93. **Diplegia:** Paralysis of any **two** corresponding extremeties—both upper or both lower.
94. **Direct pyramidal tract (ventral pyramidal tract, anterior corticospinal tract):** The uncrossed (direct) fibres of the corticospinal tract that synapse with the spinal nerves on the ipsilateral side of the body; these fibres travel down the ventral aspect of the cord.
95. **Dyskinesias:** Disorders of involuntary movement; may be the result of extrapyramidal tract lesions.
96. **Dorsospinocerebellar tract:** One of the two main tracts that bring sensory information from the periphery to the cerebellum; proprioceptive information from the upper body travels on this fibre tract; it carries messages received by the reticular nuclei in various parts of the brainstem from the cortex, spinal cord, vestibular system and red nucleus; information from this tract enters the cerebellum on the inferior cerebellar peduncle.

97. Dual innervations of organs.
98. **Dura mater:** Latin for 'hard mother', the dura mater is the most superior of the layers of the meninges; this tough, inflexible tissue forms several structures that serve to separate the cranial cavity into compartments and protect the brain from displacement, as well as forming several vein-like sinuses that carry blood back to the heart.

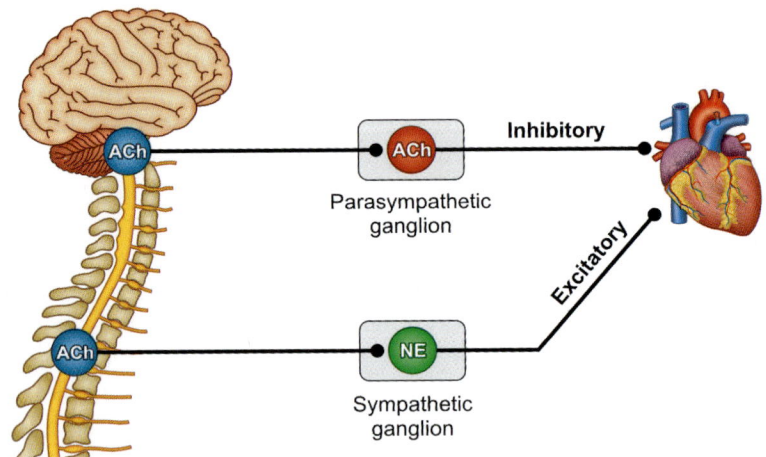

99. **Edinger-Westphall nucleus:** Supplies the parasympathetic fibres of the oculomotor nerve. Ludwig Edinger (1855–1918) and Karl Westphall (1833–1890).
100. **Ependyma:** The membranous lining of the ventricles and central canal of the spinal cord.
101. **Efferent fibres:** Nerve fibres that take messages from the brain to the peripheral nervous system; efferent fibres are almost always motor fibres.
102. **Epidural space:** A potential space that may exist between the dura mater and the skull.
103. **Erb-Duchenne paralysis:** Results from injury to the C5 and C6 roots of the brachial plexus. Wilhelm Erb (1840–1921) and GBA Duchenne (1806–1875)
104. **External granular layer:** The second most superior layer of the cortex; it is very dense and contains small granular cells and small pyramidal cells.
105. **External pyramidal layer (medial pyramidal layer):** The third most superior layer of the cortex; it contains pyramidal cells in row formation and the cell bodies of some association fibres.
106. **Extrapyramidal tract:** The system involved in automatic motor movements, gross motor movements, posture and muscle tone (in combination with the autonomic nervous system) and facial expression; it is an indirect, multisynaptic tract; the components of the extrapyramidal system include the basal ganglia, the red nucleus, substantia nigra, the reticular formation, and the cerebellum.
107. **Falx cerebelli:** Separates the lobes of the cerebellum; the falx cerebelli is formed by the dura mater.
108. **Falx cerebri:** Separates the lobes of the cerebrum; the falx cerebri is formed by the dura mater.
109. **Finger agnosia:** An inability to recognise objects through the sense of touch; may be the result of damage to the angular gyrus in the hemisphere dominant for speech and language.

110. **Fissure:** A particularly deep sulcus.
111. **Fissure of Rolando (central sulcus):** The sulcus that separates the frontal and parietal lobes.
112. **Fissure of Sylvius (lateral fissure):** The fissure that separates the frontal and temporal lobes.
113. **Flocculi (singular–flocculus):** The most ancient part of the cerebellum; the flocculi are part of flocculonodular lobe.
114. **Flocculonodular lobe:** The lobe of the cerebellum that consists of the flocculi and the nodulus; the flocculonodular lobe is involved in the maintenance of equilibrium.
115. **Foramina of Luschka:** Two lateral openings (along with the medial foramen of Magendie) which serve to connect the fourth ventricle to the subarachnoid space.
116. **Foramen of Magendie:** A medial opening (along with the lateral foramina of Luschka) which serves to connect the fourth ventricle to the subarachnoid space.
117. **Foramina of Monro (interventricular foramina):** Two openings which connect the lateral ventricles to the third ventricle.
118. **Fornix:** A subcortical component of the limbic system; the fornix is a group of fibres that arise from the hippocampus and connect the rhinencephalon to the thalamus and hypothalamus; the fornix is connected to the septal nuclei and the mammillary bodies.
119. **Fourth ventricle:** One of the four ventricles of the brain; it is filled with cerebrospinal fluid; the fourth ventricle is located between the cerebellum and the pons.
120. **Frontal lobe:** The most anterior lobe of the brain; it is bounded posteriorly by the central sulcus and inferiorly by the lateral fissure; this lobe is associated with higher cognitive functions and is involved in the control of voluntary muscle movement.
121. **Fusiform layer (multiform layer):** The sixth and most inferior layer of the cortex.
122. **GABA:** A neurotransmitter that is involved in the inhibitory function of the basal ganglia; it is a glutamate.
123. **Gait:** Gait is the style in which an individual walks. The following are abnormal types:
     - **Dancing gait**—irregular steps; cannot walk in straight line, e.g. Chorea.
     - **Stamping gait**—wide based, Rhomberg's ±ve, steps vary in length.
     - **Waddling gait**—Gower's sign –ve in muscular dystrophy, there are also winged scapulae.
     - **High stepping gait**—seen in LMN disorders associated with footdrop.
124. **Gamma neurons:** Neurons of the final common pathway (located on the ventral aspect of the spinal cord); these cells conduct slow motor impulses and their main function is to stretch muscle spindles; gamma cells are only half as numerous as alpha cells.
125. **Ganglia:** Groups of neurons located in the peripheral nervous system; the ganglia are four chains of nuclei (two on each side of the spinal cord) that make up the autonomic nervous system; the outer chains form the parasympathetic division and the inner chains form the sympathetic division.
126. **Ganglionic cells:** Neurons of the autonomic system that originate within the ganglia and project to postganglionic neurons.
127. **Ganglionic layer:** The fifth layer of the cortex; it contains small granular cells, large pyramidal cells, and the cell bodies of some association fibres (the association fibres that originate here form the Bands of Baillerger, which are two large fibre tracts).
128. **Globus pallidus:** The more medial part of the lenticular nucleus.
129. **Gyrus:** A raised fold of brain tissue.

130. **Hemiballismus:** A violent (destructive) form of motor restlessness involving one side of the body; these movements are more violent than those called choreoathetoid and involve proximal portions of extremity more than the distal. The site of lesion is subthalamic nucleus of Luys.

131. **Hemiplegia:** Spastic or flaccid paralysis of one side of the body and extremeties.

132. **Heschl's gyrus (anterior transverse temporal gyrus):** The primary auditory area; it is located in the temporal lobe.

133. **Hippocampus:** A cortical area classified as part of the limbic system; it is a gyrus located on the medial edge of the temporal lobe.

134. **Homunculus:** 'Little man'; a pedagogical device that is used to explain and demonstrate the functioning of the motor strip.

135. **Horner's syndrome:** Ptosis and constriction of the pupil result from interruption of the sympathetic innervation to the eyelids and pupil. Johann Horner (1831–1886).

136. **Hydrocephalus:** A condition that occurs when too much cerebrospinal fluid is produced and the ventricles swell, resulting in pressure being exerted on the tissue of the brain; it may be caused by tumours.

137. **Hydroencephali:** A rare birth defect in which the cerebrum is absent and the space where it should be is filled with cerebrospinal fluid; the term literally means 'water brain'.

138. **Hypothalamus:** A subcortical structure located immediately below the thalamus, part of it is also anterior to the thalamus and it forms the floor and part of the lateral walls of the third ventricle; by controlling the functioning of the pituitary gland it regulates basic biological functions (e.g. appetite, body temperature, sex drive).

139. **Infarction:** Death of tissue.

140. **Inferior cerebellar peduncles (restiform bodies):** One of the three fibre bundles called cerebellar peduncles that connect the cerebellum to the brainstem; the inferior cerebellar peduncle connects the cerebellum with the vestibular nuclei located in the lower pons and medulla, and with the reticular formation; proprioceptive information from the upper body (information that travels along the dorsospinocerebellar tract) enters the cerebellum on the inferior cerebellar peduncle.

141. **Inferior colliculi:** Structures of the midbrain that relay auditory information to the medial geniculate bodies of the thalamus.

142. **Interconnecting fibres:** Nerve fibres that connect structures within the brain; the two types of interconnecting fibres are commissural fibres and association fibres.

143. **Internal capsule:** A group of myelinated ascending and descending fibre tracts that connect the cortex to other parts of the central nervous system; although the axons that pass through it descend to the brainstem and spinal cord, the capsule itself ends within the cerebrum; the internal capsule is located between the lenticular nucleus and the caudate nucleus.

144. **Internal carotid artery:** A division of the common carotid; the internal carotid arteries supply blood to the brain; the two main branches of this artery are the anterior cerebral artery and the middle cerebral artery, other branches include the anterior communicating artery and the posterior communicating artery.

145. **Internal granular layer:** The fourth layer of the cortex; it is very thin; it contains pyramidal cells in row formation.

146. **Interneurons:** Association neurons of the spinal cord; interneurons connect the anterior and posterior horns of grey matter and are involved in the reflex arc (they function within the same segment of the spinal cord).

147. **Internuncial neurons:** Association neurons of the spinal cord; internuncial neurons project (ascend) to the brainstem and cerebellum.

148. **Island of Reil (the insula):** The cortical area that lies below the fissure of Sylvius; it is considered by some anatomists as the fifth lobe of the brain; it may be associated with the viscera.

149. **Kinesthesia:** Feedback from muscle spindles only (thus a more specific term than proprioception).

150. **Klumpke's paralysis:** Injury to the lowest root of the brachial plexus—Augusta Dejerine-Klumpke (1859–1927).

151. **Lateral aspect:** The part of the motor strip that is located on the lateral surface of the hemisphere; it is responsible for motor control of the upper body (including the larynx, face, hands, shoulders, and trunk).

152. **Lateral corticospinal tract (lateral pyramidal tract):** The fibres of the corticospinal tract that decussate at the pyramids.

153. **Lateral fissure (fissure of Sylvius):** The fissure that separates the frontal and temporal lobes.

154. **Lateral geniculate bodies:** The thalamic nuclei that receive visual information from the superior colliculi of the midbrain, process, and then transmit this information to the cortex.

155. **Lateral ventricles:** The two large ventricles (filled with cerebrospinal fluid) that have anterior horns located in the frontal lobes, inferior horns located in the temporal lobes, and which also extend posteriorly into the parietal lobes.

156. **Left-right disorientation:** An inability to distinguish the left from the right; may be the result of damage to the angular gyrus in the hemisphere dominant for speech and language.

157. **Lenticular nucleus (lentiform nucleus):** One of the two structures that make up the basal ganglia; it is composed of the globus pallidus and the putamen; the lenticular nucleus is located between the caudate nucleus and the Island of Reil with its anterior aspect attached to the head of the caudate nucleus.

158. **Limbic system (rhinencephalon):** The most ancient and primitive part of the brain; it is composed of both cortical and subcortical structures located on the medial, inferior surfaces of the cerebral hemispheres; the limbic system is involved in the processing of olfactory stimuli, emotions, motivation, and memory, and may be involved in cortical speech and language behaviour.

159. **Long association fibres:** Association fibres that connect areas, whicht are located in different lobes of the brain (e.g. the arcuate fasciculus).

160. **Longitudinal fissure (interhemispheric fissure):** The split or gap between the right and left cerebral hemispheres that is lined with cortex.

161. **Lower motor neurons:** Second order neurons; the cranial and spinal nerves; the cell bodies of the lower motor neurons are located in the neuraxis, but their axons can synapse with the muscles of the body.

162. **Lumbar puncture (spinal tap):** A diagnostic procedure in which a needle is inserted in the lower lumbar section of the vertebral canal to obtain a sample of cerebrospinal fluid; the fluid can be analyzed to assess general health.

163. **Magnum foramen:** The large opening in the occipital bone in the base of the skull.

164. **Mammillary bodies (mammillary nucleus):** Subcortical component of the limbic system (rhinencephalon); the mammillary bodies are connected to the hippocampus, the thalamus, and the fornix.

165. **Massa intermedia (thalamic adhesion):** The tissure that connects the two thalamic bodies of the thalamus.

166. **Medial aspect:** The part of the motor strip that extends down into the longitudinal cerebral fissure; it controls the movements of the body from the hips downward.

167. **Medial cut:** A section that divides the brain into right and left halves of equal size; it separates the hemispheres from each other; a medial cut is a type of sagittal cut.

168. **Medial geniculate bodies:** The thalamic nuclei that receive auditory information from the inferior colliculi of the midbrain, process, and then transmit this information to the cortex.

169. **Medulla oblongata:** The most inferior structure of the brainstem; the 'bulb'; the medulla is involved in circulation and respiration.

170. **Meninges:** Three layers of protective tissue that surrounds the neuraxis; the meninges of the brain and spinal cord are continuous and are connected through the foramen magnum.

171. **Midbrain (mesencephalon):** The superior most part of the brainstem.

172. **Middle cerebellar peduncle (brachium pontis):** The largest of the cerebellar peduncles; the middle cerebellar peduncle connects the cerebellum with the pons; through this connection the cerebellum receives a copy of the information for muscle movement that the pyramidal tract carries to lower motor neurons.

173. **Middle cerebral artery:** A branch of the internal carotids; the middle cerebral artery supplies blood to the entire lateral aspect of each hemisphere (including the lateral motor strip, lateral sensory strip, Broca's area, Wernicke's area, Heschl's gyrus, angular gyrus) and to the corpus striatum.

174. **Molecular layer:** The most superior layer of the cortex; it contains the cell bodies of neuroglial cells.

175. **Myelin:** A fatty insulating substance that covers, at regular intervals, many of the axons in the central and peripheral nervous system; myelin serves to increase the speed of transmission of impulses, by allowing them to jump from one unmyelinated segment to the next (this is called saltatory conduction).

176. **Meissner's plexus:** The nerve plexus in the submucosal layer of the intestine George Meissner (1829–1905).

177. **Neuraxis:** The term brain and spinal cord; the central nervous system.

178. **Neurons:** The nerve cells of the central and peripheral nervous systems; a neuron is composed of an axon, a soma, and dendrites (while all neurons have one soma and one axon, some neuons have many dendrites and others have none).

179. **Neocerebellum:** The posterior lobe of the cerebellum; it is considered to be the newest part of the cerebellum; it is involved in the coordination of muscle movement through the inhibition of involuntary movement, it is also involved in fine motor coordination

180. **Nodes of Ranvier:** The segments of axons between areas of myelin, which are in direct contact with extracellular fluid.

181. **Nodule (nodulus):** The narrowest and most inferior part of the vermis; it is part of the flocculonodular lobe of the cerebellum.

182. **Neurite** or **neuronal process:** The term refers to any projection from the cell body of a neuron. This projection can be either an axon or a dendrite. The term is frequently used when speaking of immature or developing neurons, especially of cells in culture, because it can be difficult to tell axons from dendrites before differentiation is complete.

183. **Olivary nuclei:** Landmarks in the medulla which lie posterior to the pyramids; the olivary nuclei are involved in the processing and relaying of auditory information.

184. **Occipital lobe:** The most posterior lobe of the brain; it is associated with vision.

185. **Olfactory pathways:** Subcortical component of the limbic system; the olfactory pathways originate in the nasal area and pass posteriorly to enter the temporal lobe at the hippocampal gyrus; the olfactory tract is immediately superior to the optic tract.

186. **Parkinson's disease:** Tremor and rigidity due to lesions of the substantia nigra; James Parkinson (1755–1824).

187. **Romberg's sign:** Ataxia when the eyes are closed because loss of position sense. Characteristic lesion involves posterior column. A patient who has a problem with proprioception (somatosensory) can still maintain balance by compensating with vestibular function and vision. In the Romberg test, the patient stands upright and asked to close his **eyes**. A loss of balance is interpreted as a positive Romberg sign. German neurologist Moritz Heinrich *Romberg* (1795–1873).

188. **Schwann cells:** The Schwann cells are a variety of **glial cell** that keep peripheral nerve fibres (both myelinated and unmyelinated) alive. In myelinated axons, **Schwann cells** form the myelin sheath.

Schwann cells (named after physiologist Theodor Schwann) or **neurolemmocytes** are the principal glia of the peripheral nervous system (PNS). Glial cells function to support neurons and in the PNS, also include satellite cells, olfactory ensheathing cells, enteric glia and glia that reside at sensory nerve endings, such as the Pacinian corpuscle. There are two types of Schwann cell, *myelinating* and *nonmyelinating*. Myelinating Schwann

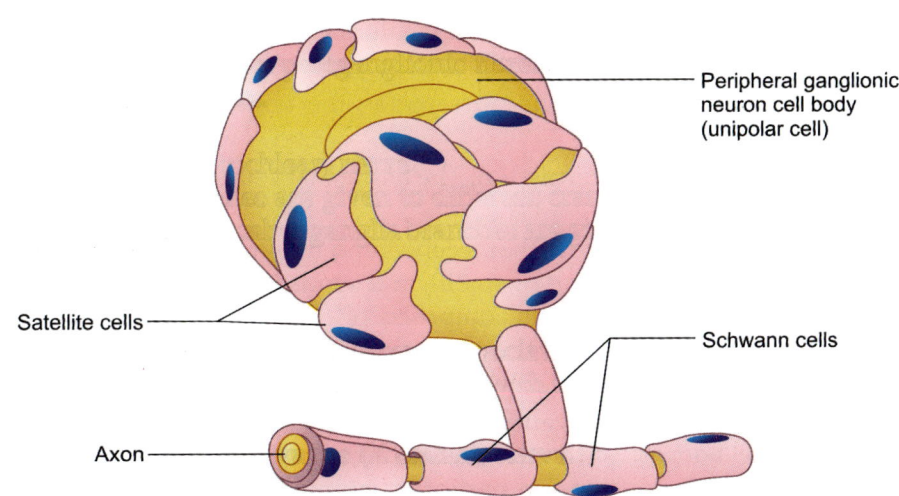

Peripheral ganglionic neuron cell body (unipolar cell)

Satellite cells

Schwann cells

Axon

cells wrap around axons of motor and sensory neurons to form the myelin sheath. The Schwann cell promoter is present in the downstream region of the human dystrophin gene that gives shortened transcript that are again synthesised in a tissue specific manner.

During the development of the peripheral nervous system, the regulatory mechanisms of myelination are controlled via feed forward interaction of specific genes, influencing transcriptional cascades and shaping the morphology of the myelinated nerve fibres.

Schwann cells are involved in many important aspects of peripheral nerve biology—the conduction of nervous impulses along axons, nerve development and regeneration, trophic support for neurons, production of the nerve extracellular matrix, modulation of neuromuscular synaptic activity, and presentation of antigens to T-lymphocytes. Charcot-Marie-Tooth disease (CMT), Guillain-Barré syndrome (GBS, acute inflammatory demyelinating polyradiculopathy type), schwannomatosis, and chronic inflammatory demyelinating polyneuropathy (CIDP), and leprosy are all neuropathies involving Schwann cells.

189. **Satellite glial cells:** The satellite glial cells are glial cells that cover the surface of nerve cell bodies in sensory, sympathetic and parasympathetic ganglia. Both satellite glial cells (SGCs) and Schwann cells (the cells that ensheathe some nerve fibres) are derived from the neural crest of the embryo during development. SGCs have been found to play a variety of roles, including control over the microenvironment of sympathetic ganglia. They are thought to have a similar role to astrocytes in the central nervous system (CNS). They supply nutrients to the surrounding neurons and also have some structural function. Satellite cells also act as protective, cushioning cells. Additionally, they express a variety of receptors that allow for a range of interactions with neuroactive chemicals. Many of these receptors and other ion channels have recently been implicated in health issues including chronic pain and herpes simplex. There is much more to be learned about these cells, and research surrounding additional properties and roles of the SGCs are ongoing.

190. **Tectospinal tract:** A tract with points of origin throughout the brainstem (especially in the midbrain) that ends in the spinal nerves; it is involved in the control of neck muscles, and visual and auditory reflexes.

191. **Tectum:** The roof of the brainstem.

192. **Temporal lobe:** The lobe of the brain that is inferior to the lateral sulcus and anterior to the occipital lobe; it is associated with auditory processing and olfaction.

193. **Tentorium cerebelli:** A fold of the dura mater, the tentorium cerebelli separates the cerebrum from the cerebellum.

194. **Thalamic adhesion (massa intermedia):** The tissue that connects the two thalamic bodies of the thalamus.

195. **Thalamus:** A subcortical structure that receives and integrates sensory information from the periphery (with the exception of smell), and sends the information to the cortex for further processing; the thalamus is composed of two thalamic bodies and the massa intermedia; it is located inferior to the caudate nucleus and the fornix and medial to the lenticular nucleus.

196. **Third ventricle:** One of the four ventricles, it contains cerebrospinal fluid; it lies between the two thalamic bodies, with the massa intermedia passing through it and the hypothalamus forming its floor and part of its lateral walls.

197. **Transitory ischemic attack:** Occurs when a part or parts of the brain are temporarily deprived of oxygen; often happens during the time after a blockage occurs when collateral circulation has not yet reached a level that supports normal functioning.

198. **Transcortical aphasia:** A type of aphasia that may occur as the result of blockages in the water shed areas of the brain.

199. **Transverse cut:** A cut that divides the brain into upper and lower sections; perpendicular to coronal, medial, and sagittal cuts.

200. **Velum interpositum:** The velum interpositum is a small membrane containing a potential space just above and anterior to the pineal gland. The velum interpositum is formed by an invagination of pia mater forming a triangular membrane the apex of which points anteriorly.

    Boundaries
    - *Superiorly*: The columns of the fornices and hippocampal commissure (psalterium) reaching as far forward as the foramen of Monro.
    - *Inferiorly*: The internal cerebral veins and tela choroidea of the third ventricle.
    - *Inferolaterally*: The thalamus.
    - *Posteriorly*: The narrow base of the triangle abuts the splenium of the corpus callosum.

    The velum varies in shape from person to person, sometimes interposed between the internal cerebral veins and splenium, and depending on whether or not there is a cavum vergae (in which case the columns of the fornices are displaced inferiorly, narrowing the velum interpositum).

    When somewhat distended by fluid it forms a small triangular (in axial section) space and is referred to as a cavum velum interpositum. If larger it is known as a cavum velum interpositum cyst. The space between the two leaves of pia contains the posterior medial choroidal arteries.

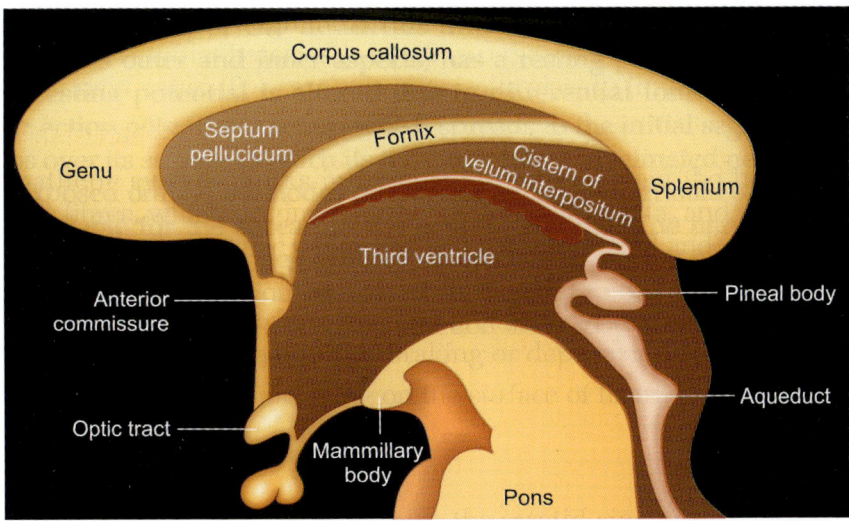

201. **Uncinate fit:** An epileptic seizure that is preceded by an olfactory hallucination.

202. **Upper motor neurons:** A type of first order neuron that carries motor impulses; the upper motor neurons remain inside the neuraxis, they synapse with lower motor neurons.

203. **Ventricles:** Four spaces within the brain that are filled with cerebrospinal fluid, they protect the brain by cushioning it and supporting its weight; they include the two lateral ventricles, the third ventricle, and the fourth ventricle.

204. **Ventrospinocerebellar tract:** One of the two main tracts that bring sensory information from the periphery to the cerebellum; it is a fibre tract that contains proprioceptive fibres from the lower body; its axons decussate and travel upward on the contralateral side of the spinal cord, then cross again and continue upward ipsilaterally, the fibres then enter the cerebellum on the superior cerebellar peduncle.

205. **Vermis:** 'worm', a thin structure that separates the hemispheres of the cerebellum from one another.

206. **Vertebral arteries:** One of the two main branches of the subclavian arteries; the two vertebral arteries ascend through the spinal column, entering the brain through the magnum foramen, at the lower border of the pons the two vertebral arteries join together to form the basilar artery (vertebral basilar artery).

207. **Vestibulocerebellar tract:** A fibre tract that brings information from the semicircular canals of the inner ear via the vestibular nucleus of the lower pons and medulla to the cerebellum; these fibres travel to the flocculi on the inferior cerebellar peduncle.

208. **Vestibulospinal tract:** A fibre tract which brings information about the body's position in space to the antigravity muscles; the fastigial nucleus of the cerebellum sends messages to the vestibular nuclei in the lower pons and midbrain, from here the information is sent to lower motor neurons in the brainstem and spinal cord.

209. **Visual agnosia:** A condition in which an individual can see a visual stimulus, but is unable to associate it with meaning or identify its function; it represents a problem with a meaning and may be a result of damage to the secondary visual areas.

210. **Watershed areas:** Areas of the brain that are located beyond the ends of the vascular systems; these areas are particularly vulnerable to problems with blood supply.

211. **Wernicke's area:** An area of the brain, located in the temporal lobe on the posterior portion of the superior temporal gyrus, that is associated with the ability to understand and produce meaningful speech; a lesion in this area will cause Wernicke's aphasia.

Index

Reader's Notes

Reader's Notes

Reader's Notes

Reader's Notes